Cardiovascular Clinics

Albert N. Brest, M.D. | Editor-in-Chief

VOLUME TWO | NUMBER ONE

Congenital Heart Disease

Daniel F. Downing, M.D. | Guest Editor

 F. A. DAVIS COMPANY, PHILADELPHIA

Cardiovascular Clinics Series:

Editor's Commentary

The 1960's witnessed remarkable advances in the diagnosis, therapy, and understanding of the natural history of many important cardiac anomalies. Many of these advances, and other important considerations relating to congenital heart disease, are detailed in the present volume. As an adult cardiologist, I can only express unabashed admiration for the extraordinary contributions made by my colleagues in pediatrics. A very special "thanks" to the Guest Editor of this volume, Dr. Dan Downing.

ALBERT N. BREST, M.D.

Contributors

Barbara J. Bourland, M.D.
*N.I.H. Fellow in Pediatric Cardiology, Department
of Pediatrics, Baylor College of Medicine and Texas
Children's Hospital, Houston, Texas*

Albert N. Brest, M.D.
*Head, Division of Cardiology, Professor of Medicine, Jefferson
Medical College and Hospital, Philadelphia, Pennsylvania*

Marie A. Capitanio, M.D.
*Associate Professor of Radiology, Temple University School
of Medicine; Associate Radiologist, St. Christopher's Hospital
for Children, Philadelphia, Pennsylvania*

Harvey L. Chernoff, M.D.
*Assistant Professor of Pediatrics, Tufts University
School of Medicine; Pediatric Cardiologist, New England
Medical Center Hospitals, Boston, Massachusetts*

Daniel F. Downing, M.D.
*Chief of Pediatric Cardiology, Deborah
Hospital, Browns Mills, New Jersey*

Eugenie F. Doyle, M.D.
*Associate Professor of Pediatrics, New York University
School of Medicine; Director of Pediatric Cardiology, New
York University Medical Center, New York, New York*

Mary Allen Engle, M.D.
*Professor of Pediatrics; Director, Pediatric Cardiology, The New
York Hospital-Cornell Medical Center, New York, New York*

Elizabeth Fisher, M.D.
*Clinical Fellow in Pediatric Cardiology, The
Willis J. Potts Children's Heart Center, The
Children's Memorial Hospital, Chicago, Illinois*

Henry Kane, M.D.
*Assistant Professor of Pediatrics; Director,
Pediatric Cardiology, Jefferson Medical College
and Hospital, Philadelphia, Pennsylvania*

John A. Kirkpatrick, M.D.
*Professor of Radiology, Temple University
School of Medicine; Radiologist, St. Christopher's
Hospital for Children, Philadelphia, Pennsylvania*

J. B. Kostis, M.D.
*Senior Fellow, Division of Cardiology, Philadelphia
General Hospital, Philadelphia, Pennsylvania*

Marshall B. Kreidberg, M.D.
*Professor of Pediatrics, Tufts University School of
Medicine; Chief, Pediatric Cardiology, New England
Medical Center Hospitals, Boston, Massachusetts*

Russell V. Lucas, Jr., M.D.
Paul S. and Faith F. Dwan Professor of Pediatric
Cardiology, Department of Pediatrics, Variety Club Heart
Hospital, University of Minnesota, Minneapolis, Minnesota

Vladir Maranhão, M.D.
Chief, Cardiac Department, Director, Cardiac Catheterization
Laboratory, Deborah Hospital, Browns Mills, New Jersey

Dwight C. McGoon, M.D.
Consultant, Section of Surgery, Mayo Clinic and Mayo Foundation;
Associate Professor of Surgery, Mayo Graduate School
of Medicine, University of Minnesota, Rochester, Minnesota

Dan G. McNamara, M.D.
Professor of Pediatrics, Baylor College of Medicine; Director of
Pediatric Cardiology, Texas Children's Hospital, Houston, Texas

A. N. Moghadam, M.D.
Associate Professor of Pediatrics, University of
Pennsylvania School of Medicine; Director,
Hemodynamics Section, and Chief
of Pediatric Cardiology, Philadelphia General
Hospital, Philadelphia, Pennsylvania

James H. Moller, M.D.
Assistant Professor of Pediatrics, Department
of Pediatrics, Variety Club Heart Hospital,
University of Minnesota, Minneapolis, Minnesota

Arthur J. Moss, M.D.
Professor and Chairman, Department of Pediatrics,
University of California, Los Angeles School of Medicine,
The Center for the Health Sciences, Los Angeles, California

Milton H. Paul, M.D.
Director, Division of Cardiology, The Willis J. Potts Children's
Heart Center, The Children's Memorial Hospital, Chicago, Illinois

Saul J. Robinson, M.D.
Clinical Professor of Pediatrics, University of
California Medical School, San Francisco, California

Monika Rutkowski, M.D.
Senior Fellow in Pediatric Cardiology, New York
University Medical Center, New York, New York

Bijan Siassi, M.D.
Department of Pediatrics, University of California,
Los Angeles School of Medicine, The Center for
the Health Sciences, Los Angeles, California

L. H. S. Van Mierop, M.D.
Professor of Pediatrics, Departments of Pediatrics
(Cardiology) and Pathology, J. Hillis Miller Health Center,
University of Florida College of Medicine, Gainesville, Florida

Robert F. Ziegler, M.D.
Physician-in-Charge, Division of Pediatric
Cardiology, Henry Ford Hospital, Detroit, Michigan

Contents

Etiology of Congenital Heart Disease

Eugenie F. Doyle, M.D., and
Monika Rutkowski, M.D.

Malformations of the cardiovascular system are among the most frequently occurring of all congenital defects.[1] Their etiology in most cases remains unknown. Recent advances in the fields of genetics, embryology, and infectious and metabolic diseases, however, have provided explanations for at least some of the many defects encountered. Most of the studies performed during recent years suggest a multifactorial relationship between environmental and genetic factors in the pathogenesis of congenital heart disease.[2-5] The factors that at present appear important in impairing cardiac development will be considered.

ENVIRONMENTAL FACTORS

Intra-uterine Infections

Intra-uterine infections may have teratogenic effects and cause cardiac malformations. This effect has not been shown for bacterial infections, but has been clearly demonstrated for viral diseases. Probably less than 10 per cent of all congenital cardiac malformations are caused by intra-uterine viral infections, including the 2 to 4 per cent caused by rubella virus.[6] The types of cardiovascular defects seen in infants whose mothers had clinical rubella in the first trimester of pregnancy have been extensively studied.[6-13] These studies showed a high incidence of patent ductus arteriosus (PDA) and some form of pulmonary artery obstruction.

Among 376 infants and children with virologically proved intra-uterine rubella who have been followed by the Rubella Project at our institution,[14] 182 (48 per cent) had congenital cardiovascular anomalies. Eighty-seven of these patients had cardiac diagnostic studies, which demonstrated patent ductus arteriosus in 78 per cent, right pulmonary artery stenosis in 70 per cent, left pulmonary artery stenosis in 56 per cent, brachiocephalic artery anomalies in 33 per cent, and coarctation of the aorta in 1 per cent. Except for valvular pulmonic stenosis, which occurred in 40 per cent, intracardiac anomalies were less common.[15]

Coxsackie B virus infections have been incriminated in the etiology of endocardial fibroelastosis.[16] Serologic evidence of an intra-uterine Coxsackie infection has been correlated with an increased incidence of congenital heart disease without a type-specific lesion.[17]

No evidence of increased congenital cardiac malformations has yet been seen with intra-uterine infections with cytomegalic inclusion disease, toxoplasmosis, chickenpox, or influenza.[6, 18] Whether the mumps virus has any pathogenetic relationship to endocardial fibroelastosis is still a matter of discussion.[19-21] Measles has been considered of possible teratogenic effect, but the data are inconclusive.[22] The correlation between Down's syndrome and viral hepatitis [23] has been seriously disputed.[24] Though vaccinia during the first trimester of pregnancy may increase fetal mortality significantly, no specific correlation with congenital heart disease has been seen.[25]

2

Radiation

The teratogenic effect of radiation depends largely on dosage and gestational age of the fetus, the most radiosensitive period being the first 16 weeks of gestation.[26] Radiation during that time may result in fetal or neonatal death, as well as in genital, skeletal, neurological, and ocular malformations.[26, 27] Specific effect on cardiovascular development is not available, however. It is generally agreed that radiation for therapeutic or diagnostic purposes should not be applied later than 10 days after the last menstrual period.[27, 28] This view is supported by the series in which a relationship between maternal X-ray exposure and increased incidence of Down's syndrome was found.[29, 30] Clinical experience suggests that in the total picture of congenital heart disease, the percentage of cases in which there is a history of maternal exposure to radiation during the first trimester is indeed low.

Metabolic Disorders

These disorders have been clearly proved to play a role in the etiology of congenital heart disease.

Diabetes mellitus

The exact mechanism of the teratogenic effect of diabetes is unknown; however, its existence is clearly demonstrated by the significantly increased incidence of lethal congenital malformations (2.9 per cent) in infants of diabetic mothers.[31] An increase in incidence of congenital cardiac malformations is reported by Driscoll and coworkers [32] who described, in their series of 95 postmortem examinations, six infants with a ventricular septal defect (VSD) and a number of more complicated anomalies. They also emphasized the tendency to cardiomegaly. A case with tetralogy of Fallot and another with cor trilocular biventriculare in a series of 140 diabetic offspring has been described.[33] The incidence of diabetes in families of infants with transposition of the great vessels appears to be higher than in families with other cardiac malformations.[34]

Phenylketonuria

Phenylketonuria may be associated with cardiovascular malformations. A family study of two female phenylketonuric patients with a total of ten offspring showed that seven of these had cardiovascular defects, usually coarctation of the aorta or patent ductus arteriosus. However, other reports on offspring of 16 phenylketonuric parents have not mentioned any cardiac malformations.[35]

Hypercalcemia

In this syndrome, supravalvular aortic stenosis, peripheral pulmonic stenosis, aortic hypoplasia, abnormal facies, faulty dentition, and varying

3

degrees of mental retardation may be associated. In spite of many reports [36-41] and animal experimental studies,[42] there is as yet no agreement as to whether this syndrome results from an increased calcium sensitivity in the mother or fetus, an overdosage of vitamin D, or a genetic defect. This syndrome may well demonstrate a multifactorial basis for cardiovascular anomalies, there being present a genetic defect that becomes potentiated by abnormal calcium metabolism. Figure 1 demonstrates a severe degree of supravalvular aortic stenosis of the diffuse type in a 4-year-old boy who also had severe stenoses in his pulmonary arterial tree. His brother had milder pulmonic stenoses.

Drugs

Many drugs cross the placenta readily and may exert a teratogenic effect on the fetus. The magnitude of the adverse effect depends on the type of drug, the dosage, and the time given. A definite relationship to congenital malformations, including cardiac anomalies, has been established for only a small number of drugs. Many more have been incriminated, but inconclusively.[43] The time of highest incidence of cardiac malformations appears to be between the 40th and 45th days after the last menstrual period.[34] Definite cardiac teratogenicity has been shown for thalidomide [44] without predilection for a specific lesion. One single case of transposition of the great vessels has been described with the use of dextroamphetamine.[43] Aminopterin and Amethopterin, both anticarcinogenic drugs, are documented to cause multiple congenital anomalies, including cardiac malformations.[45]

Drugs such as digitalis and thyroid stimulants, as well as antithyroid

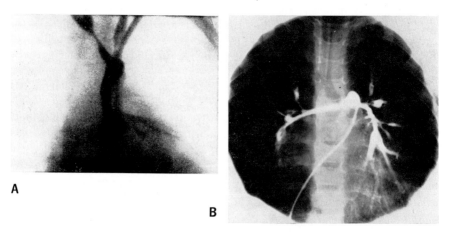

A

B

Figure 1. Supravalvular aortic stenosis syndrome. A, note the extreme degree of diffuse supravalvular aortic obstruction in this 4-year-old boy. Constriction of the right innominate artery is striking. B, severe stenosis of right and left pulmonary arteries and peripheral branches.

agents, do not exert a cardioteratogenic effect when used in therapeutic doses.[34]

Obstetric Considerations

Parental age

The association between increasing maternal age and congenital heart disease is not clearcut. Some investigators found that increased maternal age had no definite influence on congenital cardiac malformations,[3, 5] whereas others found a statistically significant correlation between maternal age and the occurrence of VSD and tetralogy of Fallot.[4] This controversy is in contrast to the clearcut relation between maternal age and occurrence of Down's syndrome.[46] Advanced paternal age appears at present of significant influence only in the group of 21/22 translocation.[47]

Prenatal factors

The history of antepartum bleeding during the first 11 weeks of gestation has been found to be associated not only with a high fetal loss rate, but also with a significantly increased risk of congenital anomalies, low birth weight, and neonatal mortality in the liveborn.[48] The exact relation between cardiac anomalies and obstetric complications is not known, though in clinical experience one frequently obtains a history of threatened spontaneous abortion in the pregnancy that resulted in an infant with congenital heart disease.

Prematurity

Prematurity apparently has some influence, whether direct or indirect, on congenital heart disease, since the incidence of PDA and VSD is increased.[34]

Geographic conditions

An increased incidence of PDA and atrial septal defect has been found in children born at high altitudes.[49]

GENETIC FACTORS

Recognized chromosomal aberrations and mutations of single genes account for approximately 6 per cent of all congenital heart disease.[2] The exact pathogenetic mechanism whereby genetic abnormalities cause congenital defects still is unknown; nevertheless, an increasing number of studies are yielding data on relationships between recognizable genetic disorders and congenital heart defects.

Chromosomal Aberrations

Chromosomal aberrations contribute probably less than 5 per cent of all cardiac malformations. The following syndromes associated with known chromosomal aberrations are presented in detail to illustrate current thoughts on possible relations between genetic and environmental factors.

Down's Syndrome

The features of this syndrome were first described by Down in 1860. The major manifestations are listed here.

Hypotonia
Severe mental retardation
Characteristic eye signs:
  Inner epicanthus folds
  Upward lateral slant
  Speckling of iris
Low nasal bridge
Protrusion of tongue

Short broad neck
Stubby hands and fingers
Simian crease pattern
Gap and/or frontal furrow,
  1st and 2nd toes
Decrease in acetabular, iliac angle
Cardiac defects

According to most series, the incidence of congenital heart disease in mongolism can be estimated as between 12 and 44 per cent.[51] Most reports agree on the high frequency of endocardial cushion defects.[52-55] (See Fig. 2.) Next in frequency are VSD, PDA, atrial septal defect, and isolated aberrant subclavian artery. Less often encountered are transposition of the great arteries, tetralogy of Fallot, truncus arteriosus, left superior vena cava, coarctation of the aorta, anomalies of the aortic and pulmonic valves, and endocardial fibroelastosis.[51, 52] Thus, a wide spectrum of cardiovascular defects has been encountered with this syndrome.

Most patients with Down's syndrome have a karyotype of 47 chromosomes with a trisomy of the G-group (21–22) chromosomes that presumably results from a nondisjunction during the meiotic process in a parental gamete, usually maternal.[56] The etiology of the nondisjunction still is uncertain. Statistics suggest some relation with maternal age (Table 1).

A relation to increased paternal age had been suspected but could not be demonstrated except for the group of 21/22 translocation.[47] An association between maternal radiation exposure and mongolism has been reported.[29, 30] An increased incidence of thyroid antibodies has been found in the mothers of the age group 17 to 34 years who had children with Down's syndrome.[58]

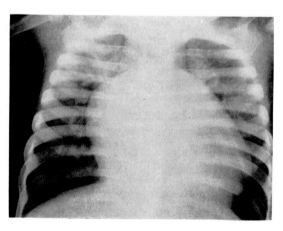

Figure 2. Down's syndrome. X ray of 9-month-old mongoloid infant in severe congestive heart failure with complete form of endocardial cushion defect.

Table 1. Risk for Down's syndrome related to maternal age

Maternal Age	Risk/live birth
15–19	1/1850
20–24	1/1600
25–29	1/1350
30–34	1/800
35–39	1/260
40–44	1/100
45–49	1/50

Trisomy 13–15

This syndrome with trisomy of the group D (13–15) was first described in 1960.[59] Its incidence is 1 per 5000 live births.[50] Forty per cent of mothers of reported affected infants were older than 35 years at the time of delivery. Most affected infants (65 per cent) were female. The most distinctive features of the syndrome are summarized in Table 2. The incidence of

Table 2. Frequency of clinical features and necropsy findings in reported cases of trisomy 13–15[50,56]

Area	Common (50% or more)	Less common occurrence
General	Apneic spells	Hypertonia, hypotonia
CNS system	Mental deficiency; deafness; minor motor seizures; agenesis of external olfactory lobes	Fusion of frontal lobes; agenesis of corpus callosum; cerebellar hypoplasia
Cranium	Sloping forehead	Microcephaly, wide sagittal sutures
Eyes	Microphthalmos, colobomata	Shallow supraorbital ridges; slanting palpebral fissures; absent eyebrows; hypertelorism
Auricles	Abnormal helices; low-set ears	
Mouth, mandible	Cleft lip, palate	Micrognathia, narrow palate
Skin	Capillary hemangioma	Localized scalp defects; loose skin at neck
Hands	Horizontal palmar crease; hyperconvex, narrow fingernails; flexion and overlapping of fingers	Retroflexed thumb; ulnar deviation of hand and fingers
Feet	Polydactyly of hands and feet; posterior prominence of heel	Dermal hallucal arch fibular pattern; syndactyly; hypoplastic toenails
Abdomen	Accessory spleen; large gallbladder; incomplete rotation of colon	Umbilical inguinal hernia; omphalocele; heterotopic pancreas tissue
Renal		Hydronephrosis; double pelvis and ureter.
Genitalia	Cryptorchidism; abnormal scrotum; partial bicornuate uterus	
Cardiac	Malformation	Rotational anomaly; VSD; ASD; PDA; anomalous venous return; bicuspid aortic valve; overriding aorta

associated heart disease is approximately 80 per cent. The most frequent anomaly is VSD; dextrorotation also has been reported.[50]

The outlook for these children is very poor, cardiac failure and bronchopneumonia being the most frequent causes of death.[50] Over 80 per cent died before the age of 6 months.[56] However, one of our patients with this syndrome, whose karyotype is seen in Figure 3, survived to age 4 despite a large VSD with pulmonary hypertension and ultimately succumbed to renal failure.

Trisomy 18

The incidence of the syndrome Trisomy 18,[60] first described in 1960,[61] is 1 per 3500 live births.[62] Seventy-eight per cent of all reported cases were females. The syndrome has been reported chiefly in Caucasians, but has been seen in Puerto Ricans, Negroes and Chinese. The mean maternal age is 34.3 years.[63] The percentage frequencies of clinical features and necropsy findings are presented in Table 3.

A high incidence of associated heart disease has been reported. In 90 per cent, a VSD was found.[64-66] The VSD was described by Townes [67] as being triangular and in the posterior membranous septum. Other associated cardiovascular lesions include PDA, patent foramen ovale, thickened valvular leaflets, bicuspid aortic and pulmonic valves,[64] double outlet right ventricle,[68] infantile arteriosclerosis,[69] and dextrocardia.[70]

The prognosis for these babies is extremely poor. Over 80 per cent have died before the age of 6 months from congestive cardiac failure, bronchopneumonia, or infections of the genitourinary tract.[66]

Cri du Chat Syndrome

This syndrome belongs to the group of chromosomal deletions, of which an increasing number have been recognized in recent years. Lejeune,[71] in 1963, reported three patients who had a peculiar cry, physical and mental retardation, microcephaly, small body size, low-set ears, antimongolian slant

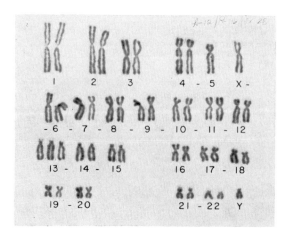

Figure 3. Karyotype of patient with trisomy 13–15. Note the extra chromosome in the D group. Patient had ventricular septal defect with severe pulmonary hypertension, extreme mental and motor retardation, low set ears, bifid 5th digits. Death at age 4 resulted from renal failure complicating extreme hydronephrosis.

8

Table 3. Frequency of clinical features and necropsy findings in reported cases of Trisomy 18[50,57,64,65]

Area	High frequency (80–100%)	Common (50–80%)	Less common occurrence (10–50%)
Growth	Birth weight < 6 lb.; failure to thrive		
CNS	Mental deficiency; muscular hypertonicity		
Cranium		Prominent occiput	Metopic sutures
Ears	Low-set, malformed		
Eyes			Ptosis; inner epicanthic fold; corneal opacities; small palpebral fissures
Mouth and mandible	Micrognathia; narrow palatal arch		Cleft lip and palate; small mouth
Hands	Fingers flexed; index finger overlaps 4th		Simian crease; single crease 5th finger; hypoplasia of fingernails; ulnar or radial deviation of hand
Feet	Hallux short or dorsi-flexed		Rocker-bottom feet
Thorax		Short sternum	Wide chest or widespread nipples
Pelvis and hips		Small pelvis; limited hip abduction	
Genitalia		Cryptorchidism	
Renal			Horseshoe kidney; double kidney; double ureter
Cardiac	VSD	PDA; PFO	ASD; bicuspid aortic valve; nodular or fibrotic thickening of valve leaflets

of the eyes, hypertelorism, and divergent strabismus. The karyotype revealed a deletion of the short arm of chromosome 5. Seven additional cases have been reported thus far. The distinctive weak, mewing cry results from weakness and underdevelopment of the larynx, with a small, soft, very mobile epiglottis; it may disappear as the child grows older.[72] The exact incidence of the syndrome is unknown. A correlation with increasing maternal age does not exist.

Heart disease occurred in two of the ten reported cases. One had a PDA;[72] the other patient,[71] an atrioventricular canal with pulmonic stenosis, transposition of the great arteries, and partial anomalous systemic venous return to the left atrium. The mortality rate in this syndrome is low compared to that of the trisomies.

Turner Syndrome

Turner[73] originally described seven female patients with short stature, webbed neck, cubitus valgus, and infantilism (Fig. 4). Subsequently,

9

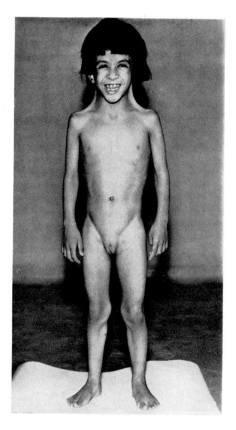

Figure 4. Turner's syndrome. Eight-year-old girl with coarctation of the aorta whose karyotype demonstrated 45 chromosomes, lacking one X chromosome. Note webbing of neck, shield-like chest.

gonadal dysgenesis also was recognized as being associated with this syndrome.[74, 75] In 1959, analysis of the karyotype of such cases revealed 45 chromosomes, including only one X chromosome.[76] Of these patients, approximately 70 per cent are chromatin negative, though others who are chromatin positive have varying forms of XO monosomy.[56] The X may be of paternal or maternal origin. The monosomy can arise from nondisjunction during oogenesis or spermatogenesis or during early mitosis. Maternal or paternal age does not seem to have any influence. The incidence of the syndrome is 1 per 2500 liveborn females.[50] The most distinctive features of the syndrome are listed below:

Short stature (less than third percentile)
Unusual facies
Low-set ears
Micrognathia
Epicanthal folds
Low posterior hairline

Webbed neck
Shield-like chest
Cubitus valgus
Skeletal abnormalities
Renal abnormalities (horseshoe kidney)
Moderate mental retardation

CARDIOVASCULAR ABNORMALITIES. The incidence of associated cardiovascular defects varies considerably, from 20[77] to 44 per cent.[78] The predominant lesions are coarctation of the aorta and pulmonic stenosis, and less commonly, subaortic and aortic stenosis, PDA, and septal defects. There appears to be a striking correlation between the finding of coarctation and chromatin-negative mass, in agreement with the general experience of increased frequency of this lesion in males. On the other hand, pulmonic stenosis was found with equal frequency in chromatin-negative and chromatin-positive Turner's syndrome.[78]

Single-Gene Mutants

Known single-gene mutants account for less than 1 per cent of all congenital cardiovascular anomalies.[2] This category can be divided into autosomal recessives and dominants and X-linked recessives and dominants. McKusick[79] has attempted to classify these varied, frequently complicated defects into specific groups according to either the pathogenetic mechanism or the recognizable noncardiac manifestations.

Disorders of Connective Tissue

These represent a group of heritable diseases with cardiac and noncardiac anomalies resulting from a defect of the collagen and/or the elastic fibers. In some, the underlying pathological mechanism has been demonstrated to be a disturbance of mucopolysaccharide metabolism; in others, it is still unknown. Apparently, the mutation of a single gene determines a substance or a metabolic process that affects many developing body structures: hence the varied manifestations of many of these structures. In Table 4 are listed the currently recognized connective tissue disorders and their major manifestations.

Complex Syndromes with Malformations of the Heart

These syndromes, all determined by a single gene mutation, feature in most cases a cardiovascular anomaly. They are presented with their major manifestations in Table 5.

Inborn Errors of Metabolism

These constitute a small group of diseases in which the basic defect, an enzyme deficiency, is responsible for cardiovascular and noncardiac anomalies. Major features are presented in Table 6.

Phakomatoses

These constitute a group of congenital syndromes affecting the central nervous system, the eye, and the skin (phakoma: Greek, spot), as well as the cardiovascular system. Table 7 includes their major manifestations.[79]

Vascular Malformations

These represent abnormalities of the arterial, venous, or lymphatic systems. Their major manifestations are listed in Table 8.

11

Table 4. Connective tissue diseases and major manifestations[79,80]

Syndrome	Pathological or biochemical defect	Cardiovascular features	Major noncardiac manifestations	Inheritance pattern
Marfan [81]	Chondroitin-sulfate C deposition in elastic media of aorta and in mitral valve	Aortic and mitral insufficiency, aortic aneurysm (diffuse or dissecting)	Long, tapered fingers, elongated body proportions, ectopia lentis, thoracic deformities	Autosomal dominant
Hurler [82–84]	Chondroitin-sulfate B, heparitin-S deposition in viscera (liver, spleen, cardiovascular & CNS), cornea	Pseudoatherosclerosis of aorta, pulmonary & coronary arteries, myocardial damage, systemic hypertension	Skeletal deformities, dwarfism, grotesque facies, corneal clouding, deafness, mental retardation	Autosomal recessive
Hunter	Chondroitin-sulfate B, heparitin-S deposition in same organs as in Hurler except cornea	Same manifestations as in Hurler, but milder	Same manifestations as in Hurler but milder; no corneal clouding	X-linked recessive
Morquio-Ullrich	Keratosulfate	Aortic insufficiency	Skeletal deformities (flat vertebrae), dwarfism, cloudy cornea, near normal IQ	Autosomal recessive
Scheie	Chondroitin-sulfate B	Aortic insufficiency	Skeletal deformities (joints), cloudy cornea, normal intellect	Autosomal recessive
Pseudoxanthoma Elasticum [85]	Elastic fiber defect	Peripheral artery occlusion (medial thickening), hypertension	Skin changes, angioid streaks in fundus, hemorrhage in GI tract and CNS	Autosomal recessive
Ehlers Danlos	Collagen fiber defect	Rupture of major arteries, dissecting aortic aneurysm, rarely cardiac defects	Hyperextensible joints, hyperelastic, friable skin, gastrointestinal diverticula, bowel rupture	Autosomal dominant
Osteogenesis Imperfecta [86]	Failure of collagen maturation	Aortic insufficiency	Increased fragility of bones, blue sclerae, deafness, dental deficiencies	Autosomal recessive

Table 5. Complex syndromes with cardiovascular anomaly

Syndrome	Cardiovascular anomaly	Major noncardiac manifestations	Inheritance pattern
Kartagener [87]	Dextrocardia	Sinusitis, bronchitis, situs inversus	Autosomal recessive
Holt-Oram [88,89]	Atrial septal defect (secundum type); ventricular septal defect, less frequent	Radial defect of the upper extremity (Fig. 5)	Autosomal dominant
Ellis-van Creveld [90,91]	Defect or absence of atrial septum	Chondrodystrophic dwarfism, ectodermal dysplasia (nails and teeth), polydactyly, partial harelip	Autosomal recessive
Laurence-Moon-Biedl [92]	Nonspecific lesions: tetralogy, single ventricle, transposition of great arteries	Obesity, polydactyly, retinitis pigmentosa, hypogonadism, renal anomalies, mental retardation	Autosomal recessive

Figure 5. Holt-Oram syndrome. X ray of the hands of a 4-year-old girl with a large secundum atrial septal defect whose mother had identical cardiac and finger lesions. Note the fingerlike bony structure of the thumb. Three phalanges are present. The thumb does not appose the index finger in the normal manner.

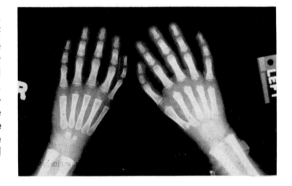

Table 6. Inborn errors of metabolism

Syndrome	Biochemical defect	Cardiovascular manifestations	Noncardiac manifestations	Inheritance pattern
Pompe (glycogen-storage disease type II)[93]	α-1,4-glucosidase deficiency	Cardiomegaly, early congestive heart failure	Hypotonia, macroglossia, death in infancy	Autosomal recessive
Homocystinuria [94]	Cystathione synthase deficiency	Thromboembolic phenomena, pulmonic and aortic regurgitation	Ectopia lentis, cataracts, malar flush, mental retardation, inguinal hernia	Autosomal recessive

13

Table 7. Phakomatoses

Syndrome	Cardiovascular manifestations	Noncardiac manifestations			Inheritance pattern
		CNS	Eye	Skin	
Tuberous sclerosis (Bourneville Pringle)	Rhabdomyoma of the heart	Convulsions, retardation, intra-cranial calcifications	Retinal phakoma	Depigmented nevi, adenoma sebaceum, subungual fibroma	Autosomal dominant
Neurofibromatosis (von Recklinghausen)	Hypertension, pheochromo-cytoma	Convulsions, retardation, peripheral-nerve and brain tumors		Café au lait, nevus, fibroma, molluscum	Autosomal dominant
von Hippel-Lindau	Hypertension, pheochromo-cytoma	Hemangioblastoma in cerebellum	Retinal angioma		Autosomal dominant
Sturge-Weber-Dimitri	Vascular anomalies of carotid and meningeal arteries	Convulsions, hemiparesis, hemianopsia, mental retarda-tion, intracranial calcifications	Glaucoma	Facial, port-wine, nevus in trigeminal nerve distribution	Autosomal dominant

14

Table 8. Vascular malformations and their manifestations

Syndrome	Anomaly	Manifestations	Inheritance pattern
Osler-Rendu-Weber (hereditary hemorrhagic teleangiectasia)[95]	A–V fistulae, telangiectases	Cutaneous lesions (face, lip), visceral lesions (pulmonary, gastrointestinal)	Autosomal dominant
Milroy (lymphedema)[96]	Hypoplasia of lymphatic vessels	Edema of the upper and lower extremities	Autosomal dominant

Neurological and Muscular Disorders

These diseases are degenerative disorders that involve the central nervous system or the skeletal muscle system and frequently also have cardiovascular manifestations.[79, 84] Their major features are presented in Table 9.

MULTIFACTORIAL ETIOLOGY OF CONGENITAL CARDIAC MALFORMATIONS

This theory holds that the vast majority of congenital cardiac defects result from the interaction of many genes with environmental factors, resulting in cardiac anomalies. The multifactorial pattern of inheritance applies to those diseases that share the following features: they are common; family aggregates can be demonstrated; the recurrence rate in siblings is 1 to 5 per cent; nonidentical twins are affected in 1 to 5 per cent; identical twins are affected in 25 to 30 per cent; and they are influenced by environmental factors.[2]

The genetic patterns of cardiovascular anomalies have been investigated in family, twin, and animal studies.

Table 9. Neurological and muscular disorders

Syndrome	Cardiovascular manifestations	Noncardiac features	Inheritance pattern
Friedreich's ataxia[97,98]	ECG changes, arrhythmias, cardiomegaly, congestive heart failure	Ataxia, nystagmus, dysarthria, musculoskeletal deformities	Autosomal recessive and dominant
Duchenne (muscular dystrophy)[99-101]	ECG changes, arrhythmias, cardiomegaly, congestive heart failure	Abnormal gait, muscular weakness, pseudohypertrophy of calf muscles	X-linked recessive
Refsum[102]	Electrocardiographic changes, arrhythmias (sudden death)	Symmetrical chronic polyneuritis, ataxia, retinitis pigmentosa, ichthyosis, deafness, skeletal deformities	Autosomal recessive
Riley-Day[103,104]	Postural hypotension, hypertensive episodes	Absence of tears and tastebuds, indifference to pain, poor motor coordination, emotional lability, excessive perspiration	Autosomal recessive

Family Studies

Family Incidence

Large surveys in the past have established the definite fact of a three- to four-fold increase in occurrence of congenital heart disease in siblings compared to the incidence in the general population.[3] The data for the incidence in siblings and parents of probands are summarized in Table 10.

The incidence in offspring of probands was approximately 2 per cent in the series of Neill.[3] Figures for specific defects were given by Nora [106]: 2.6 per cent of offspring of parents with an atrial septal defect had the same lesion, a 37 times greater incidence than for the general population; the figure for a VSD was 3.7 per cent, a 21 times increased incidence.

The incidence of consanguinity among parents of patients with congenital heart disease was 1.1 per cent according to Campbell,[4] 2.5 per cent according to Lamy,[5] and 1.7 per cent according to Fuhrmann,[107] percentages higher than normally expected. This finding was not consistent, however.[3] The one lesion unquestionably associated with consanguinity is situs inversus.[108, 4, 5] The recessive mode of inheritance for this anomaly is established.

The data for specific lesions provided by Campbell [4] and Nora [2] are summarized in Table 11. The observed frequencies of affected siblings correspond well with the predicted frequencies for multifactorial inheritance.[2]

Family Cluster Studies

In family cluster studies, attention is paid to the great number of family pedigrees with congenital heart disease, which may reveal an autosomal dominant or recessive mode of inheritance. Examples for X-linked recessive or dominant inheritance in connection with congenital heart disease have not yet been reported.[3] Family pedigrees for atrial septal defect have been described by many authors.[2-4, 109-113] Similar pedigrees have been reported for PDA,[3, 114, 115] for valvular and supravalvular aortic stenosis,[3, 116, 117] for pulmonic stenosis,[5, 118] and for tetralogy of Fallot.[3, 4] The hypertrophic muscular form of subaortic stenosis probably is transmitted by an autosomal dominant modus.[79] The disease, which affects males more severely, shows a

Table 10. Congenital heart disease in families of probands

Author	No. of Patients	Incidence of congenital heart disease (%)	
		In siblings	In parents
McKeown [105]	431	1.8	0–0.24
Campbell [4]	1227	1.7	0.3
Lamy [5]	1188	2	0
Neill [3]	1000	3	0.35
Nora [2]	1602	3.4	

Table 11. Familial incidence of specific malformations

Anomaly	Author	No. Patients	Affected Siblings (%)
Ventricular septal defect	Nora	207	4.3
	Campbell	180	3.3
Atrial septal defect	Nora	117	3.2
	Campbell	170	1.1
Patent ductus arteriosus	Nora	131	3.2
	Campbell	261	2.1
Tetralogy of Fallot	Nora	118	2.2
	Campbell	300	2.7
Aortic stenosis	Nora	101	2.6
Pulmonic stenosis	Nora	114	2.9
Coarctation of aorta	Campbell	151	0.4

great variety of expression, from a moderate degree of hypertrophy to severe left ventricular outflow tract obstruction.[4, 119–122]

The cause of endocardial fibroelastosis remains obscure. There are some cases, occurring in siblings, that suggest a recessive inheritance pattern.[123–125] In a number of families, conduction anomalies have been reported, some associated with deafness and sudden death, some only presenting with congenital A–V dissociation.[126–131]

In summary, the studies of family incidence and family clusters reveal the appearance of the same congenital defect as a recessive defect in one family, as an apparent dominant in another family, and as neither in the majority of cases.

Twin Studies

Twin studies have compared the concordance rate for cardiovascular defects in monozygotic and dizygotic twins. The results of the published twin studies are summarized in Table 12.

The low concordance rate for the monozygotic twins suggests that genetic mechanisms are not the sole determining factor in congenital heart disease.

Table 12. Cardiovascular defects in twin studies

Author	Monozygotic		Dizygotic	
	Concordant	Discordant	Concordant	Discordant
Uchida [132]		13		13
Ross [133]	2	11	2	24
Neil [3]	2	10		
Nora [2,134]	6	7	1	23
Lamy [5]		7	1	8
Campbell [135]		12		4

Animal Homologies

Congenital heart disease in animals has been studied.[2, 136, 137] A definite Mendelian pattern of inheritance has not been established, although familial occurrence of congenital heart disease in animals is further evidence for a certain genetic component in the maldevelopment. Interesting from the point of interaction between genetic and enviromental etiology are the experiments by Nora.[2] The predisposition of the A/Jax mouse to be born with an atrial septal defect is 1 per cent. If the fetus is treated with amphetamine, the incidence of congenital heart disease increases to 12 per cent, the predominant lesion being an atrial septal defect.

Discussion

In single mutant gene syndromes and chromosomal aberration syndromes, the presence or absence of the anomaly is determined by the genetic factor. The phenotypic expression is influenced only to a small degree by the environment. Further identification of chromosomal abnormalities in patients with congenital heart disease will doubtless occur with improvement of techniques for chromosomal morphological and enzymatic analysis.[138, 139] For the large group of cardiovascular defects resulting from multifactorial etiology, it is generally accepted [2, 3] that multiple genes are involved in the etiology of one anomaly, with considerable influence of environmental factors, which, if they act on the fetus at a vulnerable period in cardiac development, will result in the lesion to which he is predisposed.

FAMILY COUNSELING

Families with a child affected by congenital cardiac disease usually seek advice concerning family planning. Fortunately, the recurrence risk in most families is rather low (2 to 3 per cent). If, however, two members of a family are affected, the recurrence risk is considerably higher, and a pedigree should be obtained before further counseling. If a dominant or recessive Mendelian pattern is established, the Mendelian laws apply, and the recurrence risk for each child is equal, i.e., one of two or one of four for each further pregnancy. The advice given will certainly be influenced by the type of cardiac lesion. If parents have congenital heart disease, the risk of cardiac defects for their offspring is approximately 3 per cent.[3] Specific figures for atrial septal defect are 2.6 per cent and for VSD, 3.7 per cent.[134] The outcome for offspring of cyanotic women is, of course, less favorable because of the increased risk of spontaneous abortions.[3]

References

1. RICHARDS, M. R., MERRITT, K. K., SAMUELS, M. H., AND LANGMANN, A. G.: *Congenital malformations of the cardiovascular system in a series of 6053 infants.* Pediatrics 15:12, 1955.
2. NORA, J. J.: *Multifactorial inheritance hypothesis for the etiology of congenital heart diseases.* Circulation 38:604, 1968.

3. NEILL, C. A.: *Genetic aspects of congenital heart disease*, in Moss, A. J., and Adams, F. H.: *Heart Disease in Infants, Children and Adolescents.* The Williams & Wilkins Co., Baltimore, 1968, p. 36.

4. CAMPBELL, M.: *Causes of malformations of the heart.* Brit. Med. J. 2:895, 1965.

5. LAMY, M., deGROUCHY, G., AND SCHWEISGUTH, O.: *Genetic and non-genetic factors in the etiology of congenital heart disease. A study of 1188 cases.* Amer. J. Hum. Genet. 9:17, 1957.

6. CAMPBELL, M.: *Place of maternal rubella in the etiology of congenital heart disease.* Brit. Med. J. 1:691, 1961.

7. GIBSON, S. T., AND LEWIS, K. C.: *Congenital heart disease following maternal rubella during pregnancy.* Amer. J. Dis. Child. 83:317, 1952.

8. STUCKEY, D.: *Congenital heart defects following maternal rubella during pregnancy.* Brit. Heart J. 18:519, 1956.

9. SWAN, C.: *Rubella in pregnancy as an etiological factor in congenital malformation.* Obstet. Gynaec. Brit. Comm. 56:591, 1949.

10. ROWE, R. D.: *Maternal rubella and pulmonary artery stenoses. Report of eleven cases.* Pediatrics 32:180, 1963.

11. LYNFIELD, J., VICHITBANDHA, P., YAO, A., RODRIGUEZ-TORRES, R., KARLSON, K., AND KAUFMAN, J. H.: *Neonatal heart failure following rubella in utero.* Amer. J. Cardiol. 17:130, 1966.

12. McCUE, C. M., ROBERTSON, L. W., LESTER, R. G., AND MALICK, H. P., JR.: *Pulmonary artery coarctations. A report of 20 cases with review of 319 cases from the literature.* J. Pediat. 67:222, 1965.

13. VENABLES, A. W.: *The syndrome of pulmonary stenosis complicating maternal rubella.* Brit. Heart J. 27:49, 1965.

14. COOPER, L. Z., ZIRING, P. R., OCKERSE, A. B., FEDUN, B. A., KIELY, B., AND KRUGMAN, S.: *Rubella. Clinical manifestations and management.* Amer. J. Dis. Child. 118:18, 1969.

15. KIELY, B.: *Cardiovascular anomalies in virologically proved congenital rubella.* Abs. Amer. Pediat. Soc., April 30, 1969, p. 39.

16. FRUEHLING, L., KORN, R., LAVILLAUREIX, Y., SURJUS, A., AND FOLISEREAU, S.: *La myo-endocardite chronique fibro-élastique du nouveau-né et du nourrisson (fibro-elastose).* Ann. Anat. Path. 7:227, 1962.

17. BROWN, G., AND EVANS, T. N.: *Serologic evidence of coxsackie virus etiology of congenital heart disease.* J.A.M.A. 199:183, 1967.

18. KRUGMAN, S., AND WARD, R.: *Infectious Diseases of Children.* The C. V. Mosby Co., St. Louis, 1968.

19. NOREN, G. R., ADAMS, P., JR., AND ANDERSON, R. C.: *Positive skin reactivity to mumps virus antigen in endocardial fibroelastosis.* J. Pediat. 62:604, 1963.

20. GERSONY, W. M., KATZ, S. L., AND NADAS, A. S.: *Endocardial fibro-elastosis and the mumps virus.* Pediatrics 37:430, 1966.

21. ST. GEME, J. W., JR., NOREN, G. R., AND ADAMS, P., JR.: *Proposed embryopathic relation between mumps virus and primary endocardial fibroelastosis.* New Eng. J. Med. 275:339, 1966.

22. MANSON, M. G., LOGAN, W. P. D., AND LOY, R. M.: *Rubella and other virus infections during pregnancy.* Ministry of Health Reports on Public Health and Medical Subjects. No. 101. H.M.S.O., London.

23. STOLLER, A., AND COLLMANN, R. D.: *Incidence of infective hepatitis followed by Down's syndrome nine months later.* Lancet 2:1221, 1965.

19

24. KOGON, A., KRONMAL, R., AND PETERSON, D.: *Viral hepatitis and Down's syndrome.* Lancet 1:615, 1967.

25. McARTHUR, A.: *Congenital vaccinia and vaccinia gravidarum.* Lancet 2:1104, 1952.

26. DEKABAN, A. S.: *Abnormalities in children exposed to X-radiation during various stages of gestation: Tentative timetable of radiation injury to the human fetus,* Part I. J. Nucl. Med. 9:471, 1968.

27. BRILL, A. B., AND FORGOTSON, E. H.: *Radiation and congenital malformations.* Amer. J. Obstet. Gynec. 90:1149, 1964.

28. RUSSELL, W. L.: Proceedings of the International Conference on Peaceful Uses of Atomic Energy, Geneva 11:382–383, 401–402, 1956. United Nations, New York.

29. UCHIDA, I. A., HOLUNGA, R., AND LAWLER, C.: *Maternal radiation and chromosomal aberrations.* Lancet 2:1045, 1968.

30. SIGLER, A. T., LILIENFELD, A. M., COHEN, B. H., AND WESTLAKE, J. E.: *Radiation exposure in parents of children with mongolism (Down's syndrome).* Bull. Johns Hopkins Hosp. 117:374, 1965.

31. GELLIS, S., AND YI-YUNG HSIA, D.: *The infant of the diabetic mother.* Amer. J. Dis. Child. 97:1, 1959.

32. DRISCOLL, S. H., BENIRSCHKE, K., AND CURTIS, G.: *Neonatal deaths among infants of diabetic mothers.* Amer. J. Dis. Child. 100:818, 1960.

33. HURWITZ, D., AND HIGANO, N., *Diabetes and pregnancy.* New Eng. J. Med. 247:305, 1952.

34. NEILL, C. A.: *Pregnancy and congenital heart disease.* Postgrad. Med. 44:118, 1968.

35. STEVENSON, R. E., AND HUNTLEY, C. C.: *Congenital malformations in offspring of phenylketonuric mothers.* Pediatrics 40:33, 1967.

36. ANTIA, A. U., WILTSE, H. E., ROWE, R. D., PITT, E. L., LEVIN, S., OTTESEN, O., AND COOKE, R. E.: *Pathogenesis of the supravalvular aortic stenosis syndrome.* J. Pediat. 71:431, 1967.

37. TAUSSIG, H. B.: *Possible injury to the cardiovascular system from vitamin D.* Ann. Intern. Med. 65:1195, 1966.

38. GARCIA, R. E., FRIEDMAN, W. F., KABACK, M. M., AND ROWE, R. D.: *Idiopathic hypercalcemia and supravalvular aortic stenosis: Documentation of a new syndrome.* New Eng. J. Med. 271:117, 1964.

39. BEUREN, A. J., SCHULZE, C. H., EBERLE, P., HARMJANZ, D., AND APITZ, J.: *The syndrome of supravalvular aortic stenosis, peripheral pulmonic stenosis, mental retardation and similar facial appearance.* Amer. J. Cardiol. 13:471, 1964.

40. BLACK, J. A., AND BONHAM CARTER, R. E.: *Association between aortic stenosis and facies of severe infantile hypercalcemia.* Lancet 2:745, 1963.

41. MORROW, A. G., WALDHAUSEN, J. A., PETERS, R. L., BLOODWELL, R. D., AND BRAUNWALD, E.: *Supravalvular aortic stenosis. Clinical, hemodynamic and pathologic observations.* Circulation 20:1003, 1959.

42. FRIEDMAN, W. F., AND ROBERTS, W. C.: *Vitamin D and the supravalvular aortic stenosis syndrome. The transplacental effects of vitamin D on the aorta of the rabbit.* Circulation 34:77, 1966.

43. TAKATA, A.: *Adverse effects of drugs on the fetus.* Hospital Formulary Management 4:25, 1969.

44. LENZ, W.: *Malformations caused by drugs in pregnancy.* Amer. J. Dis. Child. 112:99, 1966.

45. COHLAN, S. Q.: *Fetal and neonatal hazards from drugs administered during pregnancy.* New York State J. Med. 64:493, 1964.

46. WRIGHT, S. W., DAY, R. W., MULLER, H., AND WEINHOUSE, R.: *The frequency of trisomy and translocation in Down's syndrome.* J. Pediat. 70:420, 1967.

47. PENROSE, L. S.: *Paternal age in mongolism.* Lancet 1:1101, 1962.

48. SHAPIRO, S., ROSS, L. J., AND LEVINE, H. S.: *Relationship of selected prenatal factors to pregnancy outcome and congenital anomalies.* Amer. J. Public Health 55:268, 1965.

49. ALZAMORA, V., ROTTA, A., BATTILANA, G., ABUGATTAS, R., RUBIO, C., BOURONCLE, J., ZAPATA, C., SANTA-MARIA, E., BINDER, T., SUBIRIA, R., PAREDES, D., PANDO, B., AND GRAHAM, G.: *On the possible influence of great altitudes on the determination of certain cardiovascular anomalies.* Pediatrics 12:259, 1952.

50. SMITH, D. W.: *Autosomal abnormalities.* Amer. J. Obstet. Gynec. 90:1055, 1964.

51. BERG, J., CROME, L., AND FRANCE, N. E.: *Congenital cardiac malformations in mongolism.* Brit. Heart J. 22:331, 1960.

52. ROWE, R. D., AND UCHIDA, I. A.: *Cardiac malformation in mongolism. A prospective study of 184 mongoloid children.* Amer. J. Med. 31:726, 1961.

53. SHERMAN, F. E.: *An Atlas of Congenital Heart Disease: Compiled from the Museum of Congenital Heart Disease at Children's Hospital of Pittsburgh.* Philadelphia, Lea & Febiger, 1963.

54. FONTANA, R. S., AND EDWARDS, J. E.: *Congenital Cardiac Disease: A Review of 357 Cases Studied Pathologically.* W. B. Saunders Co., Philadelphia, 1962.

55. ABBOTT, M. E.: *Atlas of Congenital Cardiac Disease.* American Heart Association, New York, 1936.

56. NELSON, S. E., VAUGHAN, V. C., AND McKAY, G. R.: *Textbook of Pediatrics.* W. B. Saunders Co., Philadelphia, 1969.

57. CARTER, C. O., AND EVANS, K. A.: *Risk of parents who have had one child with Down's syndrome (mongolism) having another child similarly affected.* Lancet 2:785, 1961.

58. FIALKOW, P. G.: *Thyroid antibodies, Down's syndrome and maternal age.* Nature 214:1253, 1967.

59. PATAU, K., SMITH, D. W., THERMAN, E., INHORN, S. L., AND WAGNER, H. P.: *Multiple congenital anomaly caused by an extra autosome.* Lancet 1:790, 1960.

60. SMITH, D. W.: *The no. 18 trisomy syndrome.* J. Pediat. 60:513, 1962.

61. EDWARDS, J. H., HARNDEN, D. G., CAMERON, A. H., CROSS, V. M., AND WOLFF, O. H.: *A new trisomic syndrome.* Lancet 1:787, 1960.

62. MARDEN, P. M., SMITH, D. W., AND McDONALD, M. J.: *Congenital anomalies in the newborn infant including minor variations. A study of 4412 babies by surface examination for anomalies and buccal smear for sex chromatin.* J. Pediat. 64:357, 1964.

63. HECHT, F., BRYANT, G. J., MOTULSKY, A. G., AND GIBLETT, E. R.: *The no. 17–18 (E) trisomy syndrome.* J. Pediat. 63:605, 1963.

64. LEWIS, A. J.: *The pathology of 18 trisomy.* J. Pediat. 65:92, 1964.

65. Zellweger, H., Beck, K., and Hawtrey, C. E.: *Trisomy 18.* Arch. Intern. Med. 113:598, 1964.

66. Rohde, R. A., Hodgman, J. E., and Cleland, R. S.: *Multiple congenital anomalies in the E trisomy (group 16–18) syndrome.* Pediatrics 33:258, 1964.

67. Townes, P. L., Kreutner, A., and Manning, J.: *Observations on the pathology of the trisomy 17–18 syndrome.* J. Pediat. 62:703, 1963.

68. Rogers, T. R., Hagstrom, J. W. C., and Engle, M. A.: *Origin of both great vessels from the right ventricle associated with the trisomy-18 syndrome.* Circulation 32:802, 1965.

69. Rosenfield, R. L., Breibart, S., Isaacs, H. G., Klevit, H. D., and Mellman, W. J.: *Trisomy of chromosomes 13–15 and 17–18: Its association with infantile arteriosclerosis.* Amer. J. Med. Sci. 244:763, 1962.

70. Crawford, M. D.: *Multiple congenital anomaly associated with an extra autosome.* Lancet 2:22, 1961.

71. Lejeune, J., Lafourcade, J., Berger, R., Vialatte, J., Boeswill-Wald, M., Seringe, P., and Turpin, R.: *Trois cas de délétion partielle du bras court d'un caromosome 5.* C. R. Acad. Sci. (Paris) 257:3098, 1963.

72. McCracken, J. S., and Gordon, R. R.: *"Cri Du Chat" syndrome: A new clinical and cytogenetic entity.* Lancet 1:23, 1965.

73. Turner, H. H.: *A syndrome of infantilism, congenital webbed neck and cubitus valgus.* Endocrinology 23:566, 1938.

74. Wilkins, L., and Fleischmann, W.: *Ovarian agenesis: Pathology, associated clinical symptoms and the bearing on the theories of sex differentiation.* J. Clin. Endocr. 4:357, 1944.

75. Grumbach, M. M., Van Wyk, J. J., and Wilkins, L.: *Chromosomal sex in gonadal dysgenesis (ovarian agenesis): Relationship to male pseudohermaphrodism and theories of human sex differentiation.* J. Clin. Endocrin. 15:1161, 1955.

76. Ford, C. E., Jones, K. W., Polani, P. E., De Almeida, J. C., Briggs, J. H.: *A sex-chromosome anomaly in a case of gonadal dysgenesis (Turner's syndrome).* Lancet 1:711, 1959.

77. Haddad, H. M., and Wilkins, L.: *Congenital anomalies associated with gonadal aplasia. Review of 55 cases.* Pediatrics 23:885, 1959.

78. Rainier-Pope, C. R., Cunningham, R. D., Nadas, A. S., and Crigler, J. J., Jr.: *Cardiovascular malformations in Turner's syndrome.* Pediatrics 33:919, 1964.

79. McKusick, V. A.: *A genetical view of cardiovascular disease.* Circulation 30:326, 1964.

80. McKusick, V. A.: *The genetic mucopolysaccharidoses.* Circulation 31:1, 1965.

81. Bolande, R. P.: *The nature of the connective tissue abiotrophy in the Marfan syndrome.* Lab. Invest. 12:1087, 1963.

82. Krovetz, L. J., Lorincz, A. E., and Schiebler, G. L.: *Cardiovascular manifestations of the Hurler syndrome: Hemodynamic and angiocardiographic observations in 15 patients.* Circulation 31:132, 1965.

83. Maroteaux, P., and Lamy, M.: *Hurler's disease, Morquio's disease, and related mucopolysaccharidoses.* J. Pediat. 67:312, 1965.

84. Barnett, H. L., and Einhorn, A. H.: *Pediatrics.* Appleton-Century-Crofts, New York, 1968.

85. GOODMAN, R. M., SMITH, E. W., PATON, E., BERGMAN, R., SIEGEL, C., OTTESEN, O., SHELLEY, W., PUSCH, A., AND McKUSICK, V.: *Pseudo xanthoma elasticum: A clinical and histological study.* Medicine 42: 297, 1963.

86. CRISCITIELLO, M. G., RONAN, J. A., JR., BESTERMAN, E. M. M., AND SCHOENWETTER, W.: *Cardiovascular abnormalities in osteogenesis imperfecta.* Circulation 31:255, 1965.

87. GORHAM, G. W., AND MERSELIS, J. G., JR.: *Kartagener's triad: A family study.* Bull. Johns Hopkins Hosp. 104:11, 1959.

88. HOLT, M., AND ORAM, S.: *Familial heart disease with skeletal malformations.* Brit. Heart J. 22:236, 1960.

89. MASSUMI, R. A., AND NUTTER, D. O.: *The syndrome of familial defects of heart and upper extremities (Holt-Oram syndrome).* Circulation 34:65, 1966.

90. HUSSON, G. S., AND PARKMAN, P.: *Chondroectodermal dysplasia (Ellis-van Creveld syndrome) with a complex cardiac malformation.* Pediatrics 28:285, 1961.

91. GIKNIS, F. L.: *Single atrium and the Ellis-van Creveld syndrome.* J. Pediat. 62:558, 1963.

92. McLOUGHLIN, T. G., KROVETZ, L. J., AND SCHIEBLER, G. L.: *Heart disease in the Laurence-Moon-Biedl syndrome. A review and a report of 3 brothers.* J. Pediat. 65: 388, 1964.

93. HOHN, A. R., LOWE, C. U., SOKAL, J. E., AND LAMBERT, E. C.: *Cardiac problems in the glycogenoses with specific reference to Pompe's disease.* Pediatrics 35:313, 1965.

94. SCHIMKE, R. N., McKUSICK, V. A., HUANG, T., AND POLLACK, A. D.: *Homocystinuria studies of 20 families with 38 affected members.* J.A.M.A. 193:711, 1965.

95. HODGSON, C. H., BURCHELL, H. B., GOOD, C. A., AND CLAGETT, O. T.: *Hereditary hemorrhagic teleangiectasia and pulmonary arteriovenous fistula: Survey of a large family.* New Eng. J. Med. 261:625, 1959.

96. ESTERLY, J. R., AND McKUSICK, V. A.: *Genetic and physiological studies of Milroy's Disease.* Clin. Res. 7:263, 1959.

97. EVANS, W., AND WRIGHT, G.: *The electrocardiogram in Friedreich's disease.* Brit. Heart J. 4:91, 1942.

98. BOYER, S. H., CHISHOLM, A. W., AND McKUSICK, V. A.: *Cardiac aspects of Friedreich's ataxia.* Circulation 25:493, 1962.

99. GILROY, J., CAHALAN, J. L., BERMAN, R., AND NEWMAN, M.: *Cardiac and pulmonary complications in Duchenne's progressive muscular dystrophy.* Circulation 27:484, 1963.

100. HOOEY, M. A., AND JERRY, L. M.: *The cardiomyopathy of muscular dystrophy. Report of two cases with a review of the literature.* Canad. Med. Ass. J. 90:771, 1964.

101. WELSH, J. D., LYNN, T. N., JR., AND HAASE, G. R.: *Cardiac findings in 73 patients with muscular dystrophy.* Arch. Intern. Med. 112:199, 1963.

102. RICHTERICH, R., VAN MECHELEN, P., AND ROSSI, E.: *Refsum's disease (Heredopathia Atactica Polyneuritiformis): An inborn error of lipid metabolism with storage of 3,7,11,15-tetramethyl hexadecanoic acid.* Amer. J. Med. 39:230, 1965.

103. DANCIS, J., AND SMITH, A. A.: *Current concepts, familial dysautonomia.* New Eng. J. Med. 274:207, 1966.

23

104. RILEY, C. M.: *Familial dysautonomia.* Advances Pediat. 9:157, 1957.

105. McKEOWN, T., MacMAHON, B., AND PARSONS, C. G.: *The familial incidence of congenital malformation of the heart.* Brit. Heart J. 15:273, 1953.

106. NORA, J. J., DODD, P. F., McNAMARA, D. G., HATTWICK, M. A. W., LEACHMAN, R. D., AND COOLEY, D. A.: *Risk to offspring of parents with congenital heart defects.* J.A.M.A. 209:2052, 1969.

107. FUHRMANN, W.: *Untersuchungen zur Atiologie der Angeborenen Angiokardiopathien.* Acta Genet. (Basel) 11:289, 1961.

108. COCKAYNE, E. A.: *The genetics of transposition of the viscera.* Quart. J. Med. 7:479, 1938.

109. CAMPBELL, M., AND POLANI, P. E.: *Factors in the aetiology of atrial septal defect.* Brit. Heart J. 23:477, 1961.

110. CARLETON, R. A., ABELMAN, W. H., AND HANCOCK, E. W.: *Familial occurrence of congenital heart disease. Report of three families and review of the literature.* New Eng. J. Med. 259:1237, 1958.

111. ZUCKERMAN, H. S., ZUCKERMAN, G. H., MAMMEN, R. E., AND WASSERMIL, M.: *Atrial septal defect. Familial occurrence in four generations of one family.* Amer. J. Cardiol. 9:515, 1962.

112. WEIL, M. H., AND ALLENSTEIN, B. J.: *A report of congenital heart disease in five members of one family.* New Eng. J. Med. 265:661, 1961.

113. KAHLER, R. L., BRAUNWALD, E., PLAUTH, W. H., JR., AND MORROW, A. G.: *Familial congenital heart disease. Familial occurrence of atrial septal defect with A–V conduction abnormalities; supravalvular aortic and pulmonic stenosis; and ventricular septal defect.* Amer. J. Med. 40:384, 1966.

114. BURMAN, D.: *Familial patent ductus arteriosus.* Brit. Heart J. 23:603, 1961.

115. POLANI, P. E., AND CAMPBELL, M.: *Factors in the causation of persistent ductus arteriosus.* Ann. Hum. Genet. 24:343, 1960.

116. EISENBERG, R., YOUNG, D., JACOBSEN, B., AND BOITAL, A.: *Familial supravalvular aortic stenosis.* Amer. J. Dis. Child. 108:341, 1964.

117. SISSMAN, N. J., NEILL, C. A., SPENCER, F. C., AND TAUSSIG, H. B.: *Congenital aortic stenosis.* Circulation 19:458, 1959.

118. CAMPBELL, M.: *Factors in the etiology of pulmonary stenosis.* Brit. Heart J. 24:625, 1962.

119. BATTERSBY, E. J., AND GLENNER, G. G.: *Familial cardiomyopathy.* Amer. J. Med. 30:382, 1961.

120. BRAUNWALD, E., LAMBREW, C. T., ROCKOFF, S. D., ROSS, J., AND MORROW, A. G.: *Idiopathic hypertrophic subaortic stenosis. I. A description of the disease based upon an analysis of 64 patients.* Circulation 30:(suppl. 4) 3, 1964.

121. EVANS, W.: *Familial cardiomegaly.* Brit. Heart J. 11:68, 1949.

122. PARÉ, J. A. P., FRASER, R. G., PIROZYNSKI, W. J., SHANKS, J. A., AND STUBINGTON, D.: *Hereditary cardiovascular dysplasia. A form of familial cardiomyopathy.* Amer. J. Med. 31:37, 1961.

123. NIELSEN, J. S.: *Primary endocardial fibroelastosis in three siblings.* Acta Med. Scand. 177:145, 1965.

124. VESTERMARK, S.: *Primary endocardial fibroelastosis in siblings.* Acta Paediat. Scand. 51:94, 1962.

125. Rosahn, P. D.: *Endocardial fibroelastosis: old and new concepts.* Bull. N.Y. Acad. Med. 31:453, 1955.

126. Lynch, R. J., and Engle, M. A.: *Familial congenital complete heart block.* Amer. J. Dis. Child. 102:210, 1961.

127. Connor, A. C., McFadden, J. F., Houston, B. J., and Finn, J. L.: *Familial congenital complete heart block.* Amer. J. Obstet. Gynec. 78:75, 1959.

128. Wendkos, M. H., and Study, R. S.: *Familial congenital complete A–V heart block.* Amer. Heart J. 34:138, 1947.

129. Wright, F. S., Adams, P. A., Jr., and Anderson, R. C.: *Complete atrioventricular dissociation due to complete or advanced atrioventricular heart block.* Amer. J. Dis. Child. 98:72, 1959.

130. Fraser, G. R., and Frogatt, P.: *Syndrome of congenital deafness with abnormal electrocardiogram.* Heredity 15:454, 1960.

131. Khorsandian, S., Moghadam, A. N., and Muller, O. F.: *Familial congenital A–V dissociation.* Amer. J. Cardiol. 14:118, 1964.

132. Uchida, I. A., and Rowe, R. D.: *Discordant heart anomalies in twins.* Amer. J. Hum. Genet. 9:133, 1957.

133. Ross, L. J.: *Congenital cardiovascular anomalies in twins.* Circulation 20:327, 1959.

134. Nora, J. J., Gilliland, J. C., Sommerville, R. J., and McNamara, D. G.: *Congenital heart disease in twins.* New Eng. J. Med. 277:568, 1967.

135. Campbell, M.: *Twins and congenital heart diseases.* Acta Genet. Med. 10:443, 1961.

136. Patterson, D. F.: *Congenital heart disease in the dog.* Ann. N.Y. Acad. Sci. 127:541, 1965.

137. Detweiler, D. K.: *Genetic aspects of cardiovascular diseases in animals.* Circulation 30:114, 1964.

138. German, J., Ehlers, K. H., and Engle, M. A.: *Familial congenital heart disease. II. Chromosomal studies.* Circulation 34:517, 1966.

139. Anders, J. M., Moores, E. C., and Emanuel, R.: *Chromosome studies in 156 patients with congenital heart disease.* Brit. Heart J. 27:756, 1965.

Pathology and Pathogenesis of the Common Cardiac Malformations[*]

L. H. S. Van Mierop, M.D.

[*] This work was supported by U.S. Public Health Service Grant HE10912 and Research Career Development Award 5 K3 HE21540.

By conservative count, there are some 170 anomalies involving the heart and proximal great vessels. Many of these are of little or no functional significance to the individual, and others are of such rare occurrence that they are mainly of interest and importance to superspecialists in the fields of cardiology, pathology, and embryology. The number of anomalies found in the great majority of patients, either as isolated lesions or in combinations, is relatively small. These will be discussed in the following pages. Some rare anomalies also are included, either because they are mentioned in the textbooks and for some reason have acquired an importance out of proportion to their frequency of occurrence, or because they are of theoretical importance in understanding the pathogenesis of congenital heart disease.

Of the anomalies involving the aortic arch system, only two, patent ductus arteriosus and coarctation of the aorta, are dealt with briefly. A discussion of the numerous other proximal arterial anomalies is beyond the scope of this paper. For a detailed description of the pathology and pathogenesis of these anomalies, several excellent monographs may be consulted.[1-5]

To understand congenital anomalies, it is necessary to have an adequate knowledge of normal embryology, and in a discussion on the pathogenesis of such anomalies, the use of embryological terms is unavoidable. It is, however, not possible to describe here in detail the normal development of the cardiovascular system. A detailed account has recently been given by Van Mierop.[6, 7]

Finally, it should be realized that to date no one has had the opportunity actually to observe the pathogenesis of cardiac anomalies by a systematic study of embryos with congenital heart disease in statu nascendi. Strictly speaking, therefore, the pathogenesis of congenital cardiac defects is not known. By integrating observations made on normal cardiovascular development and those made in the analysis of anomalous hearts, it is often possible, however, to deduce what the pathogenesis of an anomaly may have been. Such a working hypothesis is extremely useful provided that one remembers that it is arrived at by deduction rather than by actual observation.

PERSISTENT LEFT SUPERIOR VENA CAVA

A left superior vena cava, normally present in a number of species of lower mammals, occurs not uncommonly in man. Occasionally it is seen as an isolated anomaly; more commonly, it is associated with other cardiovascular malformations.

A persistent left superior vena cava, after being formed by the confluence of the left jugular and subclavian veins, descends into the chest parallel to the normal right superior vena cava and anterior to the left lung hilus, and always enters the markedly dilated coronary sinus along a course ordinarily occupied by the ligament and vein of Marshall (Fig. 1). The left innominate vein, if present, usually is smaller than normal or may be plexiform. The hemiazygos vein usually resembles the azygos vein anatomically and may approximate the latter in size.

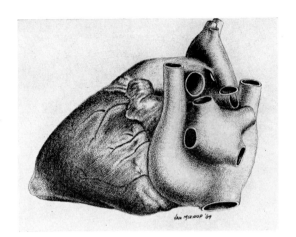

Figure 1. Persistent left superior vena cava.

The right superior vena cava usually is present as well, but it may be absent. If both cavae are present, they may be equal in size; more commonly, however, one or the other, usually the left, is somewhat smaller. Occasionally, a defect is present in the wall between the coronary sinus and the left atrium. If such a defect is large, the left superior vena cava is said to enter the left atrium.

Pathogenesis

Normally, in man, the left common cardinal vein and adjacent distal portion of the left sinus horn obliterate, and the remainder of the left sinus horn becomes the coronary sinus, which ordinarily receives only the greater and middle cardiac veins. In the normal heart, the obliterated common cardinal vein is represented by the ligament of Marshall. A persistent left superior vena cava results from persistence in toto of the left common cardinal vein and the left sinus horn. It is obvious, therefore, that such a persistent left superior vena cava always enters the coronary sinus, even though cases with an associated defect in the wall between the coronary sinus and the left atrium may give the impression that the left superior vena cava enters the left atrium directly.

ANOMALOUS PULMONARY VENOUS CONNECTION

In cases of anomalous pulmonary venous connection (APVC), some or all of the pulmonary veins discharge their blood either into major systemic veins or the coronary sinus or directly into the right atrium.

In *partial* APVC, one or more pulmonary veins empty into the proximal superior vena cava, close to the right atrium, or into the sinus portion of the right atrium itself. The involved veins almost always drain part or all of the right lung. The others empty normally into the left atrium. An atrial septal defect generally is present. Particularly common is the type of atrial septal defect referred to as the sinus venous type of atrial septal defect (discussed later). Occasionally, isolated anomalous pulmonary veins enter systemic veins

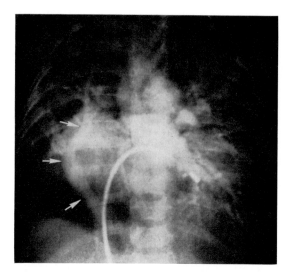

Figure 2. Levophase of a right ventricular angiocardiogram in an infant with anomalous return of the right pulmonary veins to the inferior vena cava (scimitar syndrome).

some distance from the heart. In a rare but well-known type of partial APVC, much or all of the right lung drains by way of a common vein into the proximal inferior vena cava. Because of the characteristic appearance of this vein in radiographs of the chest, this anomaly is referred to as *scimitar syndrome* (Fig. 2).

In *total* APVC, all of the pulmonary venous blood enters the systemic venous system or, rarely, the right atrium. An atrial septal defect or a patent foramen ovale always is present. Several types are distinguished, depending upon the manner in which the pulmonary venous blood enters the systemic circuit.

By far the most common form of TAPVC is that *to a persistent left superior vena cava* (Fig. 3). In this type, the right and left pulmonary veins converge to form a single vessel, which is located behind the abnormally small left atrium and runs obliquely craniad and to the left to empty into a per-

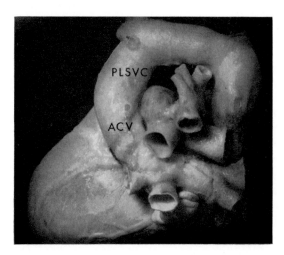

Figure 3. Total anomalous pulmonary connection to the left innominate vein by way of a persistent left superior vena cava. Posterior view. ACV, anomalous common vein. PLSVC, persistent left superior vena cava.

sistent left common cardinal vein (distal portion of a left superior vena cava). Usually the anomalous common vein runs anterior to the left lung hilus; occasionally, however, it is found between the left pulmonary artery and the left main bronchus, in which case the flow of blood may be severely interfered with, and pulmonary venous congestion results.

In TAPVC *to the coronary sinus,* the pulmonary veins join to form a very short, wide common vessel, which usually empties into the distal extremity of the hugely dilated coronary sinus (Fig. 4).

It is interesting that these two forms of TAPVC tend to occur as isolated lesions. Other types of TAPVC, e.g., to the right atrium or to several different sites, are much more commonly seen in association with other severe cardiac anomalies.

In an unusual but interesting form of TAPVC, the pulmonary veins join to form a single vessel that descends in front of the esophagus and travels with it through the esophageal hiatus to enter somewhere in the portal venous system, most commonly the left gastric vein (Fig. 5). Usually there is a stenotic area in the pre-esophageal vein just before it enters the portal venous bed. Such a stenosis causes severe pulmonary venous hypertension.

Pathogenesis

Embryologically, the intrapulmonary veins are derived from the venous plexus around the foregut and, in early embryonic life, anastomose freely with the systemic veins. After the embryonic common pulmonary vein has made its appearance as an outgrowth of the primitive left atrium and has established connections with the pulmonary venous plexus, the systemico-pulmonary venous anastomotic channels normally obliterate. If the embryonic pulmonary vein does not develop at all, if it obliterates secondarily, or if some portions of the pulmonary venous plexus fail to gain connections with the common pulmonary vein, one or more of the anastomotic channels are retained, resulting in total or partial anomalous pulmonary venous con-

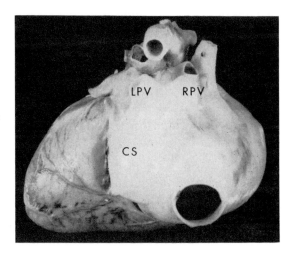

Figure 4. Total anomalous venous connection to the coronary sinus. Posterior view of the heart. CS, coronary sinus. LPV, left pulmonary vein. RPV, right pulmonary vein.

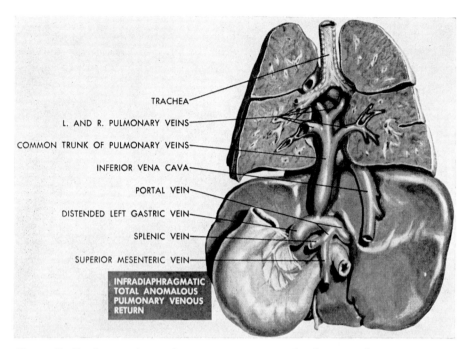

TRACHEA

L. AND R. PULMONARY VEINS

COMMON TRUNK OF PULMONARY VEINS

INFERIOR VENA CAVA

PORTAL VEIN

DISTENDED LEFT GASTRIC VEIN

SPLENIC VEIN

SUPERIOR MESENTERIC VEIN

INFRADIAPHRAGMATIC
TOTAL ANOMALOUS
PULMONARY VENOUS
RETURN

Figure 5. Total anomalous pulmonary venous connection by way of a common pre-esophageal vein to the portal venous bed. The specimen is viewed from the back, and the posterior portions of the lungs have been removed. (From Van Mierop, L. H. S.: Congenital Anomalies of the Heart.[8])

nection, the particular type depending upon which systemicopulmonary anastomotic channel or channels are retained.

ATRIAL SEPTAL DEFECTS

Atrial septal defects (ASD) are classified commonly as being of either the ostium primum or ostium secundum type. Interatrial communications resulting from persistence of the *true* ostium primum, however, are exceedingly rare, and the type of defect that is improperly called ostium primum type ASD is caused by a malformation of the atrioventricular endocardial cushions and is not an anomaly of the atrial septum proper. Its pathology and pathogenesis will be discussed later.

Two main types of true ASD may be distinguished. By far the most common is a *defect in the floor of the fossa ovalis* (Fig. 6). There may be a single opening of varying size, or multiple communications may be present. This type of ASD is one of the most common forms of congenital heart defect found as an isolated lesion. It is, however, also often seen in association with other cardiovascular anomalies.

The second important type of ASD is commonly referred to as *sinus venosus type ASD*. An interatrial communication, usually of moderately large size, is present in the posterosuperior, muscular part of the atrial sep-

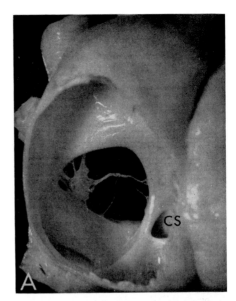

Figure 6. Atrial septal defect at the foramen. CS, Coronary sinus. In A, the septum primum has been reduced to a few strands.

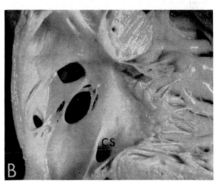

tum, just at the entrance of the superior vena cava. The defect does not have an upper rim, and the ostium of the superior vena cava tends to override the defect. Almost always, one or more of the right pulmonary veins, particularly those of the right upper lobe, enter the right atrium at or near the defect. Characteristically, the fossa ovalis is normal.

Pathogenesis

Normally, in cardiac development, before ostium primum closes, multiple perforations appear in septum primum, which coalesce to form ostium secundum. In normal development, a second, partial muscular septum (septum secundum) is formed just to the right of septum primum and overlying ostium secundum by infolding of the roof of the interseptovalvular space. The foramen ovale in septum secundum and the ostium secundum in septum primum thus form the extremities of a very oblique channel connecting the two atria. Septum primum, which until shortly after birth is

33

fibrous and diaphanously thin, acts as a flap valve that, after birth, applies itself to the much stiffer muscular septum secundum, thereby effectively preventing blood flow from left atrium to right atrium. If the normal process of resorption of septum primum is carried too far or occurs in abnormal sites, septum secundum cannot cover the large opening or multiple perforations, and an interatrial communication results. Not infrequently, ostium secundum is of normal size, but septum secundum does not develop well, in which case an interatrial communication again remains. This type of defect is always associated with other severe cardiac anomalies.

The pathogenesis of the sinus venous type of atrial septal defect is not clear at present.

ENDOCARDIAL CUSHION DEFECTS

A number of types of endocardial cushion defects (ECD) are distinguished. The pathological features shared by all to a varying degree are as follows: (1) The aortic or anterior cusp of the mitral valve is cleft, and its origin is concave towards the atrium instead of convex as in the normal heart; (2) The interventricular septum has a peculiar, scooped out appearance; (3) The left ventricular outflow tract is narrower and longer than normal; (4) The superoinferior (anteroposterior if the heart is held standing on its apex) diameter of the ventricles is increased at the base; (5) A large interatrial communication of very characteristic appearance, a ventricular communication, or both may be present.

Several forms of *partial* ECD are distinguished. All these have in common the presence of two atrioventricular ostia.

In the most common form, the anterior cusp of the mitral valve is cleft, and an interatrial communication of moderate size is present just above the atrioventricular ostia (Fig. 7). This interatrial communication typically is not a defect of the atrial septum itself but is located in the area where, in the normal heart, one finds the atrioventricular part of the cardiac septum. The origins of the anterior, cleft cusp of the mitral valve and septal cusp of the tricuspid valve are lower, i.e., located more apically, than are those in the normal heart. The muscular ventricular septum again has the characteristic scooped out appearance; however, in this type of endocardial cushion defect, an interventricular communication is not present. Fibrous tissue and chordae tendineae are found closing off the space between the border of the muscular ventricular septum and the under surface of the atrioventricular valve cusps. Transitional forms between this form of partial ECD and the complete type may be seen.

Much more uncommon is the form of partial ECD in which there is no interatrial communication. The anterior cusp of the mitral valve, while cleft to a greater or lesser extent, originates from its normal position, and there is a large interventricular communication. Again, the ventricular septum has a scooped out appearance.

The least severe form of partial ECD, in which there is a cleft of the mitral

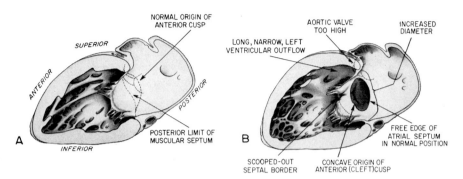

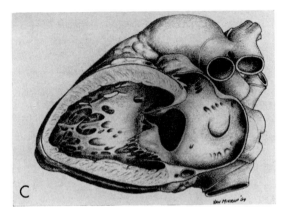

Figure 7. Endocardial cushion defect. A, left side of the cardiac septum in a normal heart; B, endocardial cushion defect, partial type, with interatrial communication and cleft mitral valve; C, Endocardial cushion defect, complete type. (A and B from Van Mierop, L. H. S., and Alley, R. D.: Management of the cleft mitral valve in endocardial cushion defects.[9])

valve but the cardiac septum is intact, is very rare. Even in these cases, the muscular ventricular septum is usually deficient, and the basilar portion of the ventricular septum, just below the atrioventricular valve, is closed by fibrous tissue.

In the *complete* type of ECD, there is a large, centrally located defect of the cardiac septum involving the atrioventricular part of the septum and the basilar portion of the ventricular septum (Fig. 7C). There is a single, large atrioventricular ostium. This single atrioventricular orifice is generally guarded by five valve cusps, three of which correspond to the normal anterior and posterior cusps of the tricuspid valve and the posterior cusp of the mitral valve. Of these, the posterior mitral cusp is not uncommonly hypoplastic or even nearly absent. The fourth and fifth, centrally located cusps usually are large, face each other, and originate from the superior and inferior borders of the common atrioventricular ostium. The left halves of these cusps together correspond to the anterior cusp of the mitral valve of the normal heart. The right halves correspond to the atrioventricular portion of the cardiac septum, the upper, central part of the ventricular septum, including its membranous part, and the anterior two thirds of the septal cusp of the tricuspid valve. The central part of the common atrioventricular ostium is at a lower level, i.e., closer to the cardiac apex, than are the medial portions of the normal tricuspid and mitral ostia. It is this downward or apical displacement that accounts for the interatrial component of the septal defect. The atrial septum itself is not necessarily abnormal. The free concave border of the atrial septum corresponds in the normal heart to the line of origin of the anterior cusp of the mitral valve. In other words, the interatrial communication corresponds largely in position to the atrioventricular part of the cardiac septum of a normal heart. Characteristically, the fossa ovalis is normal, although not uncommonly there are associated defects in this region.

Below the common atrioventricular valve, an interventricular communication of varying size is present. It involves the basilar part of the muscular ventricular septum and gives the remainder of the septum a peculiar scooped out appearance. The inferior (posterior if the heart is held on its apex) cusp of the common atrioventricular orifice usually is attached by means of short chordae tendineae to the border of the muscular septum; the superior (anterior) cusp is commonly free of the septum, but is attached by means of chordae tendineae to the medial or sometimes to the anterior papillary muscle of the right ventricle on the right side and the anterior papillary muscle of the left ventricle on the left side.

In all forms of ECD, even in the complete type, the abnormal atrioventricular valve cusps may be surprisingly well formed and competent. More commonly, however, particularly on the left side, the edges of the cusps are thickened and nodular, and the valve is incompetent. In these cases, roughened areas of endocardial thickening are seen in the left atrium, particularly on its posteromedial wall.

Pathogenesis

All forms of ECD are caused by various degrees of failure of fusion of the superior and inferior endocardial cushions of the embryonic atrioventricular canal. In normal development, after the superior and inferior endocardial cushions have fused, they bend to form an arch or bay that is convex towards the atrial side and concave towards the ventricular side. Subsequently, the atrial septum primum fuses with the dorsal or convex aspect of the fused endocardial cushions about midway between their right and left extremities. The ventricular septum, in turn, fuses with the right extremity of the fused cushions over a rather broad area. The left half of the endocardial cushions develops into the central portion of the anterior cusp of the mitral valve, the part between the areas of fusion of the septum primum and the ventricular septum becoming the atrioventricular part of the cardiac septum. The extreme right side, by a process of undermining that takes place in the ventricles and that leads to the formation of the atrioventricular valve cusps, chordae tendineae, and papillary muscles, develops into the anterior half of the septal cusp of the tricuspid valve and the adjacent part of the ventricular septum, of which the most anterior portion eventually becomes thin and fibrous: the membranous septum.

In ECD, in addition to the partial or complete failure of fusion of the two major endocardial cushions, the arch or bay usually is not formed. This failure results in an apparent downward displacement of the atrioventricular

36

valve cusps. Furthermore, the free border of septum primum cannot fuse with the endocardial cushions, so that an interatrial communication remains and the atrioventricular part of the cardiac septum is not formed. In addition, the upper part of the ventricular septum remains deficient, resulting in either an interventricular communication or a large area of fibrous rather than muscular tissue. The cleft in the mitral valve is a result of failure of fusion of the left halves of the endocardial cushions. Finally, the aortic valve in endocardial cushion defects cannot descend to assume its proper position and therefore is located somewhat higher and further to the right than in a normal heart. This arrangement, in part, accounts for the elongated left ventricular outflow tract.

ANOMALIES OF THE TRICUSPID VALVE

In *tricuspid valve atresia,* there is only rarely a recognizable, small tricuspid annulus that forms the rim of an imperforate membrane. More commonly, there is no indication at all of a tricuspid valve in the floor of the right atrium (Fig. 8A). Small tags of fibrous tissue and abortive chordae tendineae may be present on the ventricular side. A ventricular septal defect, usually quite small, almost always is present, and the right ventricle is diminutive and slitlike (Fig. 8B). The foramen ovale is patulous, or an atrial septal defect may be present. Tricuspid atresia commonly occurs with other cardiac anomalies, such as transposition of the great vessels, pulmonary valve stenosis or atresia, and ventricular inversion. In the latter case, it is, of course the left atrioventricular valve that is atretic.

In *Ebstein's anomaly of the tricuspid valve,* the right atrium is grossly dilated. The right atrioventricular ostium is quite large, but only the anterior cusp of the tricuspid valve originates normally from it. The other cusps appear to take their origin from the right ventricular wall in a more apical

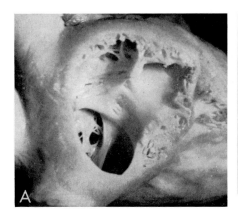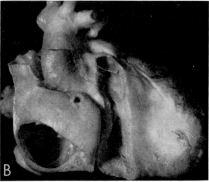

Figure 8. A, tricuspid atresia, right atrial view. There is no indication of a tricuspid valve in the floor of the atrium. Multiple fenestrations are present in the floor of the fossa ovalis, and the coronary sinus ostium is enlarged. B, The right ventricle is markedly hypoplastic and slit shaped.

position, giving the impression that the right atrioventricular annulus is displaced downward (Fig. 9). Thus, a variable part of the right ventricular inflow tract becomes "atrialized." The tricuspid valve cusps are always redundant and often have a crumpled appearance, and the chordae tendineae are usually poorly developed. Not uncommonly, the tricuspid valve apparatus resembles a crumpled sack with an opening, generally smaller than the normal tricuspid ostium, found in a constant, eccentric position near the crista supraventricularis of the right ventricle. Usually, multiple smaller openings found elsewhere in the sack represent efforts at formation of chordae tendineae. In milder cases, the wall of the atrialized portion of the right ventricle has retained its musculature. In the severest cases, however, it may be fibrous and extremely thin.

Pathogenesis

Tricuspid atresia: At some time during cardiac development, usually at an early age, but after partitioning of the atrioventricular canal has been completed, the endocardial cushion tissue around the right atrioventricular orifice fuses. The presence of a ventricular septal defect must be considered a compensatory mechanism and clearly indicates that atresia of the right

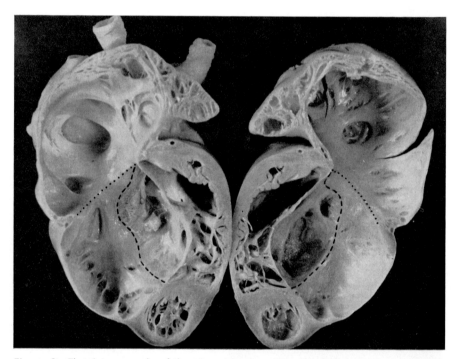

Figure 9. Ebstein's anomaly of the tricuspid valve. The dotted line indicates the position of the true tricuspid annulus; the broken line marks the "false" origin of the tricuspid valve. Note that the anterior cusp of the valve arises normally. The wall of the atrialized portion of the right ventricle has almost completely lost its musculature and has become fibrous.

atrioventricular orifice occurs at some time between fusion of the atrioventricular endocardial cushions and closure of the ventricular septum. Secondarily, the inflow portion of the right ventricle, and in most cases also the pulmonary trunk, remain extremely hypoplastic.

Ebstein's anomaly of the tricuspid valve: Embryologically, the anomaly appears to result from an abnormality in the process of undermining of the right ventricular wall, which normally leads to a liberation of the inner layer of ventricular muscle. This process should continue until the atrioventricular junction is reached. Much of the apical portion of the valve "skirt" thus formed is normally resorbed until only papillary muscles and narrow strands remain. The latter become fibrous (chordae tendineae), as do the valve cusps themselves. In Ebstein's anomaly, the process of undermining apparently is incomplete and the annulus is not reached. Perhaps because the anterior cusp of the tricuspid valve is formed very early in embryonic life, most of this cusp originates normally.

ANOMALIES OF THE MITRAL VALVE

Congenital mitral atresia and stenosis are rare. *Mitral atresia* is almost always associated with other significant cardiac anomalies. Its pathogenesis is similar to that of tricuspid atresia.

Congenital *mitral stenosis* may result from aplasia of part of the valve, in which case one of the papillary muscles and associated chordae tendineae have not developed. In other cases, the borders of the cusps and the chordae tendineae are thickened and nodular and may be fused with each other to form a stiff, narrow funnel with a central opening. Endocardial fibroelastosis of the left ventricle may be associated. The pathogenesis of this latter form of mitral stenosis is not known at present.

VENTRICULAR SEPTAL DEFECTS

Ventricular septal defects (VSD) are very common, both as isolated lesions and associated with other cardiovascular anomalies. Of the various types of VSD, those located in the *basilar portion of the ventricular septum,* beneath the aortic valve, are by far the most common. As seen from the right ventricular side, they are found behind the crista supraventricularis in the general area where, in the normal heart, the membranous portion of the interventricular septum is located. For this reason, they are generally referred to as "membranous septal defects" (Fig. 10). Because of the complex developmental history of this particular region of the septum, there is considerable variation in size, shape, and precise location of the defects. Some extend to the base of the aortic sinuses of Valsalva, while others are some distance away. The adjacent portions of the anterior and septal cusps of the tricuspid valve and the corresponding chordae tendineae commonly show "jet" lesions consisting of thickened fibrous areas. Similar patches of fibrosis may be found on the crista supraventricularis and on the anterior right ventricular wall.

Defects of the muscular portion of the ventricular septum may be single

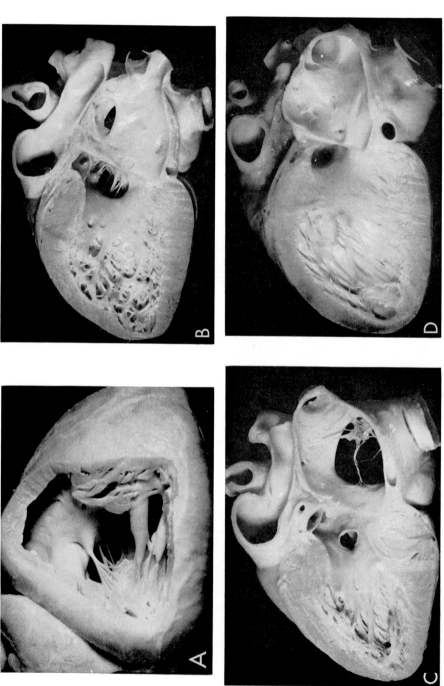

Figure 10. Basilar, infracristal ventricular septal defect. A and B, right ventricular and left septal views of a large defect caused mainly by maldevelopment of the right halves of the fused endocardial cushions. The anterior cusp of the mitral valve has been removed. A small atrial septal defect at the fossa ovalis also was present in this specimen. C, small ventricular septal defect not involving the membranous septum. This type of defect may result from failure of fusion to the right extremities of the fused endocardial cushions with the border of the ventricular septum. A large atrial septal defect at the fossa ovalis also was present in this specimen. D, small basilar septal defect located immediately below the aortic valve in the area of the membranous septum. A defect such as this probably results from a deficiency of a right extremity of the superior endocardial cushions.

or multiple, and they vary greatly in size. Most commonly, they are located in the central or apical portions of the septum (Fig. 11). Small defects in the trabeculated portion of the ventricular septum may be so well hidden among the trabeculae as to escape notice. They are generally easier to find if searched for from the left ventricular side, because the trabeculae here are less prominent and the intratrabecular spaces tend to be shallow. Large defects may be found occasionally beneath the septal cusp of the tricuspid valve in the posterobasilar portion of the septum.

A special type of defect of the muscular septum is located anterior to and above the crista supraventricularis, immediately below the pulmonary valve (Fig. 12). Commonly, this valve overrides the defect, and the pulmonary trunk can be entered easily from the left ventricle.

Other special types of defect in the basilar portion of the ventricular septum, such as that seen in tetralogy of Fallot, will be discussed elsewhere.

Pathogenesis

A number of embryological structures participate in the closure of the *basilar, subaortic portion of the ventricular septum*. Normal closure is accomplished by fusion of the right extremities of the atrioventricular endocardial cushions with the upper border of the embryonic ventricular septum and with the conus septum. Ventricular septal defects in this area result from failure of fusion between, or hypoplasia of, one or more of these structures. The exact location and size of the defect depends upon which of the contributors is deficient or develops anomalously.

Defects of the muscular septum probably result from an exaggeration of the process of diverticulation and undermining that, in normal cardiac development, leads to the formation of trabeculae carneae and keeps the ventricular septum and ventricular wall reasonably thin. Actually, even in normal embryos, small interventricular communications may be present temporarily.

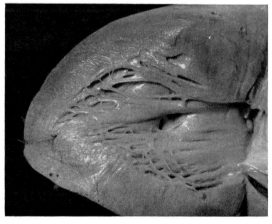

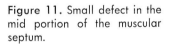

Figure 11. Small defect in the mid portion of the muscular septum.

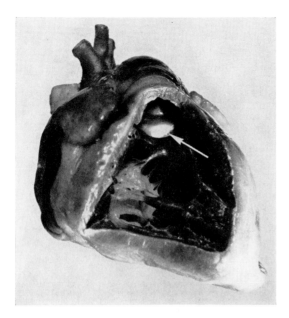

Figure 12. Large supracristal ventricular defect. In this case, the pulmonary artery overrode the defect. Note that the crista supraventricularis and the medial papillary muscle are essentially normal. This defect is caused by failure of fusion of the upper border of the conus septum with the lower border of the truncus septum; in this case, probably due to leftward displacement of the latter.

DOUBLE INLET LEFT VENTRICLE

There are a number of cardiac malformations in which only one of the two ventricles actually functions as such, e.g., tricuspid atresia and aortic atresia with intact ventricular septum. True common ventricle, the condition in which both ventricles are present but in which the ventricular septum is totally absent, is extraordinarily rare. At present, the term "single ventricle" is almost always used to indicate a very characteristic anomaly in which both atrioventricular valves empty into a large ventricle that has the general morphological characteristics of a left ventricle (Fig. 13). A septum-

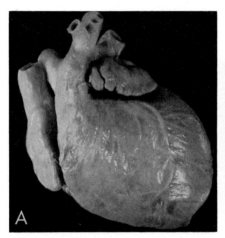
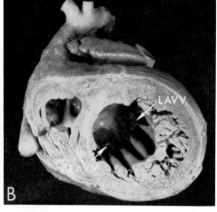

Figure 13. Double inlet left ventricle associated with transposition of the great arteries. Note the extreme rightward position of the ascending aorta and pulmonary trunk. LAVV, left atrioventricular valve. RAVV, right atrioventricular valve.

like structure of varying height, which in truth is comparable with and homologous to the normal, muscular part of the ventricular septum, separates the large ventricle from a rudimentary chamber from which one of the great arteries, usually the aorta, originates. The two atrioventricular valves are structurally similar, both resembling a normal mitral valve, one being the mirror image of the other. It is not uncommon for the right atrioventricular valve to override the interventricular communication, in which case some of its chordae tendineae insert along the upper border of the ventricular septum or on a papillary muscle in the rudimentary right ventricle. In a few cases, the great arteries are not transposed, and the pulmonary trunk arises from the rudimentary chamber. This anomaly is commonly referred to as "Holmes heart." Rarely, both great arteries may arise from the rudimentary right ventricle. Because the large chamber morphologically resembles a left ventricle, the anomaly more recently has been referred to as double inlet left ventricle, a term that has a certain appeal but is not quite accurate from a developmental point of view. Double inlet left ventricle is commonly associated with ventricular inversion, in which case the large ventricle is dextroinferior and the rudimentary outflow chamber, sinistrosuperior, with the aorta almost always arising from the rudimentary chamber.

Pathogenesis

Initially, in very young embryos in which the heart is still little more than a single, convoluted tube, the undivided atrioventricular canal empties into the embryonic ventricle (primitive left ventricle) and is located far to the left. With further development, there is a shift and enlargement of the atrioventricular canal to the right, and blood from the atrium can enter the proximal bulbus cordis (primitive right ventricle) directly, without first passing through the primitive left ventricle and primary interventricular foramen. After partitioning of the atrioventricular canal by the endocardial cushions and development of the atrial and ventricular septa, the right atrioventricular ostium connects the right atrium with the right ventricle, and the left atrioventricular ostium connects the left atrium with the left ventricle. If the embryonic atrioventricular canal retains its far leftward position, yet goes on to divide into right and left atrioventricular ostia, then both ostia continue to empty into the primitive left ventricle. The primitive right ventricle does not receive the right atrioventricular ostium and adjacent portion of the primitive left ventricle to form the definitive right ventricle. Consequently, it remains small. The communication between the large ventricular chamber and the rudimentary outflow chamber represents the persistent primary interventricular foramen of the young embryo and therefore is not a basilar VSD in the usual sense.

TETRALOGY OF FALLOT

This malformation is by far the most common type of cyanotic congenital heart disease that is compatible with life for any length of time, and cases reaching adult age are by no means exceptionally rare. The pathology is quite characteristic (Fig. 14). Cardiomegaly usually is absent, but right ventricular hypertrophy is marked, the right ventricular wall usually exceeding the left ventricular wall in thickness. A basilar ventricular septal defect of moderate to large size is present, and the always large aortic valve overrides the defect to a varying degree, giving easy access to the ascending aorta from the right ventricle. In extreme cases, the aorta appears to arise almost wholly from the right ventricle, even though fibrous continuity is maintained between the aortic and mitral valves.

The crista supraventricularis is displaced anteriorly, resulting in a stenosis of the right ventricular outflow tract. The degree of stenosis varies greatly, from a barely detectable obstruction to complete atresia. The papillary muscle of the conus characteristically is absent, and the anteromedial portion of the tricuspid valve is formed abnormally, inserting by means of chordae tendineae either along the border of the defect or onto the roof of the right ventricle adjacent to the aortic valve. The diameter of the ascending aorta generally is larger than normal.

Pulmonary valvular abnormalities are extremely common in tetralogy of Fallot. The valve may be bicuspid and/or stenotic, or atretic. The pulmonary trunk almost always is smaller than normal and, in extreme cases, may be reduced to a fibrous strand. Even in such cases, however, the right and left pulmonary arteries, while small, are almost always patent. The ductus arteriosus may be absent in tetralogy of Fallot. A right aortic arch is associated in 20 to 25 per cent of cases. In cases with very severe or total obstruction of the right ventricular outflow tract, the lungs are supplied more or less successfully with blood either by means of a patent ductus arteriosus or by multiple tortuous, thin-walled bronchial arterial collaterals, or occasionally by one or more (usually two or three) large, well-developed anomalous systemic arteries arising somewhere from the descending aorta. The caliber of such arteries may approach or even exceed that of the subclavian arteries.

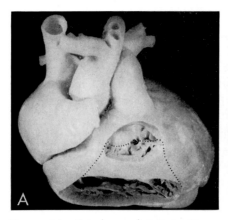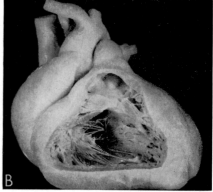

Figure 14. Tetralogy of Fallot with severe infundibular stenosis. In B, the right ventricular musculature anterior to the stenotic channel has been removed in the manner indicated by the dotted line in A.

Pathogenesis

The basic abnormality in tetralogy of Fallot appears to be an anterior displacement of varying degree of the conus septum. This displacement leads to unequal division of the conus at the expense of the right ventricular infundibulum, hence the infundibular stenosis. The displaced conus septum cannot participate in the closure of the primary interventricular foramen, which remains largely patent. Furthermore, the medial or conal papillary muscle, its chordae tendineae, and the most medial portion of the anterior cusp of the tricuspid valve, in normal development all elaborated from the free border of the conus septum, cannot be formed and, consequently, are absent. Pulmonary valvular anomalies, while commonly associated, are not an essential feature of tetralogy of Fallot.

DOUBLE OUTLET RIGHT VENTRICLE

In this anomaly, both the aorta and the pulmonary artery originate from the right ventricle (Fig. 15). The pulmonary artery is normally located, but the aorta originates from the right ventricle to the right of and posterior to the pulmonary trunk. A band of muscle separates the aortic valve from both atrioventricular valves. The aortic outlet separates the crista supraventricularis (conus septum) from the tricuspid valve, and there is no medial or conal papillary muscle. A defect in the basilar portion of the ventricular septum forms the sole outlet for the left ventricle. In some cases, the defect is anterior, in close proximity to the pulmonary valve, which overrides the defect. This special form of double outlet right ventricle is known as the Taussig-Bing complex.

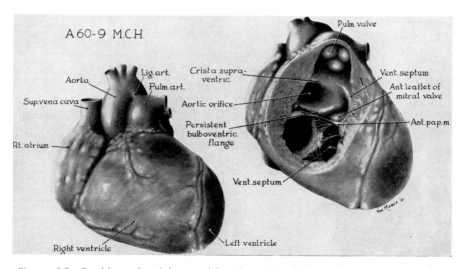

Figure 15. Double outlet right ventricle. (From Van Mierop, L. H. S., and Wiglesworth, F. W., Pathogenesis of transposition complexes, II, Anomalies due to faulty transfer of the posterior great artery.)[10]

45

Pathogenesis

In young embryos, the truncoconal portion of the heart arises laterally from the primitive right ventricle. In normal development, the truncoconal portion shifts to a more medial position, and after the formation of the truncal and conal septa, the anteromedial portion of the conus becomes the right ventricular outflow tract, while the posterior half, with completion of the ventricular septum, is greatly reduced in length in a relative sense and becomes part of the left ventricle. In double outlet right ventricle, the original embryological relations are maintained, and both halves of the conus cordis continue to arise from the right ventricle. The bulboventricular fold, which in the young embryo separates the conus cordis from the atrioventricular canal, is retained and is represented by the muscular band separating the two arterial ostia from the atrioventricular ostia. As in tetralogy of Fallot, the conus septum cannot contribute to the formation of the tricuspid valve, and the medial papillary muscle is not formed.

ANOMALIES OF THE PULMONARY VALVE

In the purest form of *bicuspid pulmonary valve,* the two cusps are of approximately equal size and the valve is not stenotic. More commonly, however, one of the two cusps is somewhat larger than the other, and a ridge or raphe of varying height is present in the floor of its corresponding sinus of Valsalva, partially dividing the sinus into two more or less equal components (Fig. 16). A bicuspid pulmonary valve may or may not be stenotic.

Stenosis of the pulmonary valve is common, both as an isolated lesion and in association with other cardiac anomalies. In the mildest cases, the valve is bicuspid or tricuspid, and there is partial fusion of one or more of the commissures (Fig. 17A). In the more severe cases, the commissures are poorly

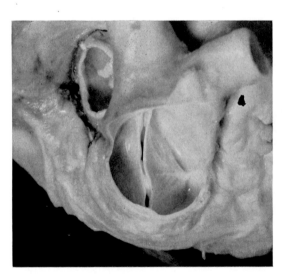

Figure 16. Bicuspid pulmonary valve. The anterior and left posterior cusp anlagen have fused to form a large single cusp containing a raphe.

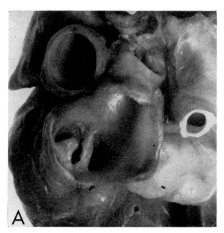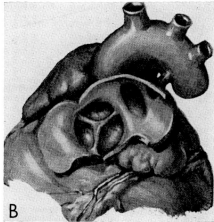

Figure 17. A, severe pulmonary stenosis because of partial fusion of all three commissures. Of these, the commissure between posterior cusps was incised surgically. The sinuses of Valsalva are hypoplastic, and the valve essentially cone shaped. B, atresia of the pulmonary valve resulting from complete fusion of the commissures. The sinuses of Valsalva and even the pulmonary valve cusps in this case were well formed. (From Van Mierop, L. H. S., Congenital Anomalies of the Heart.[8])

developed, and the valve may assume a dome-shaped appearance with a central or eccentric opening. The sinuses of Valsalva almost always are hypoplastic, sometimes to an extreme degree. In severe pulmonary valve stenosis with intact ventricular septum, the right ventricle is immensely hypertrophied. The tricuspid valve usually is distinctly smaller than normal, and its cusps and chordae tendineae are thickened. Incompetence of this valve is common. In the most severe cases of isolated pulmonic stenosis, the pulmonary trunk may be smaller than normal. In the great majority of cases, however, the diameter of the trunk (and usually also the left pulmonary artery) is increased (post-stenotic dilatation).

In *pulmonary valve atresia,* no communication at all exists between the right ventricular outflow tract and the pulmonary trunk. Occasionally, the pulmonary root is well formed, with well-developed sinuses of Valsalva and cusps, but the commissures are completely fused (Fig. 17B). More commonly, however, the pulmonary valve is dome shaped, as described above, but no opening is present, or the pulmonary root may be nonexistent, in which case the pulmonary trunk tapers down proximally to terminate blindly. In cases with an intact ventricular septum, the right ventricle is thick walled with a diminutive lumen, and the tricuspid valve is hypoplastic and often incompetent. The foramen ovale is patent, or an atrial septal defect is present.

Absence of the Pulmonary Valve. In this condition, no sinuses of Valsalva or cusps are present at all. Where the pulmonary valve should be, there is simply a ring of irregular, fibrous tags. Even though no pulmonary valve as such is present, the pulmonary trunk in the region of the nodular ring is usually smaller than normal. An absent pulmonary valve almost always is associated with a tetralogy of Fallot type of right ventricular outflow mal-formation. The infundibular stenosis, however, may be mild.

Pathogenesis

Bicuspid Pulmonary Valve. A raphe indicates that the cusp containing the raphe is derived from two anlagen that have fused at an early stage of development. A purely bicuspid valve may result from total absence of one of the cusp primordia.

Pulmonary Valve Stenosis. Pulmonary valve stenosis apparently is caused by fusion of the commissures. The earlier such fusion occurs, the more extensive it tends to be and the more hypoplastic the pulmonary root becomes. The post-stenotic dilatation is a secondary feature and is caused by turbulence created by the stenotic orifice.

The pathogenesis of *pulmonary valve atresia* is undoubtedly similar to that of pulmonary stenosis.

None of the pulmonary valve cusps have been formed at all in cases of *absence of the pulmonary valve.*

ANOMALIES OF THE AORTIC VALVE

A true *bicuspid aortic valve* is rare. In most cases, one of the cusps is somewhat larger than the other and contains a raphe. Usually the large, raphe-containing cusp is anterior, and both coronary arteries arise from the corresponding sinus of Valsalva. In some cases, the larger, raphe-containing cusp and sinus of Valsalva are homologous to the normal right anterior and the posterior cusp and sinus of Valsalva.

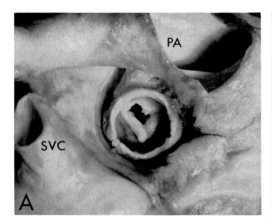
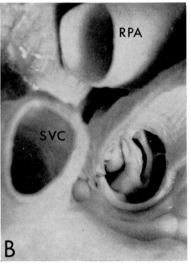

Figure 18. Aortic stenosis. In A, the valve was essentially cone shaped. Two of the rudimentary, fused commissures were incised for a short distance surgically. The valve in B is essentially bicuspid, with the left, largest cusp containing a raphe. The cusps were extremely thick and virtually immobile. A mass of fibrous tissue is present at the base of the smaller cusp, protruding into the sinus of Valsalva. PA, pulmonary artery. RPA, right pulmonary artery. SVC, superior vena cava.

48

A *stenotic aortic valve* (Fig. 18) made up of three equally developed components is extremely unusual. In most cases, the stenotic valve is bicuspid and one of the commissures is reduced to a raphe, as already mentioned. In some cases, only one commissure is somewhat developed; each of the other two is represented by a raphe, creating a so-called unicuspid aortic valve. In general, such a valve tends to be dome shaped, in which case the orifice is eccentric; in other cases, all three commissures are partly fused for a varying distance, and the narrow aortic orifice is located at the apex of the dome. Post-stenotic dilatation of the ascending aorta generally is present. Occa-

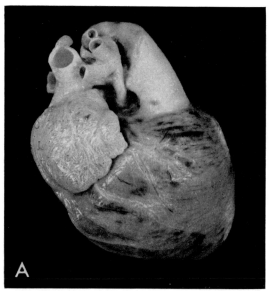

Figure 19. Aortic atresia.

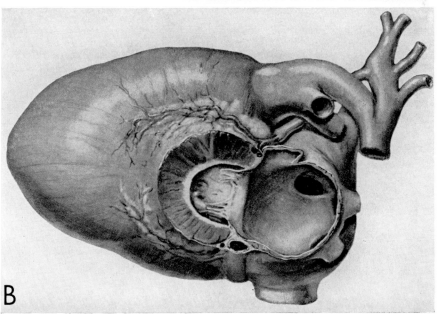

sionally, the aortic root has a narrow waist and the sinuses of Valsalva are poorly developed. Left ventricular hypertrophy is absent in cases of bicuspid and/or mildly stenotic valves. If the stenosis is severe, extreme hypertrophy of the left ventricle may be present.

In *congenital aortic atresia,* the ascending aorta is markedly hypoplastic and serves merely to bring blood to the coronary arteries (Fig. 19). The aorta always is fed by a widely patent ductus arteriosus. The ventricular septum generally is intact, and the left ventricle is diminutive or, occasionally, absent. Its endocardium is markedly fibroelastic and pearly white. The mitral valve usually is tiny, but fairly normally formed; rarely is it atretic. An atrial septal defect may be present or, more commonly, the valve of the foramen ovale (the septum primum) has prolapsed to the right.

Pathogenesis

The pathogenesis of the aortic valvular lesions is similar to that of the corresponding anomaly of the pulmonary valve.

SUBAORTIC STENOSIS

In this uncommon anomaly, a partial or complete ring of fibrous tissue is located just below the aortic valve (Fig. 20). This tissue commonly extends into the base of the aortic valve cusps, which may be somewhat thickened. Occasionally, the aortic valve is incompetent. The fibrous ring causes a subaortic stenosis of varying degree.

The degree of left ventricular hypertrophy depends upon the severity of the stenosis. If the aortic valve is incompetent, jet lesions may be found on

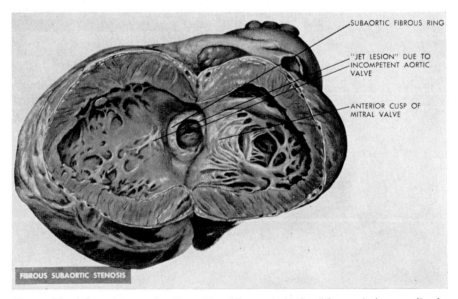

Figure 20. Subaortic stenosis. (From Van Mierop, L. H. S.: "Congenital anomalies in the heart." [8])

the ventricular septum or on the ventricular surface of the anterior cusp of the mitral valve.

The *pathogenesis* of this anomaly is not clear, but it probably results from malformation of the proximal extremity of the truncus septum where it joins the conus septum.

TRANSPOSITION OF THE GREAT ARTERIES

In this very common anomaly, the aorta arises from the heart in an anterior position, while the pulmonary trunk is posterior, and the two arterial trunks run parallel to each other (Fig. 21). In the great majority of cases, the aorta arises from a morphological right ventricle and the pulmonary trunk from a morphological left ventricle. Exceptions do occur, however, e.g., in those cases where the anomaly is associated with double outlet right ventricle and both arteries therefore arise from a morphological right ventricle.

In simple complete transposition of the great arteries, the aorta usually arises from the right ventricle in a position somewhat to the right as compared to the normal pulmonary trunk. The position of the pulmonary trunk relative to the ascending aorta is somewhat variable. When viewed from the front, with the heart in a position as in the living patient, the pulmonary trunk may be posterior and slightly to the right of, directly posterior to, or somewhat to the left and posterior to the ascending aorta. In some cases, the leftward position may be quite pronounced. Associated cardiovascular anomalies are present in over half the cases. The internal anatomy of the two ventricles in uncomplicated cases is essentially normal. At birth, there is no cardiomegaly and the wall thickness of the two ventricles is normal. If, because of the presence of associated anomalies, life is made possible for any length of time, cardiomegaly develops, the right ventricle retains its thick

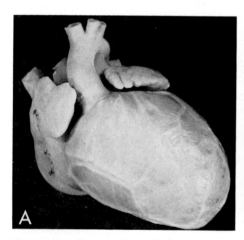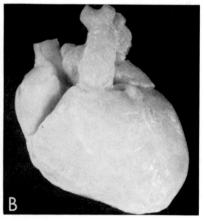

Figure 21. Transposition of the great arteries. In the specimen shown in A, the topography of the ascending aorta is typical; in B, the aorta arises from the right ventricle in a position similar to the pulmonary trunk in the normal heart. No associated anomalies were present.

wall, and the heart generally assumes a characteristic egg shape. In cases in which the only associated anomaly is a naturally occurring or surgically created atrial septal defect, the left ventricle may become quite thin walled.

Pathogenesis

The morphological similarity of hearts that have isolated transposition of the great vessels suggests that the anomaly is a simple one, i.e., caused by a single embryological error. Furthermore, since the ventricles are normally formed, the error probably takes place in the truncus arteriosus. Normally, two pairs of truncus swellings develop. Of these, the major pair executes the partitioning of the truncus, and the other, much smaller pair (the intercalated valve swellings), merely forms a pair of arterial cusps. It is possible that transposition results if the wrong truncus swellings become the major pair. In that case, the pulmonary and aortic intercalated valve swellings form the truncus septum and align themselves, respectively, with the sinistroventral and dextrodorsal conus swellings. The result is that the aorta arises from the right ventricle anteriorly, the pulmonary artery from left ventricle posteriorly. The conus septum develops normally, and therefore its derivatives (the crista supraventricularis, the medial portion of the tricuspid valve and the medial papillary muscle) are normal.

TRANSPOSITION OF THE GREAT ARTERIES WITH INVERSION OF THE VENTRICLES

As in simple complete transposition of the great vessels, the ascending aorta is anterior and parallel to the pulmonary trunk, but it arises from the left-sided ventricle and the pulmonary trunk originates from the right-sided ventricle (Fig. 22). Since, in this situation, the aorta receives arterial blood and the pulmonary artery, venous blood, this anomaly has been called corrected transposition of the great arteries. In addition to the reversed anteroposterior relationship of the great vessels, the left-right relationship of the ventricles also is reversed. The right-sided ventricle morphologically resembles a normal left ventricle (in mirror image), and its atrioventricular valve structurally resembles a mitral valve. The left-sided ventricle has the morphology of a right ventricle, again, in mirror image, and it contains a tricuspid valve. The morphology and position of the atria are normal.

The left, tricuspid, atrioventricular valve is almost always abnormal and usually incompetent. An Ebstein's anomaly of the left-sided tricuspid valve is common. Other commonly associated anomalies are ventricular septal defect, pulmonary stenosis, and double inlet (right-sided) left ventricle with a rudimentary (left-sided) right ventricular outflow chamber from which the aorta arises. The apex of the heart, in cases with ventricular inversion and situs solitus, is usually located on the left side, but in a significant number of cases, it is found more or less in the midline or even on the right side.

Pathogenesis

Corrected transposition can be thought of as resulting from a single embryological error. If, very early in embryonic life, the cardiac tube bends

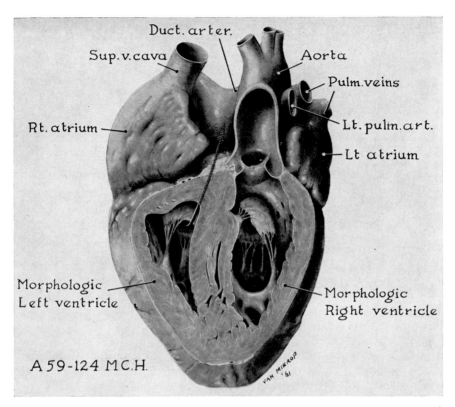

Figure 22. Inversion of the ventricles with transposition of the great arteries (corrected transposition of the great arteries). (From Van Mierop, L. H. S., and Wiglesworth, F. W., Pathogenesis of Transposition Complexes, III, True Transposition of the Great Vessels.[11])

to the left rather than to the right as it does normally, and thus the inverted bulboventricular loop internally develops normally (but in mirror image), then all structures derived from the bulboventricular part of the heart, e.g., the atrioventricular valves, the ventricles, and the proximal great arteries, become inverted. Only the intrapericardial, freely movable part of the embryonic heart can participate in the inversion; the fixed, extrapericardial portions, e.g., the atria, sinus venosus, and truncoaortic sac, cannot. Hence, the atria develop normally and are normally located. Development of the truncoaortic sac itself proceeds normally, but since partitioning of the inverted truncus arteriosus takes place in mirror image, the end result is transposition of the great arteries, with the aorta arising anteriorly from a left-sided right ventricle and the pulmonary trunk posteriorly from a right-sided left ventricle.

PERSISTENT TRUNCUS ARTERIOSUS

In this anomaly, a large, single vessel arises from the heart and gives off the coronary arteries, the pulmonary arteries, and the aortic arch (Fig. 23). The

53

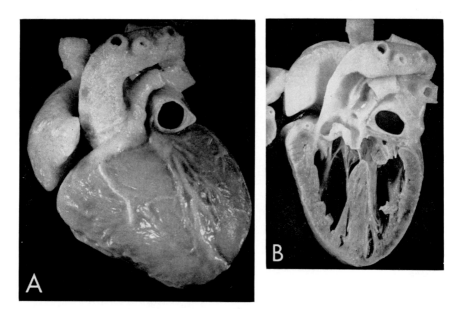

Figure 23. Persistent truncus arteriosus. In the specimen illustrated, the crista supraventricularis (conus septum) was absent.

truncal valve generally is tricuspid, but may be tetracuspid or bicuspid. A large ventricular septal defect always is present and anterior, beneath the valve. The crista supraventricularis may or may not be present.

Several types of persistent truncus arteriosus can be distinguished, depending upon the manner in which the pulmonary arteries arise from the common trunk. In the most common type, there is a short main pulmonary stem that bifurcates into a right and a left pulmonary artery. More rarely, these arteries arise independently from the trunk, or the pulmonary arteries as such are absent. The ductus arteriosus is almost always absent.

Pathogenesis

This anomaly results from a partial or complete failure of development of the truncus swellings, which at best remain hypoplastic. Consequently, partitioning of the truncus arteriosus does not take place. If, in addition to the hypoplastic truncus swellings, both intercalated valve swellings are present, all these structures may form a valve cusp, and the result is a quadricuspid valve. If one of these structures completely fails to develop, a tricuspid valve is formed; if only the intercalated valve swellings or a pair of hypoplastic truncus swellings develop, the result is a bicuspid valve. The axis of the ostium of the bicuspid valve depends upon whether it is formed by the intercalated valve swellings or by the truncal swellings. In most cases, the truncoaortic sac is partitioned normally, and the aorticopulmonary septum therefore is present, resulting in a short, common pulmonary artery arising from the major trunk. In cases where the truncoaortic sac fails to divide, the two pulmonary arteries will arise from the common trunk independently. In many cases, partitioning of the conus takes place, at least proximally. In such specimens, there is a crista supraventricularis, and the tricuspid valve and conus papillary muscle are normal. The upper border of the conus septum, however, does not find a truncus septum to fuse with. The result is a large interventricular communication above the crista supraventricularis and below the common valve. In other instances, the conus septum, and therefore the crista and medial papillary muscle, may be absent. The absence of the ductus arteriosus in the great majority of cases is probably the result of early obliteration of both distal sixth arches rather than of the right sixth arch only, since a ductus arteriosus would be superfluous in persistent truncus arteriosus. The ductus always is present and widely patent if persistent truncus arteriosus is associated with an interrupted aortic arch.

AORTICOPULMONARY SEPTAL DEFECT

In this anomaly, commonly also referred to as aorticopulmonary window, there is a communication, usually large, between the pulmonary trunk and the ascending aorta, located almost immediately above the level of the arterial valves. The arterial valves in this condition typically are normal (Fig. 24).

Pathogenesis

The anomaly is most likely caused by failure of fusion between the distal extremity of the truncus septum and the aorticopulmonary septum. It is probable that in addition, the distal portion of the truncus septum is hypoplastic; in fact, this could be the main factor.

ANOMALOUS LEFT CORONARY ARTERY

Anomalous origin of the left coronary artery from the pulmonary artery is an uncommon but serious cardiovascular malformation. The anomalous

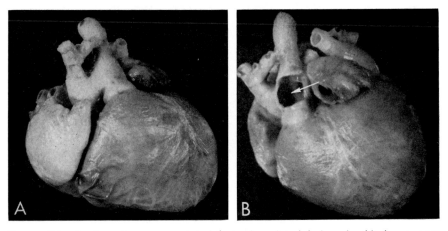

Figure 24. Aorticopulmonary septal defect. Associated lesions in this heart were coarctation of the aorta and a persistent left superior vena cava.

artery almost always arises from the left posterior sinus of Valsalva of the pulmonary trunk, and the distribution of its branches is normal. All the branches, however, are strikingly small and extremely thin walled (Fig. 25). Since the pressures in the aorta and pulmonary trunk are equal prior to birth and the oxygen saturations of the blood not very different, the anomaly is of no prenatal consequence. After birth, however, with the normally occurring fall in pulmonary arterial pressure, perfusion of the anomalous left coronary artery is rapidly reduced, resulting in myocardial ischemia, particularly of the anterolateral portions of the left ventricle. In many cases, intercoronary anastomoses develop, and the right coronary artery and its branches become extremely dilated and tortuous. The potential benefits of such collaterals for the left ventricle are, however, largely negated because of a runoff of the blood into the low-pressure pulmonary artery so that relatively little blood reaches the myocardium itself. Furthermore, most of the damage to the left ventricular myocardium already has occurred before the development of anastomoses. There is marked dilatation of the left ventricle, and the myocardium becomes fibrotic, particularly in its antero-lateral and apical portions, and mostly involving the inner layers. The endocardium becomes thickened and fibroelastotic, and calcifications may be present. Typically, there is not much thinning of the left ventricular wall.

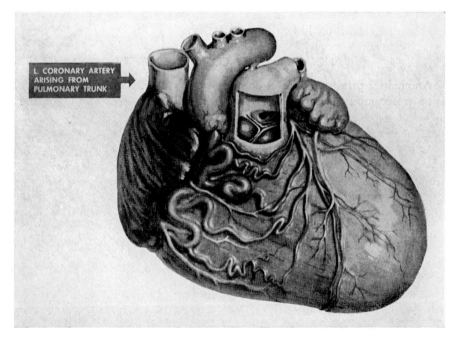

Figure 25. Anomalous origin of the left coronary artery from the pulmonary trunk. Note the extreme tortuosity and dilatation of the right coronary artery and its branches. (From Van Mierop, L. H. S., Congenital Anomalies of the Heart.[8])

Pathogenesis

Hackensellner [12] found in early embryos coronary arterial anlagen arising from both the aortic and the pulmonary arterial roots. If this is indeed the case, it is conceivable that in some instances a pulmonary anlage is retained, whereas the normal, aortic coronary arterial rudiment disappears.

PATENT DUCTUS ARTERIOSUS

This very common anomaly represents a failure of closure of an arterial channel normally present before birth. It connects the origin of the left pulmonary artery, near the bifurcation of the pulmonary trunk, with the inferior aspect of the descending aortic arch (Fig. 26). There is great variation in length and diameter of the ductus arteriosus. Occasionally it is aneurysmally dilated. Jet lesions are commonly present around the pulmonary ostium of the ductus and on the wall of the pulmonary trunk.

Pathogenesis

It is not clear why in some cases the ductus arteriosus fails to close after birth. It may be caused by a structural abnormality of the ductus wall, abnormal or absent innervation of the ductus, or both.

COARCTATION OF THE AORTA

In this condition, there is a congenital narrowing (coarctation) of the descending aorta in the vicinity of the entrance of the ductus arteriosus. The site of coarctation varies: it may be located proximal to, at the point of entrance of, or distal to the ductus arteriosus. Postductal coarctation is the lesion most commonly found in children beyond infancy and in adults. There is marked narrowing of the aorta, occasionally total occlusion, just beyond the ligamentum arteriosum. The descending aortic arch, proximal to the coarctation, commonly is hypoplastic.

The descending aorta is supplied with blood through a massive system of

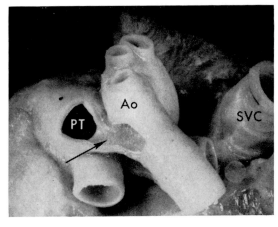

Figure 26. Patent Ductus Arteriosus. Ao, aorta. PT, pulmonary trunk. SVC, superior vena cava.

collaterals. The main collateral routes are via branches of the subclavian arteries (internal mammary, transverse scapular, and transverse cervical) and the intercostal arteries. Other collateral pathways are formed by cervical vessels at the thoracic inlet and the vertebral and anterior spinal arteries. All these vessels become quite dilated and tortuous, and the marked tortuosity of the intercostal arteries is responsible for the well-known rib notching seen in older children and adults. Aortic valve anomalies such as bicuspid aortic valve, aortic stenosis, or both are extremely common in patients with coarctation of the aorta. The reason for this curious association is not known.

Preductal coarctation is most commonly seen in infants and usually is associated with other intracardiac anomalies. The ductus arteriosus often is widely patent, in which case collateral vessels are not present or very poorly developed.

Pathogenesis

The pathogenesis of coarctation of the aorta is not clear. It has been suggested that ductal tissue extends into the wall of the aorta in this particular area and is responsible for the constriction. It is not understood, however, why coarctation of the aorta should already be present prior to birth, as it usually is.

References

1. STEWART, J. R., KINCAID, O. W., AND EDWARDS, J. E.: *An Atlas of Vascular Rings and Related Malformations of the Aortic Arch System.* Charles C Thomas, Springfield, Ill., 1964.

2. EDWARDS, J. E.: *Congenital malformations of the heart and great vessels,* in Gould, S. E.: *Pathology of the Heart.* Charles C Thomas, Springfield, Ill., 1968.

3. EDWARDS, J. E., CAREY, L. S., NEUFELD, H. N., AND LESTER, R. G.: *Congenital Heart Disease.* W. B. Saunders Co., Philadelphia, 1965.

4. HUDSON, R. E. B.: *Cardiovascular Pathology.* Williams & Wilkins Co., Baltimore, 1965, vol. 2.

5. SHERMAN, F. E.: *An Atlas of Congenital Heart Disease.* Lea & Febiger, Philadelphia, 1963.

6. VAN MIEROP, L. H. S.: *Embryology of the heart,* In Netter, F. H., *The CIBA Collection of Medical Illustrations.* CIBA Pharm. Co., Summit, N.J., 1969, vol. 5.

7. VAN MIEROP, L. H. S.: *Congenital heart disease,* in Netter, F. H., *The CIBA Collection of Medical Illustrations,* CIBA Pharm. Co., Summit, N.J., 1969, vol. 5.

8. VAN MIEROP, L. H. S.: *Congenital anomalies of the heart,* in Netter, F. H.: *The CIBA Collection of Medical Illustrations,* CIBA Pharm. Co., Summit, N.J., 1969, vol. 5.

9. VAN MIEROP, L. H. S., AND ALLEY, R. D.: *Management of the cleft mitral valve in endocardial cushion defects.* Ann. Thor. Surg. 2:416, 1966.

10. VAN MIEROP, L. H. S., AND WIGLESWORTH, F. W.: *Pathogenesis of transposition complexes, II, Anomalies due to faulty transfer of the posterior great artery.* Amer. J. Cardiol. 12:226, 1963.

58

11. VAN MIEROP, L. H. S., AND WIGLESWORTH, F. W., *Pathogenesis of transposition complexes, III, True transposition of the great vessels.* Amer. J. Cardiol. 12:233, 1963.

12. HACKENSELLNER, H. A.: *Akzessorische Kranzgefässanlagen der Arteria pulmonalis unter 63 menschlichen Embryonenserien mit einer grössten Lange von 12 bis 36 mm.* Zeitschr. Mikr. Anat. Forsch. 62:153, 1956.

Congenital Heart Disease: Clinical Approach

Marshall B. Kreidberg, M.D., and
Harvey L. Chernoff, M.D.

Deaths from congenital heart disease occur primarily in the first few months—indeed, mostly in the first 10 days—of life.[1] Thus, early diagnosis and treatment are essential if the present high mortality rate is to be decreased.

A heart murmur and congestive heart failure in an infant need no longer suggest a hopeless prognosis, but once congenital malformation of the heart is suspected, the various diagnostic possibilities should be considered carefully, and management should encompass the total clinical situation. With present-day aggressive treatment of congestive heart failure and acidosis, even infants with serious disorders may be expected to undergo diagnostic studies as well as palliative or curative surgery. Improved methods of treating those infants with pulmonary disturbances that exaggerate the abnormal hemodynamics of moderately severe congenital heart disease make proper diagnosis imperative. Correction of metabolic acidosis in the severely cyanotic infant before diagnostic cardiac catheterization and surgery has proved to be of tremendous help in lowering the mortality rate.

When the early signs of heart disease are recognized, diagnostic procedures such as cardiac catheterization and cineangiocardiography can be instituted immediately, pointing the way to more effective treatment. The responsibility for becoming aware of the signs of serious congenital heart disease in infants usually rests on the primary-care physician. He also must recognize the need for referring a patient with these signs to a pediatric cardiology service before the condition becomes advanced.

DIAGNOSTIC APPROACH

Five important signs in the neonate or infant should warn the physician of the presence of congenital malformation of the heart: (1) cyanosis, (2) tachypnea, (3) congestive heart failure, (4) cardiac murmur, and (5) abnormal heart rate.

Some correlations of signs with malformations are given here.

Severe Cyanosis
1. Transposition of the great vessels
2. Pulmonary atresia or severe stenosis with intact ventricular septum
3. Tetralogy of Fallot with severe pulmonic stenosis
4. Dextrocardia syndromes with asplenia
5. Tricuspid atresia
6. Ebstein's malformation of the tricuspid valve

Congestive Heart Failure
1. Hypoplastic left heart syndrome (aortic atresia)
2. Coarctation of the aorta
3. Ventricular septal defect
4. Patent ductus arteriosus
5. Endocardial cushion defects

   6. Total anomalous pulmonary venous return

   7. Persistent truncus arteriosus

   8. Arteriovenous fistula

   9. Double outlet right ventricle

Cardiac Murmur

   1. Innocent or insignificant or functional murmur

   2. Patent ductus arteriosus

   3. Pulmonary stenosis

   4. Aortic stenosis

   5. Ventricular septal defect

   6. Atrioventricular valve insufficiencies

   7. Arteriovenous fistula

Abnormal Heart Rate

   1. Supraventricular tachycardia

   2. Complete heart block

Cyanosis

When cyanosis has been observed in the newborn, the possibility of pulmonary disease, intracranial damage, sepsis, or hypoglycemia must be considered along with congenital heart disease.[2] The absence of a loud murmur is not necessarily reassuring, since in many serious forms of congenital heart disease, such as transposition of the great vessels, severe tetralogy of Fallot, or the malformations associated with pulmonary atresia and total anomalous pulmonary venous drainage (especially below the diaphragm), a murmur may be absent or insignificant.[3] Because of the frequent association of asplenia with severe congenital malformations of the heart, the initial evaluation should include blood studies to detect the presence of Howell-Jolly and Heinz bodies.[4-7]

Because of the rapidity with which a newborn infant with congenital heart disease and cyanosis can deteriorate, prolonged observation is unwise. If cyanosis persists after administration of 100 per cent oxygen by mask for 15 minutes, it is unlikely that the arterial desaturation results from a pulmonary disorder, and cardiac evaluation is indicated, usually by means of cardiac catheterization and angiographic studies, to establish the diagnosis.

Tachypnea

While dyspnea is a well-appreciated component of cardiac distress, the more subtle tachypnea is often overlooked. A resting respiratory rate of over 45 per minute in a full-term infant, or over 60 per minute in a premature, should arouse the suspicion of possible heart disease. Although other causes must be considered, it should be kept in mind that tachypnea may be the first indication of cardiac decompensation, appearing initially only after exertion, such as feeding. Tachypnea may be present in congenital heart disease without heart failure, especially in those conditions that cause an

63

increase in the pulmonary blood flow, as a form of compensation for the reduction in lung compliance that results from pulmonary engorgement.

Congestive Heart Failure

An early sign of congestive heart failure is a gallop rhythm in the presence of tachycardia and tachypnea. As decompensation progresses, the sounds take on a muffled quality. The liver usually becomes enlarged early in infants with congestive heart failure. If failure is progressive, overt peripheral evidence of reduced cardiac output is manifested by poor pulses, duskiness, and even collapse.

An important guide in diagnosing mild degrees of decompensation in infants, especially when the failure is of a chronic "low-grade" nature rather than a rapidly progressive one, is a history of irritability and apparent loss of appetite. The infant will take feedings avidly, but he will become fussy and stop the feeding before it is completed; or an infant may not feed well from the bottle, but take solids and liquids willingly from a spoon. Both types of children are often seen because of failure to thrive.

Prompt treatment with digoxin (Table 1), oxygen, and diuretics (Table 2) may bring about improvement in the infant with severe congestive failure. It should be kept in mind, however, that neonates who go into failure usually improve only marginally and temporarily, and that cardiac catheterization and cineangiocardiography should be instituted promptly, just as in the case of cyanotic infants, if the response to therapy is not satisfactory.

After the neonatal period, response to anticongestive measures usually is longer lasting, and the need for immediate investigation by catheterization is less urgent. Many of these infants, however, have defects that predispose them to pulmonary hypertensive vascular changes. It is necessary to follow these children closely, often catheterizing them repeatedly until the time of surgical correction, to insure that they are not developing irreversible pulmonary vascular changes.[9]

Table 1. Dosage schedules for digoxin * (adapted from Kreidberg et al.[8])

Route of administration	Onset of effect (min.)	Interval before maximum effect (hr.)	Total calculated digitalizing dose		
			Patients < 2 yr. mg/kg	Patients > 2 yr. weighing < 30 kg. (mg./kg.)	Patients > 2 yr. weighing > 30 kg.‡ (mg.)
Intravenous	5–10	2–4	0.075 †	0.04 †	0.75–2.0 †
Intramuscular	15–60	4–6	0.075 †	0.04 †	0.75–2.0 †
Subcutaneous	15–60	4–6	0.075 †	0.04 †	0.75–2.0 †
Oral	120	4–6	1½ times parenteral †	1½ times parenteral †	1½ times parenteral †

* Maintenance dosage in all cases is 1/10 to 1/8 of actual digitalizing dose every 12 hours.
† Half given immediately and one fourth 4–8 and 8–16 hours later.
‡ Mature adolescents may require up to 3.0 mg.

Table 2. Cardiovascular drug therapy

Drug	Dosage	Comment
Ethacrynic acid	1.0 mg./kg. (I.V.) as single dose	Special care should be taken not to infiltrate perivascular tissues. May be repeated in 24 hr.
Sodium bicarbonate	Initial dose 2.0 mEq./kg. at a rate of 1 mEq. (approx. 1.0 cc.) per sec. Succeeding doses 1.0 mEq./kg. at same rate	Repeat as often as every 5 minutes, as indicated by pH of arterial samples
Morphine	0.05–0.1 mg./kg. (IV or IM)	Lower dosage may be repeated in 5–10 minutes if needed.
Isoproterenol	1.0 mg. in 150 cc. 5% D/W	Infusion rate must be carefully controlled, preferably by constant infusion pump. Rate determined by response. Goal is pulse rate over 100 but not over 160, systolic blood pressure of 90–100 mm. Hg. Overdose manifested by hyperdynamic precordium, elevated BP, and pulse over 160.

Cardiac Murmurs

One must accept the fact that not all murmurs heard in the neonatal period or the first year of life are indicative of important malformations. Clinical judgment and knowledge will help to distinguish the significant from the insignificant murmur.

The intensity of an organic murmur may not be as significant as its quality. The harsh, long ejection systolic murmur of pulmonic or aortic stenosis or the pansystolic murmur of tricuspid or mitral insufficiency should warn the physician of more serious possibilities, since in these infants, cardiac decompensation may develop in the first few days of life. In congenital heart disease, especially in the neonate, the absence of a murmur or the presence of one that appears insignificant may be misleading. In the presence of a moderately large patent ductus or ventricular septal defect, flows may not reach a level to generate murmurs for the first few weeks of life. During this period, the normal, high neonatal pulmonary resistance restricts flow through the lungs, thereby preventing large flows from left to right.[9] As pulmonary resistance falls, the murmurs take on the characteristics usually associated with the defects.

A type of functional murmur primarily found in infants is a blowing ejection murmur of grade II–III/VI intensity, heard along the lower left sternal border. The murmur, if it occupies most of systole, may be confused with that of an interventricular septal defect. The innocence of this murmur is suggested by the absence of a thrill, normal X ray and electrocardiographic findings, and a gradual decrease in intensity during the first few months of life, with the murmur disappearing in the first year in the majority of cases.

Abnormal Heart Rate

A heart rate greater than 200 per minute suggests the possibility of supraventricular tachycardia. In almost all instances, some form of intervention will be required, since infants with such tachycardia rapidly develop cardiac decompensation. While standard electrocardiographic techniques usually can distinguish supraventricular from ventricular tachycardia, differentiation may necessitate the use of a high-speed electrocardiographic recorder and specialized leads, e.g., esophageal leads. A Wolff–Parkinson–White pattern, frequently seen in children with paroxysmal atrial tachycardia, suggests that the tachycardia will recur.[9]

A small number of neonates, especially the premature, may have a resting pulse slightly under 200. As with tachypnea, however, inappropriate tachycardia suggests an underlying cardiac etiology with possible early decompensation.

In infants, bradycardia is much less common than tachycardia. A slow heart rate combined with signs of congestive heart failure indicates a grave prognosis. Heart rates of 80 to 90 per minute occasionally occur in normal neonates. An electrocardiogram will show whether this slow rate is of sinus origin rather than a function of an abnormal pacemaker site or atrioventricular block. Infants with total heart block may have rates ranging as low as 30 to 50 per minute.[10] Such children may not manifest signs of decompensation early, yet show motor retardation as they become older. Increasing the rate to a more normal level may produce dramatic developmental progress. The method of achieving an increase in heart rate will depend on the etiology of the heart block. In congenital complete atrioventricular dissociation, for example, an electrical pacemaker may be indicated. Recently we have treated with a pacemaker an 8-month-old infant with complete block and rates in the thirties. The results are gratifying. The child, formerly irritable, pale, and failing to develop normally, is now alert, active, and happy and appears healthy and normal for his age.

DISCUSSION

If any of the five warning signs of heart disease is noted in an infant, the minimal initial diagnostic procedures should include an electrocardiogram and posteroanterior and lateral views of the chest. In some radiology departments, an anteroposterior view is taken. The patient should be in the upright position and the X-ray tube should be positioned to permit an accurate estimate of heart size. If the electrocardiogram and chest films are normal and the murmur is not loud, there are instances in which the murmur may disappear spontaneously within the first few days or weeks of life.

The interpretation of pulmonary vascularity and cardiac size and shape takes on increased significance in the cyanotic newborn. All too frequently, the observer who is not experienced with evaluating X rays of neonates fails to appreciate the slight decrease in vascularity that often is the only abnormal finding. The lack of distinguishing features by X ray can be seen in

Figure 1. The cyanotic infant with a small heart, decreased pulmonary vascular markings, and insignificant or absent murmur may have a very serious cardiac malformation.

The need for prompt referral of the cyanotic infant is increasingly evident when it is realized that cardiac catheterization techniques may have therapeutic value in frequently occurring conditions, such as transposition of the great vessels, total anomalous pulmonary venous return, tricuspid atresia or other hypoplastic right ventricle syndromes, and hypoplastic left heart syndrome,[11] where free communication between the right atrium and left atrium is helpful (Table 3). Enlargement of interatrial communication by balloon septostomy (Rashkind procedure [12]) may prove lifesaving by allowing free mixing of oxygenated and unoxygenated blood or by decompressing an overloaded circuit or left atrium. When the studies are carried out early, the umbilical vessels still are patent and can provide nonsurgical access for cardiac and aortic catheters. This possibility is of importance not only from the standpoint of potential ease and speed of catheter insertion, but also because this route offers other considerable advantages. The umbilical vein will accept catheters as large as 8F. In a newborn, the 4F catheter is the largest that one can usually insert by cutdown without sacrificing the femoral vein. The insertion of a balloon catheter is much less difficult through the larger umbilical vessel. Cannulation of the systemic arterial system in small infants is a difficult surgical procedure. It involves isolation of the vessel to be cannulated, arteriotomy, and repair of the artery following the procedure. The latter often is made difficult not only because of the small size of the artery, but also because the artery may go into spasm because of manipulation of the catheter.

In the newborn with patent umbilical vessels, the problems of arteriotomy are eliminated. It is relatively simple to cannulate the umbilical artery and to pass a soft catheter into the aorta. This catheter can be manipulated to the arch and into the ventricle from which it arises. It also frequently can be passed through a patent ductus arteriosus into the pulmonary artery and thence into the right ventricle. Catheterization of the systemic arterial system allows evaluation of hemodynamics and angiographic studies and permits the very important frequent determinations of arterial pH. This free access to arterial blood samples cannot be overstressed. Venous or capillary blood samples do not sufficiently mirror the arterial pH to permit accurate evaluation of therapy of the acidosis in the sick cyanotic newborn.

Another important advantage of using the umbilical vessels is appreciated when one considers the usual clinical course of the cyanotic newborn. These children usually will undergo at least one more catheterization after the newborn period, when they are being evaluated for more definitive surgical procedures or if they are developing difficulty. If the patient undergoes surgery during late infancy or in childhood, he will almost certainly require recatheterization at some time following the surgical procedure to evaluate the results. The use of the umbilical route in infancy leaves both saphenous veins available for these later studies.

An aspect not well appreciated by those unaccustomed to dealing with infants with cyanotic heart disease is the profound alteration in acid-base balance. In severe forms, a profound degree of acidosis accompanies the low arterial oxygen content. Even in the newborn with only mild distress, an arterial pH of 6.9 to 7.2 is not uncommon. When palliation is delayed, it becomes increasingly difficult to correct the acid-base imbalance, and procedures are less well tolerated. Frequent arterial blood gas and pH determinations may be required to assess the infant's response to therapy, either medical or surgical.

The high levels of acidosis that accompany cyanosis are secondary to the severe tissue hypoxia that exists. Arterial oxygen tension ranging from the

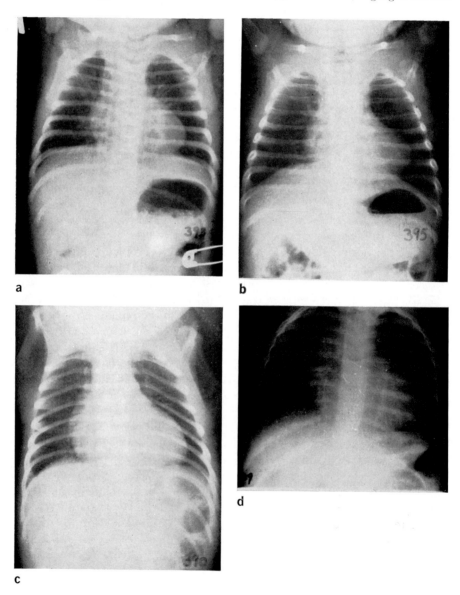

a

b

c

d

Table 3. Frequency of malformations, in 100 consecutive newborns with heart defects, that may be temporarily palliated by balloon septostomy (adapted from Rowe and Mehrizi [11])

Transposition of the great vessels	14%
Tricuspid atresia and hypoplastic right ventricle syndrome	7%
Total anomalous pulmonary venous return	4%
Hypoplastic left heart syndrome	4%

high teens to the low or mid twenties is not at all unusual. In the first few hours of life, these extraordinary variations from the normal seem to be tolerated quite well. In a matter of hours, however, the infant becomes unable to compensate for these severe changes, and his condition rapidly deteriorates, a process that can be exceedingly difficult to reverse. If a diagnosis has already been made, it often is possible to carry out some form of palliation (balloon septostomy or surgery) to increase the oxygen content of the systemic circulation and thereby correct the high acidosis. During the period of acidosis, liberal but judicious use of sodium bicarbonate is helpful (Table 2). We have not found any advantage in using tromethamine (THAM).

Morphine is of little use in the progressively ill cyanotic infant. This agent has been employed to relieve the acute hypoxic spells that cyanotic infants may experience. When the condition of the cyanotic newborn is rapidly deteriorating, the morphine plays a decreasingly effective role.

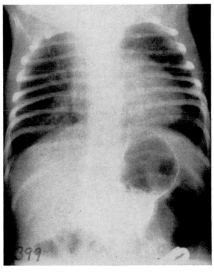
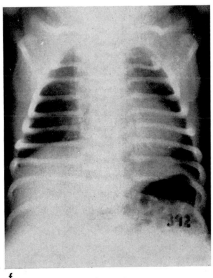

e   f

Figure 1. Posteroanterior teleoroentgenograms in neonates, illustrating the similar appearances of some anomalies. Diagnoses confirmed by cardiac catheterization and cineangiography. (a) Transposition of the great vessels, with intact ventricular septum, (b) tetralogy of Fallot, (c) pulmonic stenosis, (d) pulmonary arterial hypoplasia, (e) tetralogy of Fallot, (f) tricuspid atresia.

After a downward course has begun, the approach must be considerably more energetic. In addition to an attempt to increase the arterial oxygen content and to buffer the acidosis, it is necessary to support the failing cardiovascular system, which progresses rapidly to a state of peripheral vascular collapse. If the circulation can be maintained by drugs such as isoproterenol (Isuprel), it may still be possible to make a catheterization diagnosis.

As an example, a cyanotic infant 12 hours old entered the hospital in severe distress and responded reasonably well to supportive therapy with oxygen by mask and sodium bicarbonate by vein. Shortly after admission, a clinical diagnosis of transposition was suggested. While the infant was being prepared and draped for cardiac catheterization, his condition deteriorated rapidly. This deterioration was not preceded by a fall in body temperature. A check showed that the face mask was in place and oxygen flow was good. The umbilical vein was immediately catheterized and sodium bicarbonate administered, but improvement was only slight. Isoproterenol was infused with greater improvement, but the child's condition still was very poor.

A small injection of contrast medium established the diagnosis of transposition. The left atrial blood was fully saturated. The superior vena cava and right atrial oxygen saturations were very low. The umbilical catheter was removed and a balloon catheter was passed via the umbilical vein into the right atrium and through the patent foramen ovale into the left atrium. The infant at this point was flaccid, with barely palpable peripheral pulses and poor respiration. The balloon was inflated and the septum torn three times within a period of less than 3 minutes. On the third pull, the full balloon passed through the septum without resistance. Thereafter, improvement was gratifying. Muscle tone again became evident. The cyanotic color improved from a very deep to a mild degree. Respirations became deeper and the infant started to cry. The oxygen saturation in the superior vena cava rose from 40 to 68 per cent. The arterial pH had increased from 6.89 to 7.1 by the time the infant was transferred to the ward. Infusions of sodium bicarbonate were continued at frequent intervals.

The dramatic changes that an infant may show—both favorable and unfavorable—underscore the need for early diagnosis to prevent the progression of pathophysiological changes to an irreversible level. The decision in the cyanotic infant, then, is clear: all such infants should be referred immediately.

Like the cyanotic, the acyanotic infant in distress requires prompt referral. The child who has a moderate or large left-to-right shunt or obstructive lesion but appears healthy may present a more difficult decision. The physician hesitates to recommend consultation, knowing that this recommendation will cause family anxiety. Parents, and even some physicians, may find it difficult to accept the need for consultation when a child has no overt symptoms. While there may be no urgency for early consultation, serial visits afford the consultant a better opportunity to discover the subtle signs that may indicate impending problems.

70

A brief review of the changes in pulmonary circulation during the neo-natal period may help to explain the early course of certain common acyanotic congenital heart defects and also the production of a murmur that may be noted shortly after an infant has gone home from the newborn nursery.

In the first few hours after birth, the pulmonary resistance is still very high, resulting in a blood pressure in the pulmonary arterial tree at systemic levels. As might be expected, the pressure in the ventricles is about equal. Even with a patent ductus or interventricular septal defect, there may be no murmurs audible because the flow is not of sufficient velocity to create the turbulence that produces a murmur. The second sound at the base is loud and accentuated, a characteristic sign in pulmonary hypertension.

Only when the pulmonary resistance falls, which is the natural course of events in the pulmonary arterial tree, will there be a left-to-right gradient sufficient to result in increased flow across the defects, with the production of an audible murmur. The fall in pulmonary resistance reaches a low point at about 6 weeks of age. It is not unusual, therefore, for congestive heart failure to be first manifested at about this age.

Any infant or child with a left-to-right shunt in whom there is auscultatory evidence of a loud and increasingly intense second pulmonic sound may have pulmonary hypertension and require early correction. This auscultatory finding is, in most instances, associated with electrocardiographic, vectorcardiographic, and X-ray evidence of combined ventricular hypertrophy, often with evidence on serial studies of progressive increase in the size of the right ventricle. The clinical and laboratory findings may coexist or may be singly more prominent. In either instance, prompt referral is warranted, since the findings can mean that irreversible changes are taking place in the pulmonary arterial tree. Repeated studies, including catheterization, may be required to determine the optimal time for surgical intervention.

A physician who examines large numbers of children is aware that many cardiac murmurs seem to be without clinical significance. Auscultation by pediatric cardiologists from our group as a part of a program (Head Start) of preschool examinations in Boston disclosed an incidence of innocent murmurs of about 80 per cent. Studies reported in the literature [13, 14] indicate that such murmurs are present in about 50 per cent of children.

Although clinical differentiation can be difficult, certain criteria can be used to distinguish between murmurs unrelated to significant heart disease and those that suggest the presence of a significant lesion. The so-called innocent murmur in children usually shows the following characteristics: (1) low intensity (grade I–II/VI) unassociated with a thrill, (2) localization to a small area, (3) short duration, (4) coarse vibratory quality, and (5) no history of the murmur being present since infancy and no evidence compatible with acquired heart disease.

Murmurs in children with no prior history of these sounds may be noted during periods of increased cardiac output associated with fever, excitement, nervous tension, or exercise. In most instances, these murmurs decrease or disappear when the cardiac output returns to the resting state. In the absence of symptoms, a grade I–II/VI, short ejection systolic murmur (not pansystolic) rarely indicates significant heart disease unless it is localized over the apex. Systolic murmurs that disappear on inspiration are usually functional or insignificant.

The venous hum is a to-and-fro murmur best heard in the infraclavicular areas and up into the neck, and occasionally in the sternal notch. It is thought to have its origin at the junction of the jugular and subclavian veins. The murmur, when continuous, may be confused with the bruit of patent ductus arteriosus, although it is soft and lacks the machinery-like characteristic of a ductus. Graf and associates reported its presence in 50 per cent of children under 9 years of age and in 30 per cent between 12 and 15 years.[15]

Venous hums are best heard when the child is erect with the head extended. The hum may decrease or disappear when pressure is applied to the jugular vein or when the child lies down or turns his head to the side opposite the murmur. It is important to recognize this characteristic when children are examined in the erect position, as is often done during auscultation in the schools.

The sternal notch venous hum initially may have an ejection systolic quality, causing it to be confused with a valvular defect. This hum, too, may be reduced by placing the child in the supine position. It often can be increased when the neck is extended. Like other children with innocent murmurs, those with venous hums show no X-ray or electrocardiographic findings to suggest cardiac disease.

With the exception of venous hums, the most frequently noted innocent murmur is probably the so-called vibratory systolic murmur, which is heard best along the lower left sternal border and usually is not audible beyond the apex. This murmur occasionally is of grade III/VI intensity and is low pitched. It usually is coarser in quality and shorter in duration than the murmur of mitral insufficiency. When the murmur does occasionally radiate beyond the apex, the possibility of rheumatic mitral involvement should be investigated. A 20-year follow-up of so-called innocent vibratory ejection murmurs by Marienfeld and co-workers confirms the assumption that this type of murmur is not significant.[16]

A group of murmurs, possibly representing structural anatomic changes, is heard frequently in the axillae and back. They are of grade I–III/VI intensity and may become louder with increase in the cardiac output. These sounds probably are generated by flow through narrowings in the pulmonary arterial vasculature, especially in the peripheral areas. Except in rare instances, these peripheral pulmonary stenoses cause no hemodynamic derangements in childhood. Occasionally there may be stenoses at the bifurcation of the main pulmonary artery of sufficient degree to cause a murmur and thrill in the sternal notch, but even in these children there may be no hemodynamic alterations. This group, nevertheless, deserves close follow-up to be sure that the murmur truly is innocent and does not represent a bicuspid aortic valve (which with time can become stenotic) or supravalvular aortic or pulmonic stenosis.

The so-called hemic murmur, while not representing a cardiovascular anomaly, does represent a pathological state. It is caused by increased flow of blood across the cardiac valves and through vessels, resulting from the hypervolemia and increased cardiac output associated with anemia. It usually is accompanied by a mild increase in heart rate and the expected clinical manifestations of anemia. The hemic murmur usually is widespread, although it may be present most prominently in the pulmonic and mitral areas. The quality is predominantly blowing, and the intensity increases with any further accelerations in cardiac output.

When a heart murmur is heard, it is best to inform the parents promptly rather than to let them discover its existence unexpectedly and become unduly concerned. It is important for the physician to explain fully the significance of the murmur and to offer appropriate reassurance so that no unnecessary limitations are placed on the child's activities, either by the parents or by school officials, unless it is warranted.

In examining the child beyond infancy, it is important to be aware of the possibility of a murmur developing in areas previously silent. This may be due to a bicuspid aortic valve that is undergoing progressive changes or to increasing hypertrophy of the subvalvular area. With growth, the cardiac output becomes greater. A valve that does not present a critical narrowing early may become significantly obstructive.

Each time the child is seen, all auscultatory areas should be examined. This should include, in addition to the classical four precordial sites—aortic (second right intercostal space, right sternal border), pulmonic (second left intercostal space, left sternal border), fourth left intercostal space, left sternal border and apex—the third left intercostal space, left sternal border, the sternal notch, neck, axillae, and back.

The possibility of aortic stenosis must always be kept in mind in children; its reported occurrence is 3 to 6 per cent.[9] It should be remembered, also, that aortic stenosis is one of the rare situations that can be responsible for sudden death in children. The child with aortic stenosis will be asymptomatic and active until the critical point of inadequate perfusion of the coronary arteries is reached. When this occurs, there may be chest pain (angina), or, if the heart's requirements for oxygen are severely limited, ventricular fibrillation may occur. As the child approaches this stage, there usually are electrocardiographic and vectorcardiographic findings of left ventricular hypertrophy with ST-segment and T-wave changes.

A further clue to the existence of aortic stenosis in children is the blood pressure and the quality of the pulse. In aortic stenosis, there is a decrease in the pulse pressure. The murmur of aortic stenosis in some patients may be heard in the antecubital fossa and may be mistaken for the Korotkoff sounds, thereby resulting in a fallacious reading and a paradoxical diagnosis of aortic insufficiency or patent ductus arteriosus (because of the erroneously interpreted low diastolic reading). The palpatory determination of blood pressure before auscultation eliminates this confusion. In addition, the pulse in patients with aortic stenosis feels thin and thready. It is not enough just to feel the femoral pulses, since this practice may lead to the erroneous impression of a normal pulse in children who are not thin.

The murmur of aortic stenosis offers a particular problem. The classical, harsh ejection systolic murmur may be present for the first time during the period from 5 years of age to adolescence. Children with this defect may have no distinguishing murmurs early. The physician following the child may not auscult the cardiac areas carefully, since the patient has not had a murmur and there is no interval illness suggesting rheumatic fever. When the child is seen by a physician who does not know him, all the cardiac auscultatory sites are examined and a murmur is discovered.

Further confusion may arise if the child falls into the group of those with aortic stenosis who have a murmur heard best over the apex. Of those with aortic stenosis, 20 per cent may have a murmur limited to this area.[17] In a hurried examination, a murmur developing in this location might be confused with that resulting from a small interventricular septal defect that did not seem to warrant consultation, since the X ray and electrocardiograms may be interpreted as normal. Only a high level of suspicion will alert the physician to define clearly the duration of the murmur and to appreciate that the murmur is heard best at the apical area rather than along the sternal border, as is the case in ventricular septal defect. Unfortunately, this is easier said than done in children in whom the heart rate may be fast and the distance between apex and sternum small.

Another pitfall in the diagnosis of aortic stenosis is the lack of appreciation that the murmur may be heard in the third left intercostal space along the left sternal border. The murmur of aortic stenosis in the third left intercostal space easily may be misconstrued in children and adolescents as an innocent murmur. This is especially true when the X rays of the chest show no increase in cardiac silhouette (Fig. 2).

If a physician has any question about the interpretation of the clinical, electrocardiographic, or X-ray findings in the child he is following, and therefore cannot make a confident decision about a course of action, consultation with a pediatric cardiologist is indicated.

A query frequently made, especially in localities not close to medical centers, is whether or not a child can be followed by a nonpediatric cardiologist. Although many cardiologists specializing in adult disorders care for adolescents with cardiac problems, proficiency in evaluating and treating the needs of infants and children with heart disease requires the specific training of a pediatric cardiologist. The initial diagnosis and response to therapy in the pediatric age group must be reviewed continually. Therapy is not successful unless the child progresses in a reasonable manner through the developmental milestones. The pediatric cardiologist's knowledge of growth and development qualifies him to evaluate the response to treatment. He also has a better understanding of the complex effect that illness in a child has on the patient and the entire family.

74

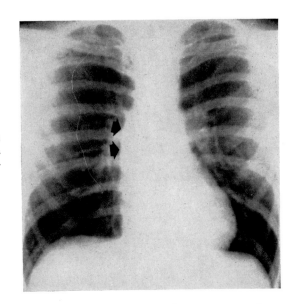

Figure 2. Chest X ray in a patient with aortic stenosis. Arrows point to prominent ascending aortic shadow.

Most pediatric cardiologists are situated in large medical centers where multidisciplined services are available. Specially trained nurses are able to teach parents how to administer medications, how to count the infant's or child's pulse and respiration, and in special instances, how to administer emergency treatment. In addition, social workers can help the family to deal with the anxieties that often accompany serious illness in children, and to arrange for financial aid.

The primary medical care of children with heart disease is carried out not by the consulting cardiologist, but by the physician who sees the child routinely. It is the primary-care physician who bears the responsibility for emergencies in addition to total management. He is also the one upon whom the family relies for interpretation of the consultant's findings and for continuing support.

To sustain this role, the primary-care physician must be kept informed of the consultant's findings and opinions, of any treatment that has been instituted or planned, of any anticipated complications or potential emergencies, and of the course recommended if emergencies do occur. Only when the family physician is aware of the physical findings of the consultant will he be able to determine whether or not unexpected changes are occurring. For this reason, it is essential that he receive prompt reports detailing the consultant's findings.

If travel to the pediatric cardiologist is not feasible, the primary-care physician can carry out some of the necessary follow-up, sending his findings and the laboratory, X-ray, and electrocardiographic reports to the consultant. This is not an optimal solution, but in some situations, it may be satisfactory. Only rare instances exist, however, in which children with heart disease cannot have the benefit of consultation with cardiologists specifically trained to deal with their complex problems.

References

1. MEHRIZI, A., HIRSH, M. S., AND TAUSSIG, H. B.: *Congenital heart disease in the neonatal period.* J. Pediat. 65:271, 1964.

2. CRAIG, W. S.: *Admissions and readmissions from district to special baby-care unit of a maternity hospital.* Brit. Med. J. 2:1139, 1962.

3. OBER, W. B., AND MOORE, T. E.: *Congenital cardiac malformations in the neonatal period: An autopsy study.* New Eng. J. Med. 253:271, 1955.

4. AGULAR, M. J., STEPHENS, H. B., AND CRANE, J. T.: *Syndrome of congenital absence of the spleen with associated cardiovascular and gastro-enteric anomalies.* Circulation 14:520, 1956.

5. GILBERT, E. F., NISHIMURA, K., AND WEDUM, B. B.: *Congenital malformations of the heart associated with splenic agenesis. With a report of five cases.* Circulation 17:72, 1958.

6. IVEMARK, B. I.: *Implications of agenesis of the spleen on the pathogenesis of cono-truncus anomalies in childhood. An analysis of the heart malformations in the splenic agenesis syndrome, with fourteen new cases.* Acta Paediat. 44 (suppl.):104, 1955.

7. RUTTENBERG, H. D., NEUFELD, H. N., LUCAS, R. V., JR., CAREY, L. S., ADAMS, P., JR., ANDERSON, R. C., AND EDWARDS, J. E.: *Syndrome of congenital cardiac disease with asplenia. Distinction from other forms of congenital cyanotic cardiac disease.* Amer. J. Cardiol. 13:387, 1964.

8. KREIDBERG, M. B., CHERNOFF, H. L., AND LOPEZ, W. L.: *Treatment of cardiac failure in infancy and childhood.* New Eng. J. Med. 268:23, 1963.

9. KEITH, J. D., ROWE, R. D., AND VLAD, P.: *Heart Disease in Infancy and Childhood,* ed. 2. The Macmillan Co., New York, 1967.

10. SCHAFFER, A. J.: *Diseases of the Newborn.* W. B. Saunders Co., Philadelphia, 1965.

11. ROWE, R. D., AND MEHRIZI, A.: *The Neonate with Congenital Heart Disease. Major Problems in Clinical Pediatrics.* W. B. Saunders Co., Philadelphia, 1968, vol. 5.

12. RASHKIND, W. J., AND MILLER, W. W.: *Creation of an atrial septal defect without thoracotomy: A palliative approach to complete transposition of the great vessels.* J.A.M.A. 196:991, 1966.

13. FREIDMAN, S., ROBIE, W. A., AND HARRIS, I. N.: *Occurrence of innocent adventitious sounds in childhood.* Pediatrics 3:782, 1949.

14. GIBSON, S.: *Clinical significance of heart murmurs in children.* Med. Clin. N. Amer. 30:35, 1946.

15. GRAF, W., MOLLER, T., AND MANNHEIMER, E.: *Continuous murmur: Incidence and characteristics in different parts of the human body.* Acta Med. Scand. 196 (suppl.):167, 1947.

16. MARIENFELD, C. J., TELLES, N., SILHERA, J., AND NORDSIECK, M.: *A 20-year follow-up study of "innocent" murmurs.* Pediatrics 30:42, 1962.

17. BERGERON, J., ABELMANN, W. H., VASQUEZ-MELAW, H., AND ELLIS, L. B.: *Aortic stenosis: Clinical manifestations and course of the disease. Review of one hundred proved cases.* Arch. Intern. Med. 94:911, 1954.

Diagnosis of Congenital Heart Disease: Clues from the History and Physical Examination

Saul J. Robinson, M.D.

Congenital heart defects are now being diagnosed with increasing frequency during infancy and early childhood. While the first hint of a congenital cardiac defect, e.g., cyanosis, murmur, tachycardia, tachypnea, or hepatomegaly, may be detected by the physician during a routine examination, the initial signs may not clearly reflect heart involvement. Furthermore, the usual complaints of the adult with a heart problem, such as angina or dyspnea, are not elicited.

HISTORY

An important element in history-taking is the reliability of the informant. Mothers are remarkable in their ability to sense that "something is wrong." Fathers usually have far less frequent contact with the child and rarely remember symptoms, past illnesses, immunizations, or other pertinent points in a history. Any physician who has tried to establish the diagnosis on a child *without* a reliable history from a parent can testify to its importance. The late Stanley Gibson[1] stated that the proper history represented approximately 80 per cent in establishing a diagnosis of a congenital cardiac abnormality, the physical examination 10 per cent, and the laboratory procedures the remainder. W. Proctor Harvey[2] gives to the history at least the same importance as to the physical examination, the radiological examination, the electrocardiogram, and other laboratory procedures in his "five fingered approach" to diagnosis.

The Chief Complaint

The complaint that first brings an infant or young child with a congenital heart problem to a physician rarely points directly to the heart. The most common complaints are failure to thrive, frequent vomiting, excessive fatigability while taking the bottle or with any activity, undue perspiration, or rapid respirations. Sometimes the mother has noted an unusual sensation over the infant's chest or a marked pounding of the heart while holding him close to her chest or bathing him.

Fatigability

This complaint may be difficult to assess. Comparison with peers is most difficult. The child who is easily fatigued may quietly leave his play with others and seek some less strenuous activity without suggestion from his parents. True fatigability must be differentiated from the restrictions of activity imposed on the child (by either parents or physician) after the discovery of a heart murmur.

Syncope

Loss of consciousness as a sign of cardiac disease may be confused with other causes of syncope. Convulsive seizures in infants caused by a dysrhythmia or bradyrhythmia, such as Adams-Stokes syndrome, may be ascribed to a primary neurological disorder and treated as such. The child with severe aortic stenosis may have syncopal or dizzy spells that may be diagnosed as epilepsy, and the child with pulmonic stenosis or tetralogy of Fallot may have hypoxic spells that also are misdiagnosed.

Cyanosis

Cyanosis may be a difficult sign to elicit from a parent. True cyanosis may be confused with the slight blueness around the mouth of many normal infants. Mottling of the skin from cold or even a labile circulation may be described as cyanosis. True cyanosis is most commonly noted on the lips and nails. Harlequinism, a unique difference in color of either the two sides of the body or the upper and lower parts of the body, is a temporary phenomenon often confused with cyanosis resulting from heart disease.

The time of onset of cyanosis is an important clue to the type of cardiac abnormality. For example, in transposition of the great vessels, cyanosis may appear early in the neonatal period, as contrasted to the frequently tardy appearance of cyanosis after several months of age in the child with tetralogy of Fallot. Again, repeated questioning of the parents may convince the mother that she is missing something, and by suggestion, cause her to give a positive answer when the question regarding cyanosis is asked.

Failure To Thrive

The inability to gain weight may result from a heart condition: however, a rapid or sudden weight gain is not always cause for delight, as it may indicate the retention of fluid with the onset of severe congestive failure. It is important to measure the height and weight gain in infants and children.

It is difficult to determine the true relationship between a cardiac defect and failure to grow. Episodes of congestive failure and/or intercurrent pulmonary infections may be more frequent causes of retarded growth than is the congenital cardiac defect itself.

Frequent Respiratory Infections

Frequent respiratory infections most often accompany abnormalities associated with large left-to-right shunts, particularly in infants. Pneumonia and atelectasis are particularly common in infants with large shunts or with large hearts or vessels that may impinge on the bronchi or pulmonary parenchyma. The cardiac abnormality is not always the cause of such a problem, however. There may be an associated allergy or an increased susceptibility to infections in children who may coincidentally have a minor cardiac defect that in itself does not contribute to the illness.

Headaches

Unless there is a known tendency to mimic someone in the household with headaches, a complaint of headache in a child is a valid one. The exclusion of eye defects, chronic sinusitis, or allergic rhinorrhea is important. In a cyanotic child, the complaint of headache, even without fever or obvious neurological findings, may indicate a cerebral abscess or impending cerebral thrombosis. In a noncyanotic child, it may be the result of hypertension secondary to coarctation of the aorta.

Murmurs

A murmur heard by a physician is the usual reason for the referral of a child to a cardiologist for a definitive diagnosis. The time of onset of such a murmur and its relationship to a preceding infection are important in the differential diagnosis between acquired and congenital cardiac disease and may sometimes be the only way by which one can determine whether a mitral or aortic valve anomaly is congenital or acquired. Confusion sometimes exists as to the time when a murmur was first heard. If the informant states that the murmur was heard at birth, it is important to determine whether the murmur really was detected at that time by a physician, or was suggested as being of congenital origin by a physician, although discovered at a much later age. It is also important to know the frequency of examination of the cardiovascular system prior to the discovery of the murmur. If the murmur was discovered by a "new physician," an attempt should be made to determine whether it was heard previously.

The onset of a murmur may have important relationship to the type of cardiac abnormality. The murmur of a ventricular septal defect or a patent ductus arteriosus may not become obvious or typical until about 4 to 6 weeks of age, as the pressure gradient between the left and right ventricle normally increases along with the decreasing pulmonary artery and right ventricular pressures. The murmur of pulmonic stenosis is more commonly heard at birth or soon thereafter.

Family History

The family history is extremely important in the assessment and diagnosis of a congenital cardiac defect. The presence of both cardiac and noncardiac defects in other members of the family may reflect a tendency toward such abnormalities and offer a clue as to the nature of the cardiac defect. For example, a strong family history of diabetes may be a clue to transposition of the great vessels or hypoplastic left heart syndrome. Some familial diseases have a strong cardiac accompaniment, e.g. Freidreich's ataxia (myocarditis), Marfan's syndrome (involvement of the aorta or mitral valve structures), Hunter-Hurler's syndrome (involvement of the mitral or tricuspid valve or a coronary artery obstruction), Ellis-van Creveld syndrome (a single atrium or atrial septal defect), Laurence-Moon-Biedl-Bardet syndrome (aortic or pulmonic stenosis), or the cardiac type of glycogen storage disease (myocardiopathy). A history of early death in several members of a family may suggest familial myocardiopathy, hypertrophic subaortic stenosis or, if associated with deafness or syncope, a syndrome associated with a prolonged Q-T interval.

80

The nature of the cardiac defect in other members of the family may also give a clue to the presence of a similar lesion in the patient, although it is of interest that discordancy is more frequent in siblings than is concordancy. Many identical twins do not show identical cardiac abnormalities; one may have none, or the defect may be of a different type. It is likely that a child will have the same type of cardiac abnormality as the mother rather than that of a sibling.

As more careful studies of family history of children with cardiac abnormalities are made, it seems obvious that there are many instances of congenital cardiac abnormalities that may not be revealed by the informant in a routine history.

Prenatal History

The mother who has had rubella during pregnancy may have an infant who demonstrates a congenital cardiac defect of a unique type, usually a patent ductus and/or pulmonary artery branch stenosis. There is growing evidence that other infections, especially of the viral type, cause congenital cardiac defects. The presence of a cardiac abnormality in the mother increases the probability of a cardiac defect in her infant, as well as the possibility that it will be a similar lesion. Surgical correction of cardiac lesions, which permits individuals to survive and bear children, may result in a higher incidence of offspring with cardiac defects.

Drugs

Drugs may cause isolated cardiac abnormalities or a syndrome associated with a cardiac defect. Administration of thalidomide may result in phocomelia and a cardiac defect; and even tranquilizers, anti-emetics and anti-allergic drugs have been suggested as causes of congenital defects. A careful history of drug ingestion by the mother during pregnancy, both by prescription and by self-administration, is important.

Altitude

The altitude in which the mother resided during pregnancy may be a factor in determining the type of cardiac abnormality present, usually a patent ductus arteriosus.[3]

Birth and Delivery

The type of birth and the method of delivery are essential points in history-taking. It is important to know what the infant weighed at birth and whether it was premature or small for date of delivery, as there seems to be a higher incidence of congenital cardiac abnormalities in premature infants, and such infections as rubella give rise to a high incidence of small although full-term infants. The nature of the delivery, the condition of the infant at birth, the type of resuscitative measures used, and whether the infant was kept in an incubator after delivery or retained in the hospital for a longer period of time than usual may give some insight as to whether a cardiac abnormality was suspected at the time, particularly if the parents are aware of an X ray of the chest or an electrocardiogram taken at the time.

Feeding Problems

Feeding problems are so much a part of the presenting signs of a congenital cardiac abnormality, particularly one associated with congestive failure, that it is important to know what the feeding history of the patient was in the early weeks of life, as well as weight gain or loss. It is not only vomiting in infants who subsequently have been noted to have coarctation of the aorta that seems significant to this observer, but also the number of scars resulting from a "Ramstedt operation" for pyloric stenosis in these children.

Immunizations

A careful history of regular immunizations may indicate the frequency and care with which the infant's health was supervised.

Discussion

Anyone who has "computerized" history-taking or has delegated this task to an unskilled person will soon realize the many omissions that may occur if only routine questions are asked of the informant without prodding by someone skilled in history-taking. The necessity for persistence in querying a parent with many children and some haziness as to past events, as well as the importance of separating the parents' observations from the comments of referring physicians, seems obvious. There must be real communication between informant and physician. An interpreter may be required if a language barrier exists.

The history obtained from a 14-, 15-, or 16-year-old child unaccompanied by a responsible parent may be only a series of omissions. However, the reliability of such an informant should not be excluded for supplemental information; e.g., the history of chest pain can be fortified immeasurably by asking the child to indicate the site and intensity of the pain. The subjective description is sometimes very dramatic in implicating a disorder of rate or rhythm, and a story of "my heart turned over" as noted with extrasystoles, or "my heart was beating in my throat," or "my heart seemed to be running away" may be important clues to the presence of certain dysrhythmias.

PHYSICAL EXAMINATION

Successful examination for heart disease in an infant or child under the age of 3 years depends greatly upon his cooperation. Removing the clothes prior to the doctor's entry into the room and then wrapping the infant loosely in a blanket until the physician appears is far better than disturbing him for this procedure, particularly if he has been sleeping. It is suggested also that any infant or small child who still takes the bottle should not be fed just before the examination, enabling the physician to use the bottle to keep the infant quiet. It is amazing what a hungry infant being fed will permit one to do. There is a variety of other procedures to help such an examination. Music has a particularly sedative effect on some infants, the mother or the father usually knows of a favorite toy or device to keep the infant happy, and almost always there is something that will capture the infant's attention for the length of time necessary to make a thorough cardiac examination.

The examination must be comprehensive and include the entire body. Extracardiac manifestations may be important clues to the presence of the anatomical cardiac abnormality; furthermore, a murmur is not the most significant finding in determining the presence or absence of a cardiac abnormality in the neonate.[4] Taussig[5] stated that a month in the life of an infant is like a year in the life of a child, and physical findings and symptoms change remarkably in the first few months of life. For example, the murmur of a ventricular septal defect may make its first appearance at 6 weeks of age in an infant who apparently has had normal cardiac findings at birth and at the time of discharge from the hospital.

Associated Abnormalities

Congenital lesions frequently are multiple, and the presence of various stigmata may suggest the type of congenital cardiac abnormality as well as its congenital rather than acquired nature. The recognition of certain syndromes may give definite evidence as to the type of cardiac abnormality present. An infant's small size for date of delivery, associated with cataracts, deafness, and microcephaly, indicates rubella syndrome, almost always accompanied by a patent ductus arteriosus and/or pulmonary artery branch stenosis, or less commonly with other cardiac lesions. Down's syndrome, which includes epicanthal eye folds, small fifth finger, and protruding tongue, is associated with a congenital cardiac abnormality in a significant number of cases, the lesion usually being some type of endocardial cushion defect. A tall child with long fingers, dislocated lens, and other manifestations of Marfan's syndrome may well have an aortic arch anomaly or aortic or mitral insufficiency. Polythelia (accessory nipples) often is associated with congenital cardiac defects and pulmonary hypertension.

Many syndromes are associated with measurable chromosomal abnormalities. Infants with a trisomy 13 syndrome usually have a cleft palate, small jaw, low-set ears, rocker-bottom feet, and polydactyly, and frequently they have a patent ductus arteriosus and/or ventricular septal defect with pulmonary hypertension. Infants with a trisomy 16–18 syndrome usually have a ventricular septal defect with pulmonary hypertension. Individuals with a modification of the short arm of chromosome 18 may have an atrial septal defect. Turner's syndrome (X–O with ovarian dysgenesis) usually is accompanied by coarctation of the aorta and/or pulmonic stenosis, and, less often, other cardiac lesions. The presence of pulmonic stenosis, in turn, may be a clue to a pseudo- or male Turner's syndrome in the absence of a demonstrable chromosome abnormality, even though not accompanied by the web neck or short stature noted in the classical form. Hunter-Hurler's syndrome, recognized by the short stature of the child, corneal opacity, hepatosplenomegaly, and kyphoscoliosis, may have a mitral or tricuspid valve deformity. Ellis-van Creveld syndrome is manifested by short stature, unusual upper lip, polydactyly, and often an atrial septal defect or a single atrium. The Holt-Oram syndrome, recognized by absent thumbs and chest deformity, may have an associated atrial septal defect with severe pulmonary vascular disease and some dysrhythmia, such as atrial flutter or fibrillation. Abnormalities of the forearm frequently are associated with ventricular septal defects. Many more forms of the "hand-heart" syndrome have been described in the literature. The Williams' syndrome is characterized by short stature, strabismus, absent nasal bridge, round face, dove-like voice, and mild mental retardation, and additionally supravalvular aortic stenosis,[6] multiple pulmonary branch stenoses,[7] and unequal intensity of the radial pulses.

General Appearance

The general behavior and appearance of the infant or child before he is subjected to the classical cardiac examination are important in determining the severity of a cardiac illness; thus, he may be quiet and peaceful or show the continuous activity, irritability, and crying that accompany congestive failure or hypoxia. A child may squat while being observed, a position most frequently noted in children with tetralogy of Fallot, especially after exercise. An infant may be comfortable only high on his mother's shoulder ("he only rests when I carry him this way"), thus simulating the orthopneic position. This preference suggests congestive failure.

The child with a mild cardiac abnormality, such as an atrial septal defect or ventricular septal defect of small size, or an obstructive lesion, such as aortic stenosis or pulmonic stenosis of mild severity, may have no observable extracardiac signs, may be well nourished and happy and have no complaints.

Tachypnea and Tachycardia

Tachypnea and tachycardia are difficult to evaluate in the infant, particularly in one that is moving or crying, and their significance depends on whether the infant is quiet or is sucking vigorously on the bottle or pacifier, or on the presence of a respiratory infection or fever, any of which can increase the respiratory and heart rates. (A resting or sleeping rate of 45 respirations per minute in an infant or 60 per minute in the premature baby may be considered the upper limits of normal.)

Cyanosis

Cyanosis is difficult to assess even to an experienced observer, and especially in the newborn nursery. The propensity for blue walls, blue window coverings, and blue blankets that completely cover the infant makes the diagnosis more difficult. Since there must be at least 5 grams of reduced hemoglobin in the peripheral capillaries for cyanosis to be present,[8] the anemic or jaundiced infant may have considerable oxygen unsaturation without clinical detection. The location of cyanotic areas over the body may pinpoint a cardiac abnormality. Cyanosis of the nails of the feet (not resulting from dependency of the extremities) without accompanying blueness of the nails of the hands and associated with a loud second sound may indicate the presence of a patent ductus arteriosus with flow from the pulmonary artery to the descending aorta. Cyanosis of the nails of the hands unaccompanied by cyanosis of the feet may indicate a transposition of the great vessels with a reverse-flow ductus.

Expiratory Grunt

An expiratory grunt is an important manifestation of the respiratory distress syndrome but also may indicate either pericarditis or congestive failure or may be secondary to a tachyrhythmia.

Chest Deformity

Chest deformity is present with many heart problems. An increased antero-posterior diameter or a protrusion of the left chest (or right chest in dextro-cardia) may be caused by an enlarged heart, usually an enlarged right ventricle. However, it should be remembered that chest deformity may accompany a cardiac abnormality without necessarily being the result of it. In addition, it is surprising how frequently chest deformities, particularly pectus excavatum, give rise to murmurs, widely duplicated second sounds, and unusual electrocardiographic and radiological findings without the demonstration of a cardiac abnormality by thorough physiological and angiographic studies.[9]

Mental Status

A child with cyanotic heart disease may appear mentally retarded and even have a head that is larger than normal, simulating hydrocephalus; however, there is nothing more dramatic than the reversal of these two findings in a child who has had a palliative or corrective procedure on his heart, particularly the child with a tetralogy of Fallot. Nevertheless, in many syndromes with accompanying congenital cardiac abnormalities, a true mental retardation is a significant part.

Skin Lesions

Small hemangiomas of the skin in an infant in congestive failure may offer a clue to hemangioendothelioma of the liver [10] or even a hemangioma of the heart. Telangiectasia of the tongue and mucous membranes may represent a syndrome associated with multiple pulmonary arteriovenous fistulae. Café-au-lait spots may indicate neurofibromatosis and, in turn, pulmonary stenosis.

Eyes, Ears, Nose, and Throat

Examination of the eyes, ears, nose, and throat is an essential part of any examination, but it is best to defer this portion of the examination until the heart and abdomen have been evaluated to obtain the cooperation of the infant or child. It is of interest that hypertelorism and flushed cheeks sometimes are found in association with pulmonic stenosis.

Abdominal Examination

Palpation of the abdomen will determine the presence of an enlarged liver or spleen, as well as any pulsations of the liver. In the younger child, the hepatojugular reflux is difficult to obtain. The abnormal location of the liver or stomach may indicate a mixed levocardia with its multiple and highly complicated cardiac findings.

Peripheral Vessels

Palpation of peripheral vessels, particularly the comparative intensity of arterial pulsations in the upper and lower extremities, is important in the differential diagnosis of coarctation of the aorta. Bounding pulses suggest some type of A–V shunt, such as a patent ductus arteriosus, and small or weak pulses may reflect either a hypoplastic left heart syndrome or aortic stenosis. In infants, the only clue to the presence of a patent ductus may be a loud second sound and bounding peripheral arterial pulses. Pulsating vessels over the scapula may indicate the collateral circulation of coarctation of the aorta, and it is interesting how frequently the axillary and brachial vessels are visibly pulsatile in this condition. Accurate inspection of neck veins is difficult if not impossible in infants or children. The type and quality of carotid and jugular waves have the same significance as those in the adult. The visible presence of rapidly oscillating carotid or of suprasternal notch pulsations may be a clue to a tachyrhythmia. Unequal arm pulses may indicate localized obstruction of a subclavian artery or the presence of a supravalvular aortic stenosis. An absent radial pulse may reflect a prior palliative operation, such as a Blalock-Taussig anastomosis with sacrifice of the subclavian artery, and may result ultimately in an extremity both shorter and narrower in diameter than the opposite one. Partial occlusion of a femoral artery following a diagnostic or cannulization procedure may have a similar effect on a lower extremity.

Palpation

It is difficult to observe an apex impulse on the smaller child; nevertheless, its isolation by observation or palpation is important in determining the location of the apex and in obtaining a crude estimate of cardiac size.

A tap palpated over the second left interspace is evidence of pulmonary hypertension. A right ventricular heave along the sternal border indicates the presence of either a right ventricular volume or pressure overload, as may occur with an atrial septal defect, pulmonic stenosis with intact septum, or tetralogy of Fallot.

A strong, palpable, and visible apical impulse may indicate left ventricular dominance; but in a thin-chested child, this finding may be normal, especially if the child is examined in the left lateral position. A pubertal or prepubertal girl may have a strong apical impulse caused by excitement alone and unaccompanied by significant heart disease.

Thrills

Thrills are the palpable manifestations of the maximal point of intensity of an organic murmur. Rarely, an insignificant thrill may be palpated just above the clavicle in association with a loud venous hum. More often, however, a thrill represents an organic murmur. It is quite difficult to palpate the carotid artery of the infant or small child without considerable effort, but one is amply rewarded when his efforts detect the thrill of valvular aortic stenosis over the right carotid artery and the second right interspace. A thrill and strong pulsation over that portion of the aorta in the suprasternal notch may be found with coarctation of the aorta. A systolic thrill in the second left interspace is present in all except the mildest degrees of valvular pulmonic stenosis. Subvalvular and infundibular pulmonic stenosis may manifest a thrill over the third and fourth left interspaces; and the latter may also be the location of the thrill and murmur of subaortic stenosis. A thrill over the fourth left interspace usually accompanies a ventricular septal defect, unless the defect is very small or the infant is in congestive failure. In infants, the thrill and murmur of ventricular septal defect is located more commonly over the xiphoid process. Detection of the maximal intensity of a thrill and murmur over the fourth right interspace suggests the presence of a left ventricular-right atrial shunt. A diastolic thrill is palpated over the apex in mitral stenosis and over the fourth left interspace in Ebstein's disease. The continuous thrill of a patent ductus arteriosus usually is palpated over the second left interspace, but in infants and small children, it may present over the fourth left interspace, the apex, or even the left axilla.

Auscultation

A properly fitted stethoscope with both a diaphragm and bell chest piece is essential for proper auscultation. The diastolic murmur of aortic insufficiency rarely is heard if only the bell is utilized, and conversely, the "flow" diastolic murmur over the apex in large ventricular septal defects can be heard only when the bell is used.

Leatham,[11] McKusick,[12] and many others have contributed greatly to our understanding of the auscultatory findings in congenital heart defects. Evaluation of signs and murmurs presupposes that the heart and great vessels are in their usual position.

Heart Sounds

Our understanding of the normal function of cardiac valves has been of great help in the proper evaluation of cardiac defects. The first heart sound consists essentially of closure of the mitral and subsequently the tricuspid valve. Under normal conditions, it is relatively impossible for the human ear to differentiate these two components, even though a slight asynchrony does exist. Not only is the human ear unable to detect such splitting, but the louder mitral closure usually overwhelms the softer tricuspid valve closure. An audible splitting of the first sound actually may represent a systolic ejection click following a single first heart sound or, in adults, a preceding atrial sound associated with severe heart disease. The first heart sound may be increased in intensity with anemia, hyperthyroidism, exercise, and emotional states (all examples of a high output state) and in mitral stenosis. It may be intermittently increased in complete heart block and with an abnormally short P–R interval. It may be decreased in shock or any disorder that lowers cardiac output or myocardial efficiency.

The second heart sound has received greater attention in the differential diagnosis of congenital cardiac defects, and its importance and proper assessment are at least of equal diagnostic value with the murmurs in infants and children. The two components of the second heart sound, heard best over the second left interspace, represent closure of the semilunar valves, i.e. aortic valve closure followed in 0.02 to 0.05 second by pulmonic valve closure. Although usually heard best over the second left interspace, the second sound occasionally is heard better over the third left interspace, especially if a murmur obscures the sounds in the usual place. Aortic valve closure is greater in intensity than is pulmonic valve closure in adults; in children, probably up to late adolescence, pulmonary closure may be slightly greater in intensity. Splitting of the second sound is increased at the onset of inspiration and decreased on expiration, such splitting being more easily detected in children than in adults. The sound of aortic closure is increased in intensity by systemic hypertension and that of pulmonary closure by pulmonary hypertension. The aortic second sound, however, usually is not decreased or absent in children with valvular aortic stenosis. Pulmonary valve closure intensity decreases with increasing severity of valvular pulmonic stenosis, while width of the splitting of the sounds increases.[13] With very severe pulmonic stenosis, the pulmonary valve closure may be so soft and the aortic valve closure so overwhelmed by the murmur that no second sound is heard (absent P_2). Increased splitting of the second sound also may occur with right bundle branch block and/or atrial septal defect. In the latter, the intensity of the second portion of the second sound usually remains normal, and splitting may be fixed, i.e., there may be no change in the width of the split with inspiration or expiration. Fixed splitting is noted commonly with atrial septal defects, but this phenomenon has been described also in about 25 per cent of apparently normal children. "Paradoxical splitting," in which splitting decreases or may disappear with inspiration and may actually increase with expiration, sometimes is present in severe aortic stenosis, in patent ductus (where it usually is overwhelmed by the murmur), and in left bundle branch block (a rare finding in congenital cardiac abnormalities in children). The presence of a single second sound is an extremely valuable finding in the differentiation of congenital cardiac abnormalities. It is present in truncus arteriosus (only one set of semilunar valves), in tetralogy of Fallot (usually an inaudible pulmonary valve closure), tricuspid atresia (with hypoplastic pulmonary artery system and tiny right ventricle), and transposition of the great vessels (displacement of the respective valves). The "Eisenmenger group" may have a loud, single second sound because reverberation of the pulmonary valve closure overwhelms the relatively soft aortic closure.

A third sound may normally be present over the apex in children, whereas its presence in older persons usually signifies severe heart disease.

Ejection Click

The ejection systolic click has assumed increasing importance in the differential diagnosis of certain congenital abnormalities. It is heard approximately 0.12 second after the first heart sound, if present. It may be the result of tensing of the aortic or pulmonary root at the onset of injection; it may be caused by the opening snap of the semilunar valves accompanying aortic or pulmonic stenosis or by marked dilatation of the proximal aorta or main pulmonary artery. Children with coarctation of the aorta or with hyperthyroidism may demonstrate an ejection click. A loud ejection click may be heard over the precordium after an episode of pleuritis, pericarditis, or pneumonia, and a mid or late systolic ejection click accompanied by a late apical systolic murmur may be associated with mild mitral insufficiency caused by aberrant insertion of the chordae tendinae or some other type of papillary muscle dysfunction.[14] The differential diagnosis between atrial septal defect and valvular pulmonic stenosis may sometimes be established by the presence or absence of a click, unless the atrial septal defect is accompanied by an anatomical narrowing of the pulmonary valve. A loud ejection click over the second left interspace is present in mild or moderate valvular pulmonic stenosis. It increases in intensity with inspiration and is somewhat high pitched. With more severe pulmonic stenosis, the ejection click may disappear as the valve loses its mobility, and thus its "opening snap." An ejection click rarely is heard with subvalvular or supravalvular pulmonary stenosis, although in tetralogy of Fallot with infundibular stenosis, a click may arise from the dilated aortic root. The ejection click rarely is heard in any type of aortic stenosis other than the valvular variety.[15]

Murmurs

A murmur still represents the most commonly detected physical finding in the diagnosis of congenital cardiac abnormality, except in the neonate. In the more serious types of cardiac abnormalities presenting themselves in infants, such as pulmonary atresia or transposition of the great vessels with a patent foramen ovale (incidentally, conditions that need early diagnosis and surgical intervention for survival), the presence of a murmur early is most unusual. On the other hand, the continuous murmur of patent ductus arteriosus may be heard for a brief time after birth. Other cardiac abnormalities that present with soft or even inaudible murmurs are total anomalous venous return with pulmonary venous obstruction, coarctation of the aorta, or a septal defect in which the pulmonary artery pressures have not as yet decreased to permit an appreciable gradient. In fact, many murmurs heard in the newborn period may result from tardy physiological changes such as delayed closure of a patent ductus arteriosus (particularly in a premature infant) or temporary mitral or tricuspid insufficiency, rather than from a permanent and serious cardiac defect. After the age of 4 to 6 weeks, a murmur more frequently accompanies a congenital abnormality. In tetralogy of Fallot, the systolic murmur heard over the third or fourth left interspace usually represents infundibular pulmonic stenosis, since pure right-to-left shunts do not give rise to murmurs. As the pulmonary stenosis of a tetralogy of Fallot becomes more severe, the associated murmur becomes shorter and softer and may disappear if secondary pulmonary atresia occurs (blood then being transported to the lungs by means of either a patent ductus or some type of iatrogenic shunt operation or collateral circulation).

Ejection murmurs begin well after the first sound and only after the semilunar valves open, and become soft and inaudible before the semilunar valves close. They reach their greatest intensity in mid-systole. Ejection murmurs are best identified with pulmonic or aortic stenosis, atrial septal defect, and even small ventricular septal defects. Sometimes the differentiation between an ejection and pansystolic murmur is most difficult. The pansystolic murmur begins and ends with the first and second sounds and is of essentially equal intensity throughout; it is best heard when mitral or tricuspid insufficiency or ventricular septal defect is present. An early systolic murmur may be heard with small ventricular septal defects, since muscular contraction closes the defect in late systole. A late systolic murmur accompanied by a click over the apex, previously considered extracardiac and sometimes associated with a "honk," now is reasonably well established as the result of some type of mild mitral valve insufficiency secondary to abnormal insertion of the chordae tendinae or papillary muscle dysfunction or a billowing mitral valve. It is heard most frequently in young girls and may be associated with T-wave changes over the left precordial leads. Although in most instances benign (there have been instances of sudden death associated with this anomaly), it does have a predilection for bacterial endocarditis if the usual prophylactic measures are ignored. An ejection systolic murmur is heard best over the second right interspace in valvular aortic stenosis, somewhat higher and transmitted into the neck vessels in supravalvular aortic stenosis. Sometimes this murmur is heard over the third and even the fourth left interspace in subvalvular aortic stenosis, especially idiopathic hypertrophic subaortic stenosis.

Valvular pulmonic stenosis gives rise to an ejection systolic murmur heard best over the second left interspace. The murmur of infundibular pulmonic stenosis is usually heard best in the third or fourth left interspace and may be difficult to differentiate by location alone from that of a ventricular septal defect. The pansystolic murmur of ventricular septal defect is heard best over the fourth left interspace, and in infants, over the xiphoid process. The murmur of tricuspid insufficiency is heard over the fourth left interspace and may be difficult to differentiate from that of a ventricular septal defect. The murmur of mitral insufficiency is heard over the apex and transmitted to the left axilla. The murmur of coarctation of the aorta may be almost inaudible over the anterior chest but may be heard well in the left axilla and over both scapular regions. It sometimes sounds almost "separate" from the heart sounds, while in the more severe types of coarctation, it may be continuous, and in infants, no murmur may be audible.

The "innocent murmur" is one that has no significant effect on the future development and activity of the child, although it is quite possible that such a murmur may result from some very mild change in the structure of the heart or great vessels. The innocent murmur most commonly heard may be present in as many as 65 per cent of children (100 per cent according to Mannheimer [16]) and is a low-pitched, vibratory systolic murmur heard along the left sternal border toward the apex, but not beyond. It occasionally is accompanied by a short, sharp systolic murmur over the clavicle and into the neck. It may change in quality and intensity with position and may assume a different quality with each examination. It usually increases in intensity in the presence of fever, exercise, or emotional stress. Many such murmurs disappear at about 14 years of age. Although the murmur appears most commonly at about 3 to 5 years of age, it may be heard as early as 1 month of age and even at birth. Its importance lies in the consternation it may cause when discovered, failure to explain its proper significance to parents, and the tendency of both physician and parents to restrict unduly a child who has such a murmur. Another type of innocent murmur is one best heard in adolescence. It is an ejection systolic murmur heard over the second left interspace, detected more easily in recumbency, and almost disappearing when the child sits up and holds his shoulders back. It also may increase with exercise or with emotion, so that under these conditions, even the most experienced observer may wish to withhold judgement as to its significance until further examination. It usually is associated with either normal or slightly increased intensity of the second sound, depending upon the emotional state of the child. Its association with a normal electrocardiogram and a radiologically normal heart size and shape adds assurance as to its innocent nature. When associated with prominence of the pulmonary artery segment, the murmur may result from idiopathic dilatation of the pulmonary artery.

The venous hum is a continuous sound that can be demonstrated over the second right interspace and into the neck vessels in virtually all children from 3 to 10 years of age, especially if the head is extended. It sometimes is heard over the second left interspace and may be confused with the murmur of patent ductus arteriosus. It disappears in recumbency or when the internal jugular vein is occluded.

Although Liebman and Soods [17] recently described an "innocent diastolic murmur," the presence of most diastolic murmurs represents some form of organic pathology of the heart. Aortic insufficiency may be congenital in origin, either as an isolated lesion or accompanying aortic stenosis. It usually is present after the relief of congenital aortic stenosis by surgical intervention.

Of considerable importance is the aortic insufficiency that may develop in a child with a ventricular septal defect of a unique type, involving one of the cusps of the aortic valve. Children with this lesion have the clinical signs of a small ventricular septal defect up to the age of 3 years and may then present with the diastolic murmur of aortic insufficiency.

Congenital mitral stenosis and even tricuspid stenosis are being recognized with increasing frequency, the former at times with coarctation of the aorta, and the latter with a small right ventricle and pulmonary atresia. The classical presystolic murmur, loud first sound, opening snap, and rumbling diastolic murmur are the same as the signs recognized in the acquired type. A diastolic murmur may be heard in association with the systolic murmur of mitral insufficiency in children, and may also be heard in individuals with aortic insufficiency (Austin Flint murmur). Children with severe pulmonary arterial obstructive disease (Eisenmenger syndrome) may present with the diastolic murmur of pulmonary insufficiency over the second left interspace (Graham Steell murmur). A soft, short diastolic murmur is present over the fourth left interspace in individuals with an atrial septal defect of the secundum type; it may be of low grade intensity, but without it, the diagnosis of atrial septal defect must remain in doubt. A mid-diastolic murmur over the apex is heard in children with large ventricular septal defects and has been an accurate indication of a pulmonic-to-systemic flow ratio greater than 2:1. It is heard only if the bell portion of the stethoscope is used.

Defects of the mitral valve frequently are associated with an endocardial cushion defect of the ostium primum type, in which case a sibilant pansystolic and short diastolic murmur are heard over the apex.

A systolic and diastolic murmur may be present in a great number of congenital cardiac lesions. The classical continuous murmur of patent ductus is a crescendo-decrescendo murmur in the second left interspace, sometimes heard even better and atypically over the third and fourth left interspaces in infants and children up to the age of 3 years. It reaches its greatest intensity at the second sound. It may be inaudible or at least undiscovered in infancy and early childhood, and conversely, may be present as a physiological phenomenon for a few hours after birth. The classical manifestations may be modified by increased pulmonary artery pressure, obliterating the diastolic component or even the entire murmur. It is heard best in recumbency.

A to-and-fro murmur is a separate systolic and long diastolic murmur most often heard in children with ventricular septal defect and aortic insufficiency. The only manifestation of an anomalous coronary artery entering a pulmonary artery, right atrium, or right ventricle may be a soft continous murmur over the fourth left or fourth right interspace. The seesaw murmur of an absent pulmonary valve has an equal systolic and diastolic phase that is easily recognized. The murmur of an aortico-pulmonary window is loud and very close to the ear, and its differentiation from a patent ductus arteriosus sometimes is impossible. Other causes of murmurs heard in both systole and diastole are listed below.[18]

1. Venous hum
2. Ruptured sinus of Valsalva

3. Truncus arteriosus
4. Aortic stenosis and insufficiency
5. Total anomalous venous return into right superior vena cava
6. Pulmonary stenosis and insufficiency
7. Aberrant right pulmonary artery located between the trachea and esophagus
8. Collateral circulation associated with pulmonary atresia (bronchial collaterals)
9. Coarctation of the aorta
10. Arteriovenous fistula of the lung
11. Mitral stenosis and insufficiency
12. Tricuspid stenosis and insufficiency
13. Blalock-Taussig anastomosis, Potts-Smith-Gibson anastomosis, and the Waterston procedure
14. Pulmonary artery coarctation
15. Coronary artery-coronary vein fistula
16. Pericardial friction rub
17. Pleural friction rub
18. Banding of the pulmonary artery
19. Absent pulmonary valve
20. Hilar glands impinging upon the pulmonary artery
21. Anomalous left coronary artery arising from the pulmonary artery
22. Atrial septal defect with mitral stenosis
23. Right pulmonary artery entering the left atrium

Continuous murmurs sometimes are heard better over the back than over the anterior chest, particularly in children with total anomalous venous return, truncus arteriosus, or pulmonary atresia with collateral circulation.

Blood Pressure

The determination of blood pressures in infants and young children is most difficult, and yet the advent of improved techniques in taking blood pressures in infants and the availability of properly fitting cuffs has been rewarded by a virtual cornucopia of early diagnoses of coarctation of the aorta in infants and children before the development of cerebral vascular accidents, bacterial endocarditis, or congestive failure, and even prior to the appearance of rib notching. Although other congenital cardiac abnormalities may be present, they do not exclude the presence of a coarctation of the aorta. Palpation of the femoral pulses (or the posterior tibial or dorsalis pedis pulses in older girls) and comparison in the intensity and timing of the radial with the femoral pulse is important but inadequate in excluding a coarctation of the aorta without careful determination of blood pressures in the arms and legs. The auscultatory method of taking blood pressures with a sphygmomanometer is preferable. A properly fitting cuff covering two thirds to three fourths of the width between the shoulder and the elbow is essential for accuracy. A cuff that is too wide gives an erroneously wide pulse pressure; one that is too narrow demonstrates unduly high systolic and diastolic pressures. The simultaneous flush method may be used in infants, but has obvious limitations; until the age of 9 months, the mean pressure determined by the flush method of the legs may be as much as 10 mm. Hg below that of the arms in the absence of a coarctation of the aorta.[19] The use of an oscillometric method for determination of blood pressure may be performed either by means of an oscillometer or by using the maximal fluctuation of the needle in an aneroid manometer to indicate systolic blood pressure. The estimation of blood pressure must be done with the infant or child quiet. There is a striking increase in both systolic and diastolic pressures with crying, vigorous sucking on the nipple, or any movement. Apprehension in the older child may cause the blood pressure to rise to significant and apparently abnormal levels until the apprehension is allayed.

CONCLUSION

A properly taken history and thorough physical examination reveal the presence and type of congenital abnormality with remarkable accuracy. In association with electrocardiographic and roentgenological studies of the chest, a proper diagnosis is established in the majority of cases.

References

1. GIBSON, S.: Personal communication.
2. HARVEY, W. P.: *Some newer or poorly recognized findings on clinical auscultation.* Mod. Conc. Cardiov. Dis. 37:85, 1968.
3. ALZAMORA, C. V., BATTILANA, G., ABRIGATTOS, R., AND SISLER, S.: *Patent ductus and high altitude.* Amer. J. Cardiol. 5:761, 1960.
4. ROWE, R. D., AND MEHRIZI, A.: *The Neonate with Congenital Heart Disease.* W. B. Saunders Co., Philadelphia, Toronto, 1968.
5. TAUSSIG, H. B.: *The management of heart disease in infants.* Audio-Digest 13:2, 1967.
6. WILLIAMS, J. C. P., BARRATT-BOYES, B. D., AND LOWE, J. B.: *Supravalvular aortic stenosis.* Circulation 24:1311, 1961.
7. WATSON, G. H.: *Supravalvular and aortic stenosis coexisting.* Brit. Heart J. 25:817, 1963.
8. LUNDSGAARD, C.: *Studies on cyanosis.* J. Exp. Med. 30:259, 1919.
9. SEGAL, B. L., AND LIKOFF, W.: *Auscultation of the Heart.* Grune & Stratton, Inc., New York, 1965.
10. WINTERS, R. W., ROBINSON, S. J., AND BATES, G.: *Hemangioma of the liver with heart failure.* Pediatrics 14:117, 1954.
11. LEATHAM, A.: *Splitting of the first and second heart sounds.* Lancet 2:607, 1954.
12. McKUSICK, V. A.: *Cardiovascular Sound in Health and Disease.* The Williams & Wilkins Co., Baltimore, 1958.
13. LEATHAM, A., AND WEITZMAN, D.: *Auscultatory and phonocardiographic signs of pulmonic stenosis.* Brit. Heart J. 19:303, 1957.
14. PHILLIPS, J. H., BURCH, G. G., AND DEPASQUALE, N. P.: *The syndrome of papillary muscle dysfunction: Its clinical recognition.* Ann. Int. Med. 59:508, 1963.

15. HANCOCK, E. W.: *Origin of the ejection sound in aortic stenosis.* Clin. Res. 13:209, 1965.

16. MANNHEIMER, G.: *Phonocardiography in Children. Advances in Pediatrics.* Year Book Medical Publishers, Inc., Chicago, 1955.

17. LIEBMAN, J., AND SOODS, S.: *Diastolic murmurs in apparently normal children.* Circulation 38:755, 1968.

18. ROBINSON, S. J., ABRAMS, H. L., AND KAPLAN, H. S.: *Congenital Heart Disease: An Illustrated Diagnostic Approach,* ed. 2. McGraw-Hill Book Company, New York, 1965.

19. MOSS, A. J., AND ADAMS, F. H.: *Flush blood pressure and intraarterial pressure: A comparison of methods in infants.* Amer. J. Dis. Child. 107:489, 1964.

Electrocardiographic Clues
in the Diagnosis
of Congenital Heart Disease

Robert F. Ziegler, M.D.

When one considers the diagnosis of congenital heart disease, it is important to remember that this diagnosis must be physiological as well as anatomical, quantitative as well as qualitative. The structural designation "interventricular septal defect," for example, is almost meaningless, because the malformation may be small or large, may involve a left-to-right, right-to-left, or bi-directional shunt or none at all, may be associated with normal, low, or high pulmonary artery pressure and vascular resistance, and may be operable or inoperable. Similarly, and in the knowledge that the electrocardiogram is capable of providing both anatomical and physiological clues, one must go beyond the simple description of the "typical" appearance of the electrocardiogram in interventricular septal defect or pulmonary stenosis and must attempt to analyze the electrical activity of the heart in terms of its correlation with the resulting intracardiac pressure-flow dynamics. Other important and supplementary diagnostic clues are, of course, provided by physical and X-ray or fluoroscopic examination.

The electrocardiogram traditionally has been and for the most part continues to be regarded as one of several clinical means for determining the presence of structural cardiac chamber enlargement, variously and nonspecifically designated "hypertrophy," "preponderance," etc. The particular portion of the electrocardiogram most often considered diagnostic of enlargement has been, again traditionally, the initial ventricular deflections or QRS complex, whatever their current mode of projection and recording. The validity of this point of view is not to be denied, nor its potential importance minimized; yet it does have some significant limitations and qualifications, especially in pediatric cardiology. The following should be listed.

1. The difficulty of differentiating accurately between so-called normal or physiological and pathologic right ventricular preponderance or enlargement in the newborn and early infant periods

2. The fact that in the newborn period, the rate at which hemodynamic changes occur is neither accurately nor synchronously reflected in the progressive changes recorded in the initial ventricular deflections (QRS) of the electrocardiogram

3. The general failure of the QRS complex alone to correlate accurately or proportionately with different qualitative types or quantitative degrees of measured hemodynamic workloads

4. The known presence of a significantly increased ventricular workload without commensurate, possibly even detectable electrocardiographic (QRS) evidence, often without certain radiographic cardiomegaly, and, most particularly in infants, with or without anatomically demonstrable cardiac chamber enlargement

5. The significant fact that, while average measurements of the initial ventricular deflections may appear diagnostically different between normal and right or left ventricular enlargement, the statistical distributions for the two groups of data, especially in infants, are frequently such as to render individual measurements nondiagnostic because of the extent of overlapping

6. The diagnostic problem presented by the balancing of electrical forces and its effect on the detection and proportionate quantitation of combined right- and left-sided cardiac chamber enlargement

From these various critically qualifying statements, one must not mistakenly conclude either that more such anatomic information could necessarily be provided by the use of other lead systems or methods of recording or that the whole electrocardiogram simply possesses no such inherent diagnostic capacity. Experience has shown, on the contrary, that the precordial lead T-wave pattern, *properly and precisely qualified,* contributes significantly toward an inferential knowledge of abnormal ventricular function, if not also structure, and that the greatest relative value of the T-wave contribution occurs precisely when that of QRS is least. On this basis, it has been shown that the electrocardiogram, in its entirety, actually is capable of providing the most sensitive and accurate clinical index to the presence, type, and degree of increased single or combined cardiac chamber physiological work and, if used over a sufficient period of time, its resulting and appropriate structural dimensions.[1]

The following discussion will be concerned primarily with diagnostic clues presented by precordial lead T-wave patterns, not as isolated electrical phenomena, but in their relations to the remainder of the electrocardiogram, most particularly the QRS complexes.[2] For the sake of practical emphasis, typically diagnostic patterns will be illustrated for the most part from representative right (V_1) and left (V_6) precordial leads.

T-WAVE PATTERNS

General Statement

The T wave of the electrocardiogram represents the electrical events accompanying ventricular repolarization. These events may be influenced by various functional factors that do not necessarily affect other portions of the electrocardiogram, the resulting alterations of wave form being referred to as "primary." The T wave also is dependent on the immediately preceding electrical events of ventricular depolarization, represented by the QRS complex, and these patterns are referred to as "secondary." In the clinical, including hemodynamic, interpretation of precordial lead T-wave patterns, it is essential to differentiate the relative roles of these two electrophysiological mechanisms.[3] One must apply the ventricular gradient principle, not analyzing the T wave as an isolated, necessarily independent, electrocardiographic deflection, but always comparing it with its accompanying QRS complex. In only this way can one come to learn whether a given T-wave pattern reflects primary hemodynamic changes or whether it simply is secondary to associated abnormalities of QRS and thereby signifies anatomic hypertrophy or dilatation, coronary artery insufficiency, abnormalities of intraventricular conduction, and so forth. By definition, and for greatest objective accuracy, this comparison must be made in terms of the net areas inscribed under the respective initial and final ventricular deflections.[3, 4]

For most practical clinical considerations, however, the same relationship can be approximated more easily and reasonably satisfactorily by comparing the amplitudes of deflections (the simple direction and amplitude of T, the amplitude of R expressed either as an R:S ratio or as a percentage of the total RS amplitude). This is the first and really most important electrocardiographic qualification in the interpretation of precordial lead T-wave patterns.

Another important question of precordial lead T-wave interpretation must be raised: that of whether and to what extent the T wave on one side is determined by or determines that on the opposite side of the precordium. Under what circumstances is the whole precordial lead T-wave pattern the expression of a single vectorial force,[5-7] dominated by either right or left side, and when may it represent two mutually independent right- and left-sided forces? Either of these situations may occur. The specific circumstances and interpretations will be presented in the discussion to follow.

Right Precordial Lead Patterns

One of the most useful electrocardiographic clues, one that contributes inferential hemodynamic information toward a complete clinical diagnosis, is T-wave positivity in right precordial (epicardial derivative) leads. It has been claimed and demonstrated that under the proper circumstances, this feature is practically pathognomonic of right ventricular hypertension.[8] The value of this sign derives not only from its accuracy and reliability, but also from its sensitivity. It is likely to be diagnostic when virtually every other clinical (including radiographic and electrocardiographic, with specific reference to the QRS complex) and even pathological evidence may be entirely lacking. The only other way of gaining such physiological information is directly by cardiac catheterization. The qualifying conditions should be listed:

1. That the patient's age be more than 1 or 2 days, before which time pulmonary artery and right ventricular pressure and pressure-work are relatively high
2. That there be no other abnormality, such as of blood electrolytes, to account for similar or other significant electrocardiographic changes
3. That the malformation, as is most often the case in this age group, be of a mechanical sort, the myocardium being otherwise normal and capable of responding predictably to the increased physiological workload
4. That, as virtually the only other electrocardiographic condition, the R-wave amplitude in the same right precordial leads be at least 30 to 35 per cent of the total RS amplitude (R:S ratio of approximately one), so that the net area inscribed under the QRS complex is near zero, thereby permitting the primary T-wave abnormality to be in evidence.[1, 2, 8]

Some practical clinical applications, drawn from a breadth of observations encompassing all the diverse situations in which right ventricular hypertension occurs, should constitute self-evidence of the diagnostic importance of this simple electrocardiographic sign.

In the first instance, right precordial lead T-wave positivity in the newborn and its subsequent primary inversion after the first day or two after birth signals the normal course of pulmonary artery and right venticular pressure and pressure-work during the progession of the pulmonary vasculature from the fetal to the mature postnatal pattern (Fig. 1). Persistence of positivity beyond this time must be considered more abnormal (Fig. 3) the longer it persists and the more it occurs in conjunction with other clinical signs of cardiovascular disease, such as cyanosis. On the other hand, normal progression to right precordial lead T-wave negativity constitutes very important evidence against congenital heart disease (of the sort producing increased right ventricular work-strain, at any rate) when evaluating other suspicious signs, such as cyanosis, edema, murmurs, and possible radiographic cardiomegaly or X-ray abnormalities of pulmonary vasculature or parenchyma (Fig. 2).

Next, when the presence of pathological right ventricular hypertension is well established by fixed and nonreversible right precordial lead T-wave positivity (nonreversible, that is, except as the ventricular gradient effect of an increasing positive area inscribed under the accompanying QRS complexes), two different sorts of observations must be made.

1. The electrocardiographic T-wave evidence of right ventricular hypertension appears to be largely independent of contralateral or left-sided factors.
2. The differential diagnostic, prognostic, and therapeutic importance of right ventricular hypertension must be established in conjunction with all other data concerning the complete central circulation. These basic relationships are shown in Figure 15.

To circumscribe somewhat more completely this important matter of right precordial lead T-wave positivity, two basic issues deserve emphasis. The first question is: In what situations does right precordial lead T-wave positivity *not* of itself signify right ventricular hypertension?

Electrocardiographically, the principal answer is that right ventricular hypertension is not signified when the R-wave amplitude in lead V_1 is only 20 to 25 per cent or less of the total amplitude of RS in this lead and, perhaps more particularly, when this R:RS ratio decreases still more in leads further to the right (V_3R and V_4R). Hemodynamically and anatomically, this situation with respect to the QRS configuration is defined by an increasingly dominant left ventricular workload and size. This dominance is normal with increasing age, particularly beyond the first decade, but abnormal within the first 10 or so years of life (Fig. 12 B, C). This change accounts for the decreasing diagnostic value of this T-wave sign in older subjects and in those pathological situations in which there is either obstructive or primary myocardial left ventricular disease. An equivalent proportion between left

101

and right ventricular size or dominance is not so likely to occur in shunt situations such as patent ductus arteriosus or interventricular septal defect.

There are two additional circumstances in which right precordial lead T-wave positivity is not of itself indicative of right ventricular hypertension. One is left bundle branch block (either true or "false," i.e., Wolff-Parkinson-White syndrome); the other is the distinctive electrocardiographic pattern associated with at least one form of idiopathic left ventricular hypertrophy.

The second question is: When may right ventricular hypertension actually be present, but *without* diagnostic right precordial lead T-wave positivity? Several sorts of situations are again to be envisioned. In one such situation, according to purely electrocardiographic description, there is associated right bundle branch block; or the amplitude of R, expressed as a percentage of RS in the same right precordial leads, has increased to 85 to 100 per cent, usually together with an absolute increased amplitude and area as well (Figs. 4D, 5). Looking again at the underlying hemodynamic implications, this (positive) QRS and (negative) T-wave combination correlates well with an advanced quantitative degree of increased right ventricular (pressure) work, frequently with the superimposition of right bundle branch block and the addition of increased right atrial work and size.

Two other electrocardiographic circumstances warrant mention with regard to this T-wave problem. First is the QRS configuration and ventricular gradient effect on the homolateral, right side of the precordium. As already noted, for T-wave positivity to be primary and thus indicative of right ventricular hypertension, the R:RS ratio must be 30 to 35 per cent or greater (Fig. 4A, B, C). When R:RS is less than this, as with a predominant left ventricular mass (whether normal by age or abnormal by malformation and work required), the influence of QRS is such as to make T-wave positivity secondary and therefore not hemodynamically diagnostic. The other circumstance is positivity of the T-wave pattern on the contralateral or left side of the precordium. If the pattern is strongly positive, as in so-called diastolic-overloading of the left ventricle, it may tend toward domination of the entire precordial lead pattern, the positivity on the left and reciprocal negativity on the right representing together a single vectorial force of repolarization.[10, 11] Seldom, however, does this configuration really obliterate the primary and independent T-wave positivity of right ventricular hypertension, unless in combination with the associated QRS pattern just described.

Left Precordial Lead Patterns

Abnormal T-wave positivity in leads from the right side of the precordium is relatively easy to detect clinically and interpret hemodynamically, because except for the first day or two of postnatal life, this deflection normally is negative throughout the pediatric age range. In leads from the left side of the precordium (epicardial derivation) this same phenomenon of abnormally increased T-wave positivity is more difficult to recognize, since this deflection already is normally positive in these leads and also has a considerable range of variation in amplitude. However, abnormally increased positivity of T does also occur over the left ventricle, but under two different hemodynamic circumstances.

Analogously with the right side, increased positivity of T may occur *primarily,* that is, independently of associated changes of QRS, as in compensated left ventricular hypertension (systemic arterial hypertension, coarctation of the aorta, and aortic stenosis) (Fig. 10B). It also may occur typically in so-called diastolic loading or increased volume-flow work and enlargement (volume hypertrophy), as in interventricular septal defect and in patent ductus arteriosus (Fig. 7A); in this hemodynamic circumstance, the T-wave changes may be considered *secondary* rather than primary, since they are associated with and probably dependent on a proportionate increase in the positive amplitude of QRS in the same leads. This proportionately increased positivity of both QRS and T also may be observed occasionally in young subjects without other evidence of organic heart disease, which simply shows again that the electrocardiogram must be interpreted in the perspective of all other available clinical and radiographic data. In left ventricular outflow obstruction, for example, the clinical diagnosis should be easy and obvious, the electrocardiogram serving to quantitate the level of increased left ventricular pressure-work. In the shunt situation, there should be a shunt murmur, radiographic enlargement of the heart, and evidence of increased volume of pulmonary blood flow, together with electrocardiographic evidence of left atrial as well as left ventricular enlargement. In the third situation, the heart simply is normal by all clinical and perhaps laboratory methods of examination.

From the hemodynamic point of view, inverted T waves in leads facing the epicardial surface of the *right* ventricle may be normal, as is most frequently the case, or they may be abnormal in the sense of coexisting with increased right ventricular work (either pressure-work or volume-work); but they may reflect secondarily, in application of the ventricular gradient principle, an increased positive amplitude and area of QRS. The latter may represent either the quantitative degree of enlargement alone or hypertrophy (with or without dilatation) plus associated right bundle branch block (Fig. 14 A & B). T-wave negativity in leads from the left side of the precordium, however, is quite another matter. Other than for such non-hemodynamic circumstances as pericarditis, coronary artery insufficiency with or without myocardial infarction, etc., this negativity may be observed in certain basic types of situations, summarized here.

Left Precordial, but Right Epicardial T-wave Patterns. With massive right ventricular enlargement, the right-sided chest leads usually are characterized by 100 per cent positivity of QRS, usually with some degree (often complete) of right bundle branch block, and secondary inversion of T. Furthermore, with this degree of enlargement, the left ventricle may be rotated posteriorly to the extent that right epicardial potential variations extend leftward to precordial lead positions V_5 and V_6 (Fig. 5). That T-wave

103

inversion in these leads is not left ventricular in origin may be suspected from the absence of normal Q waves (but no other evidence of left bundle branch block) and substantiated by the appearance of both Q and positive T waves in leads farther to the left and posterior (V_7 and V_8), the latter derived from the epicardial surface of the displaced left ventricle.

Transient, Neonatal T-Wave Inversion in the Normal Heart. The only time at which left precordial lead T-wave inversion may be considered *normal* is during the first few hours after birth,[9] and then only if it is transient and reversible to a permanently normal positive deflection in these leads (Fig. 1A). This sequence of changes apparently is independent of the right precordial lead T-wave positivity that also is normal to the newborn period. The mechanism of the left ventricular T-wave changes, probably not really known, has been variously given. One possible factor, suggested at least by the next and abnormal circumstance to be listed, is that of a transiently low systemic arterial resistance and left ventricular pressure during the newborn period.

Transposition with Normal Pulmonary Vascular Dynamics. In complete transposition of the great vessels, with a reversal of the usual, normal hemodynamic patterns of ventricular pressure-work (but, to be sure, with a lower than normal systemic and coronary artery oxygen saturation), the left precordial lead T-waves frequently are observed to be inverted, perhaps "normally," when pulmonary artery resistance and pressure and left ventricular pressure-work are low, as is the case with closed septa (Fig. 9 A, B, C). Analogously with the electrical behavior of the right ventricle, left ventricular T waves become uniformly positive with varying degrees of left ventricular hypertension, as with an accompanying interventricular septal defect and either pulmonary stenosis or pulmonary hypertension.

Increased Left Ventricular Pressure-Work. In increased left ventricular pressure-work, T-wave inversion in left epicardial leads has mainly *quantitative* significance. Analogously with right ventricular hypertension, the first and primary T-wave evidence of left ventricular hypertension (and compensated hypertrophy) is increased positivity of T without accompanying or necessarily diagnostic changes of QRS (Fig. 10B). Then, with an increasing workload and its resulting anatomical enlargement, the left precordial T waves tend to become less positive and finally inverted (Fig. 10C), usually in accompaniment either with an increasing positive amplitude and delayed inscription time of RS (resulting in an increased positive net area inscribed under the QRS complex) or with left bundle branch block. It is also important to remember that both aortic stenosis and coarctation of the aorta, the two most common forms of left ventricular outflow obstruction and increased pressure-work, not infrequently produce the physiological and electrocardiographic picture of prominent, if not predominant, right rather than left ventricular work-strain and enlargement, particularly during the newborn and early infant periods (Figs. 10A; 11A, B).

Increased Left Ventricular Volume-Flow Work. Left precordial lead T-wave inversion in the situation of increased volume of pulmonary venous return to the left heart (atrium and ventricle) has both quantitative and qualitative or differential diagnostic application. As already noted, one of the typical electrocardiographic responses to this hemodynamic workload is increased positivity of left ventricular QRS and T waves. In uncomplicated patent ductus arteriosus, in contrast to interventricular septal defect, these T waves are not infrequently inverted, presumably as the combined result of increased volume-flow work (so-called volume hypertrophy) and the decreased coronary artery perfusion made possible by a large volume aortic-pulmonary shunt together with a lowered aortic diastolic pressure (Fig. 13A). Although left precordial lead T-wave inversion occasionally is observed in the electrocardiograms of infants with high-flow interventricular septal defects, its occurrence is such as to suggest at least the presence of some complicating left-sided defect, such as coarctation of the aorta, aortic stenosis or insufficiency, mitral insufficiency, subendocardial fibroelastosis, and so forth (Fig. 14B). Along with other available clinical information, inversion may then prove a valuable differential diagnostic sign; it insures the fact that any existing pulmonary artery hypertension, no matter how high (though not, of course, above systemic levels), must result predominantly from shunt volume rather than from pulmonary vascular resistance; since it is representative of a large shunt volume, it constitutes one sign among others pointing toward the need for early surgical correction.

Some additional comments concerning the whole precordial lead T-wave pattern, particularly in patent ductus arteriosus, seem appropriate at this point (Figs. 6, 8). When the T wave in left epicardial leads is inverted (high-flow patent ductus arteriosus and occasionally interventricular septal defect), one might suppose that positivity of this deflection on the opposite or right side of the precordium simply reflects, secondarily, the inverse pattern, as though these were polar aspects of a single T-wave vector, dominated in this situation by the negative left side. Such, however, seems not to be the case, since it has been shown that right precordial lead T-wave positivity in this hemodynamic circumstance occurs only with significant right ventricular (reflecting pulmonary arterial) hypertension,[12] in necessary association with the appropriate QRS pattern previously defined (R = 30 to 35 per cent or more of RS–V_1) and considered consistent with so-called biventricular hypertrophy. If, on the other hand, the QRS pattern is completely dominated by the left side, as in obstructive or nonhemodynamic left ventricular enlargement, and R = 20 per cent of RS–V_1 or less, then T-wave positivity in the right precordial leads is *not* primary and does not of itself hemodynamically imply right ventricular hypertension (even though such might actually exist) (Fig. 12C).

Nonhemodynamic Left Ventricular Enlargement. Left precordial lead T-wave inversion is a frequent though not necessarily an absolute electrocardiographic accompaniment of nonhemodynamic left ventricular enlargement. Actually, there are a number of different electrocardiographic patterns, just as there are a number of different pathologic and perhaps hemodynamic entities. In relatively few instances only may this diagnosis be made on the basis of the electrocardiogram alone. More often, it is a matter of combining several sorts of information and proportions (or disproportions), somewhat as follows:

1. A type or degree of left ventricular enlargement disproportionate to right
2. T-wave abnormalities disproportionate to QRS
3. Overall heart size (X ray) disproportionate to the degree and pattern of increased pulmonary vascularity
4. Absence of typical or presence of atypical clinical signs, such as murmurs, peripheral pulse amplitude, congestive failure

SUMMARY AND CONCLUSIONS

Selective preference has been given in this discussion to the value of hemodynamic implications of precordial lead T-wave patterns, properly qualified by the characteristics of the associated initial ventricular deflections (QRS) and supplemented by other clinical and radiographic information.

In this perspective, representative right and left precordial (epicardial) lead T/QRS patterns provide the most sensitive and accurate clinical clue to the presence, the hemodynamic type, and the quantitative degree of single as well as combined cardiac chamber physiological work and anatomical size.

Among the various clinical applications of this type of diagnostic electrocardiographic information, the following should be listed:

1. The provision of important clues toward the establishment of a qualitative and quantitative differential diagnosis, especially in terms of so-called mechanical malformations (obstruction or shunt) and the predictable myocardial response to the resulting functional workloads
2. Important implications in the differentiation between increased *volume* of blood flow and increased vascular *resistance* in the pathogenesis of pulmonary artery hypertension
3. Practical qualitative and quantitative clues to the possibility and the need, respectively, for surgical correction of the malformation in question
4. A warning of the possibility of otherwise unsuspected atypical or complicating features in what might have seemed to be a simple and straightforward diagnostic situation. Further technical diagnostic procedures, such as venous or arterial cardiac catheterization and selective cineangiocardiography, may be indicated
5. The provision of one among several possible clues toward the detection and differentiation (including diagnostic, prognostic, and therapeutic) of primary myocardial, nonhemodynamic (especially left ventricular) disease, with its resulting cardiac enlargement and possibly failure

The electrocardiogram, in particular the right and left precordial lead T/QRS pattern, is capable in most instances of determining that the heart, especially in infants and children, is hemodynamically if not structurally normal. This determination is of great clinical importance when it becomes necessary, as is relatively frequent, particularly in infants, to evaluate the pathogenesis of such signs as cyanosis, heart murmurs, unusual cardiac rate or rhythm, various sorts of respiratory distress, peripheral edema, hepatomegaly, or supposed cardiac enlargement.

There are relatively infrequent exceptions to the precordial lead patterns and their permissible hemodynamic implications as proposed and qualified in this presentation. There may not always be strict and universal agreement regarding electrophysiological explanations. Nevertheless, the practical clinical usefulness of such diagnostic clues as are outlined here still is beyond question.

References

1. ZIEGLER, R. F.: *The clinical contribution of electrocardiography in mechanical malformations of the cardiovascular system.* Amer. Heart J. 58:504, 1959.

2. ZIEGLER, R. F.: *The T-wave of the electrocardiogram: methods of measurement and interpretation,* in: Cassels, D. E. (ed.): *The Heart and Circulation in the Newborn Infant.* Grune & Stratton, New York, 1966.

3. WILSON, F. N., MacLEOD, A. G., BARKER, P. S., AND JOHNSTON, F. D.: *The determination and the significance of the areas of the ventricular deflections of the electrocardiogram.* Amer. Heart J. 10:46, 1934.

4. MASCARENHAS, A. S., AND LANDULFO, J.: *AS Areas Manifestas De QRS–T Do Electrocardiograma Precordial.* Arch. del Inst. de Cardiol. de Mexico, Parts I, II; XVII: 86, 100; 1948.

5. CASTELLANOS, A. JR., LEMBERG, L., AND CASTELLANOS, A.: *The vectorcardiographic significance of upright T waves in V_1 and V_2 during the first months of life.* J. Pediat. 62:827, 1963.

6. CASTELLANOS, A., LEMBERG, L., GOSSELIN, A., AND CASTELLANOS, A., JR.: *Combined ventricular enlargement during the first months of life. A vectorcardiographic study of the T-loop.* Amer. J. Cardiol. 13:767, 1964.

7. HAMBY, R. I., HOFFMAN, I., AND GLASSMAN, E.: *The T loop in right ventricular hypertrophy.* Dis. Chest 55:105, 1969.

8. ZIEGLER, R. F.: *The importance of positive T waves in the right precordial electrocardiogram during the first year of life.* Amer. Heart J. 52:533, 1956.

9. HAIT, G., AND GASUL, B. M.: *The evolution and significance of T wave changes in the normal newborn during the first seven days of life.* Amer. J. Cardiol. 12:494, 1963.

10. CABRERA, E., AND GAXIOLA, A.: *A critical re-evaluation of systolic and diastolic overloading patterns.* Prog. Cardiov. Dis. II:219, 1959.

11. CABRERA, E., AND MONROY, J. R.: *Systolic and diastolic loading of the heart. II. Electrocardiographic data.* Amer. Heart J. 43:669, 1952.

12. ZIEGLER, R. F.: *The importance of patent ductus arteriosus in infants.* Amer. Heart J. 43:553, 1952.

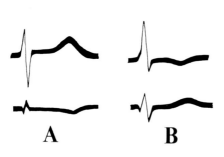

Figure 1. In this and in all subsequent illustrations, V_1 is shown above and V_6 below, both redrawn by pantographic enlargement of simultaneously inscribed leads from actual electrocardiograms selected for their representative value. In this report, no attention is given to absolute measurements, much more importance being attached to patterns. These two sets of precordial leads are from a normal infant; A at 3 hours after birth, and B at the age of 3 days. The progression of a positive to a negative $T-V_1$ evidences decreasing right ventricular and pulmonary arterial pressure. Note also the transient negativity of $T-V_6$ in the immediate newborn period.

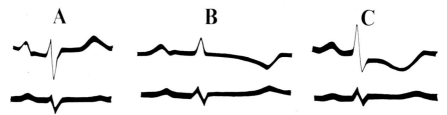

Figure 2. Three sets of simultaneous precordial leads V_1 and V_6 from a normal infant presenting with cyanosis, radiographic cardiomegaly, and polycythemia. In A, at 23 hours, the electrocardiogram and its hemodynamic inferences could be either normal or not, depending on its further course of change. At 5 days, (B) right-sided hemodynamics are normal, but there is evidence of hypocalcemia by virtue of a prolonged QT interval. In C, at 11 days, all is normal except for some continuing, though subsiding, "cyanosis," no longer of any cardiac concern. It is of further interest to note the progressive changes in V_1 without comparable or reciprocal changes in V_6, suggesting that the dominant effects may be attributed to right ventricular activity.

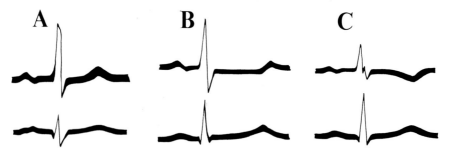

Figure 3. Three sets of simultaneous precordial leads V_1 and V_6 from the same subject. A, age 10 days. Diagnosis: patent ductus arteriosus with pure pulmonary resistance hypertension, absence of shunt, systemic and pulmonary pressures measured as equal. Electrocardiogram: uncomplicated right ventricular hypertension. B, age 1 month. Two weeks postoperative following ductus closure. Electrocardiogram and implied hemodynamics: subsiding pulmonary artery and right ventricular hypertension. C, age 3 months. Normal. This infant was first referred for simple tachycardia; there were no murmurs, no cyanosis, a virtually normal chest X ray. Abnormal electrocardiogram at 10 days showed T-wave positivity in lead V_1. Cardiac catheterization demonstrated presence of patent ductus arteriosus. Early surgical closure offered the only possible chance for subsequent return of pulmonary vascular resistance to normal. This surgical course was successful.

Figure 4. Precordial lead patterns of simple right ventricular obstruction and hypertension in four increasingly severe cases of congenital pulmonary valvular stenosis. A, age 5 years. Right ventricular pressure 40/0–10 mm. Hg; pulmonary artery pressure 20/10 mm. Hg. The T wave in lead V_1, which normally should be fairly deeply inverted, presents a $+ - +$ configuration, with a slightly positive net area. The amplitude of R in this lead is approximately 35 per cent of RS, which permits this slight T wave positivity (or less than normal negativity) to imply mild right ventricular hypertension. B, age 3 years. Right ventricular pressure 58/0; pulmonary artery pressure 20/10. There is no evidence of right ventricular hypertrophy in the QRS complexes, which are normal. The T-wave positivity in lead V_1, with an R:S ratio of one, is pathognomonic of significant right ventricular hypertension. C, age 3 months. Right ventricular pressure 64/0; pulmonary artery pressure 12/5. Right ventricular hypertension and hypertrophy are in evidence in both QRS and T-wave configurations. D, age 4 years. Right ventricular pressure 180/6. The QRS pattern clearly indicates marked right ventricular hypertrophy. The T-wave inversion in lead V_1 is now secondary (ventricular gradient) to the large positive amplitude and area inscribed under the R wave in this lead. This is not the pattern of QRS–T that would be seen in a comparably advanced quantitative degree of increased volume-flow right ventricular work and enlargement.

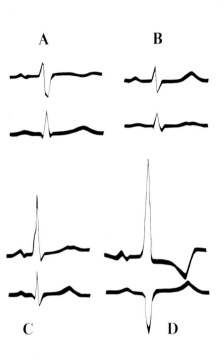

Figure 5. An instance of severe, near terminal, primary obliterative pulmonary endarteritis in a girl aged 17 years. The heart was large and peripheral pulmonary vascularity markedly diminished on X ray examination. The electrocardiogram shows very marked right-sided enlargement, atrial and ventricular, with right epicardial potential variations being apparent by leftward extension as far at least as V_6. An apparently true initial Q wave in V_1 probably is evidence of right ventricular dilatation, which, together with massive hypertrophy, was present anatomically.

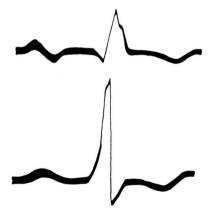

109

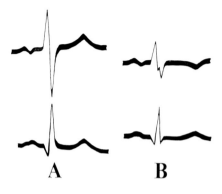

A   B

Figure 6. Preoperative (A) and 2 weeks postoperative (B) electrocardiograms in a 4½-month-old baby with a large patent ductus arteriosus and reversible pulmonary artery flow hypertension, evidenced electrocardiographically by T-wave positivity in lead V_1, diagnostic of right ventricular and therefore pulmonary artery hypertension, normal after surgical correction; left atrial and left ventricular enlargement, resulting from the increased volume of pulmonary venous return to the left heart.

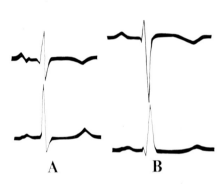

A   B

Figure 7. Two sets of precordial leads V_1 and V_6 from patients of age 4 months (A) and 8 years (B), both with uncomplicated left-to-right shunting (aorta to pulmonary artery via a patent ductus arteriosus) and without significant pulmonary hypertension. Both electrocardiograms show increased volume of pulmonary venous return to the left heart: (1) left atrial enlargement and (2) incomplete left bundle branch block as presumptive of left ventricular volume-hypertrophy. Also, particularly in A, there is increased positive amplitude of both QRS and T in lead V_6, the ST segment and T wave in B probably being modified secondarily by the left intraventricular conduction delay. Amplification and simultaneous lead recording permits the proper visualization and interpretation of the low-voltage P and Q components of the electrocardiogram.

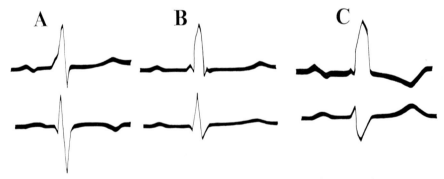

A   B   C

Figure 8. Electrocardiograms of three children with anatomically uncomplicated patent ductus arteriosus but irreversible pulmonary resistance hypertension, ages 4 years (A), 11 years (B), and 12 years (C). Right ventricular hypertension and hypertrophy are evident in all cases by both QRS and T-wave criteria. Right precordial lead T-wave positivity is preserved in A and B, reversed in C by the ventricular gradient effect of superimposed right bundle branch block and increased positive area of QRS (possibly also anatomic right ventricular dilatation). The left side is normal in each case, except for the unexplained T-wave inversion in lead V_6 in (A). This child did survive surgical closure of the ductus, but without any subsidence of the fixed level of pulmonary resistance and pressure.

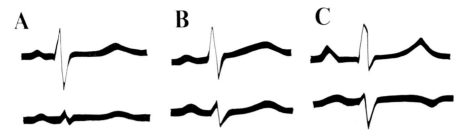

Figure 9. Three sets of precordial leads V_1 and V_6 in the same subject with complete transposition of the great vessels: A, at 2 days of age; B, at 1 month; and C, at 16 months. The positive T wave in lead V_1 is evidence at all ages of right ventricular hypertension, supporting aortic pressure and systemic arterial circulation and resistance. At 2 days, this positivity might have been normal, had it regressed soon thereafter. At 1 month of age, cardiac catheterization and angiocardiographic studies demonstrated the presence of an interventricular septal defect with which one might assume some degree of increased pulmonary vascular resistance and left ventricular hypertension. At 16 months, repeat catheterization proved that the interventricular septal defect had spontaneously closed, with a directly measured left ventricular pressure (via patent foramen ovale and mitral valve) of only 26/0 mm. Hg (mean 12); and the left ventricular T wave is now inverted. This evidence suggests a T-wave progression equivalent to that observed in similar hemodynamic circumstances on the right when the root position of the great vessels is normal.

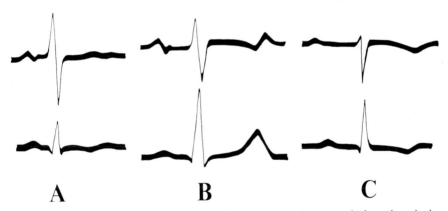

Figure 10. Three representative precordial lead patterns in congenital aortic valvular stenosis. In A, age 6 weeks, two presumably primary and independent T-wave patterns indicate (in V_1) right ventricular hypertension (52/0–12 mm. Hg) and (in V_6) left ventricular enlargement, strain, or possibly at least relative ischemia. This pattern is *not* that of biventricular hypertrophy as seen in shunt situations, but is fairly characteristic of this obstructive malformation, though only in the early infant period. In B, age 2 years, the pattern of primary increased positivity of T in lead V_6, without otherwise diagnostic QRS or P-wave abnormalities, is practically pathognomonic of compensated left ventricular hypertension up to fairly marked levels of quantitative severity (in this instance 200/0–8 mm. Hg) but without dilatation or coronary insufficiency. In C, age 3 years, the progression to T-wave negativity in lead V_6 indicates the need for surgical correction. Before this quantitative situation, marked electrocardiographically by left epicardial lead T-wave inversion, there would appear to be only very minimal risk of either serious clinical symptoms or sudden death.

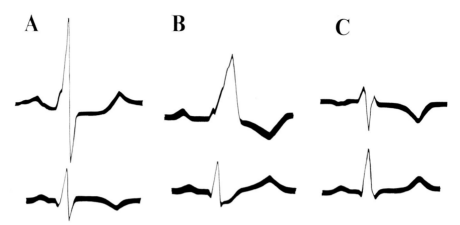

Figure 11. Simultaneous precordial leads V_1 and V_6 in three infants with coarctation of the aorta as the single anatomic malformation, each presenting a different hemodynamic and electrocardiographic picture. A, 2 months of age, presented with massive cardiac enlargement—combined right- and left-sided by electrocardiogram—and clinical congestive heart failure. Right ventricular pressure measured 75/0–4 mm. Hg. The aortic insertion of the closed ductus was distal to the site of the coarctation. The degree of right ventricular hypertension, evidenced in lead V_1 and measured directly by cardiac catheterization, as well as the T-wave inversion in lead V_6, both strongly indicate early surgical correction, which was accomplished successfully in this case. In B, age 3 months, is shown a not uncommon pattern of right bundle branch block plus right ventricular enlargement (probably combined hypertrophy and dilatation), indicating the neonatal hemodynamics of proximal aortic insertion of the fetal ductus. A significant limitation of the electrocardiogram must be pointed out here: the time lapse between electrical and hemodynamic events. From direct catheter measurement, right ventricular pressure had returned to almost normal from what must have been a more markedly elevated level in the newborn period. Also in evidence was a so-called Bernheim effect, indicating a degree of left ventricular hypertrophy also not evidenced in this electrocardiogram. In C, age 6 months, is shown a precordial lead pattern considered typical of uncomplicated coarctation at all subsequent ages. It is believed to derive from the early neonatal pattern of right ventricular enlargement and right bundle branch block resulting from the hemodynamic pattern associated with proximal aortic insertion of the fetal ductus.

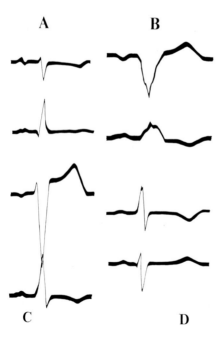

Figure 12. Electrocardiograms representing four forms of nonhemodynamic left ventricular enlargement. A, 4 months. Subendocardial fibroelastosis of the left atrium and left ventricle. B, 3 years. Idiopathic left ventricular hypertrophic subaortic obstruction. C, 5 years. Idiopathic, nonobstructive left ventricular hypertrophy. D, 7 years. Diffuse left ventricular rhabdomyomatosis with subvalvular outflow obstruction. None of these electrocardiographic patterns would be appropriate to usual hemodynamic situations such as obstruction or shunt. Only one, D, may be considered practically pathognomonic, although complete left bundle branch block as in B is most likely to occur in some form of primary myocardial disease such as idiopathic hypertrophy or subendocardial fibroelastosis, particularly in combination with coronary artery anomalies.

Figure 13. Two reasonably representative precordial lead patterns of high-flow patent ductus arteriosus (A) and interventricular septal defect (B), and the differential left precordial lead T-wave behavior described in the text. In A, age 3 months, there is a large shunt volume but without significant pulmonary hypertension (42/22 mm. Hg), with a negative T–V$_1$. This factor permits fairly marked lowering of aortic diastolic pressure, which, in turn, is believed to favor the inversion of T–V$_6$. In B, age 4 months, there is an equally large shunt volume but with pulmonary artery and right ventricular hypertension (80/42 and 80/0–13 mm. Hg, respectively). Combined right and left ventricular and left atrial enlargement are apparent in the electrocardiogram, together with the pattern of apparently incomplete left bundle branch block.

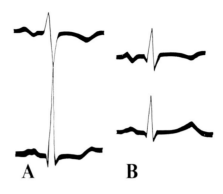

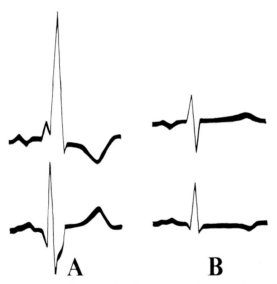

Figure 14. These two sets of precordial leads V$_1$ and V$_6$ are from the same patient. In A, age 5 months, the original diagnosis was interventricular septal defect together with coarctation of the aorta and a distal patent ductus arteriosus. In B, age 6 months, the coarctation had been repaired and the ductus closed, leaving a large left-to-right shunt through the interventricular septal defect and resulting pulmonary artery (flow) hypertension. The basic electrocardiographic pattern is that shown in B, with normal intraventricular conduction and combined right and left ventricular hypertrophy: positive T–V$_1$ as independent, primary evidence of right ventricular hypertension; negative T–V$_6$, also independent and primary evidence of left ventricular enlargement, probably of mixed hemodynamic type, and atypical for uncomplicated interventricular septal defect. The P-wave pattern in both instances is typical of left atrial enlargement, consistent with increased volume of pulmonary blood flow and venous return to the left heart. Of additional interest is the modification of this basic pattern by the superimposition of right bundle branch block (A). Both primary right and left ventricular T-wave patterns have been modified by the ventricular gradient effect of the right intraventricular conduction abnormality so that they now are secondary to the pattern of QRS. Further, it seems likely that the T-wave pattern in the two opposite precordial leads V$_1$ and V$_6$ in this latter situation does represent opposite poles of a single T-wave vector instead of the two independent vectors as described in B.

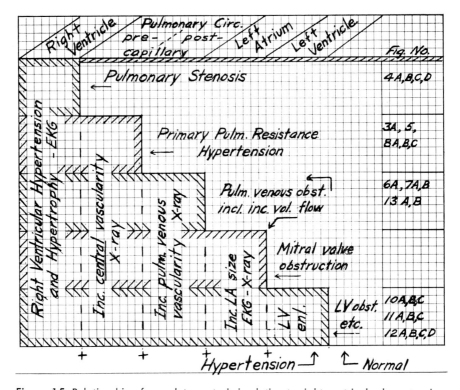

Figure 15. Relationship of complete central circulation to right ventricular hypertension.

The Roentgen Diagnosis
of Congenital Heart Disease

John A. Kirkpatrick, M.D., and
Marie A. Capitanio, M.D.

The roentgen examination of the chest of a patient with congenital heart disease is a readily available method by which significant information about the heart, the great vessels, and the intrapulmonary vasculature can be obtained expediently and with no real risk to the patient. The evaluation and interpretation of the radiological examination is dependent upon an understanding of normal cardiovascular anatomy and physiology and of how these are altered in the presence of a congenital anomaly. Its value is enhanced by the degree to which the information obtained is correlated with the history, physical examination, electrocardiogram, and other laboratory data.

There are general principles to be considered in the roentgen diagnosis of congenital heart disease. First, there is a spectrum of severity of any lesion, simple or complex, and a normal examination does not exclude the presence of congenital heart disease. Second, ventricles that are obstructed by a narrow outlet or valve or distal stenosis respond to the load by hypertrophy, and hypertrophy of a ventricle is not likely to cause an alteration in the size or shape of the heart until failure and dilatation ensue. Third, chambers, particularly the ventricles, and vessels that carry more blood than is normal, as in a shunt, hypertrophy and dilate, resulting in cardiac enlargement, a reflection of enlargement of specific chambers. Fourth, the evaluation of the great vessels and intrapulmonary vasculature is essential and must be correlated with the size and configuration of the heart. Fifth, a heart that is normal may appear enlarged in the presence of anomalies of the thoracic cage, such as a pectus excavatum deformity or asphyxiating thoracic dystrophy, and interstitial inflammatory disease of the lungs may be confused with alterations of the pulmonary vasculature.

The basic roentgen examination of the chest should include those projections that permit visualization of the chambers of the heart in such a way that their enlargement is detectable, as well as allow for the evaluation of the size, contour, and position of the great vessels and the intrapulmonary vasculature. The usual examination consists of posteroanterior, lateral, and right and left lateral oblique projections. Barium in the esophagus will aid in these assessments and is included as part of the study. Fluoroscopy is an adjunctive procedure and should be used to answer specific questions that arise after evaluation of the radiographs, particularly questions that relate to pulsations or to respirations.

A ROENTGEN CLASSIFICATION OF CONGENITAL HEART DISEASE

In an attempt to bring some order to the radiological evaluation of patients with congenital heart disease, a classification based on the appearance of the intrapulmonary vasculature and of the size and configuration of the heart has been found helpful. Though this method will not result in a specific diagnosis, it will offer an appropriate differential diagnosis. Moreover, within any one group, there may be specific roentgen findings that will narrow the diagnosis.

116

The intrapulmonary vasculature may present in one of four ways: (1) normal; (2) decreased, as in a right-to-left shunt; (3) arterial engorgement, as in a left-to-right shunt; and (4) lymphatic and pulmonary venous congestion, as in obstructing lesions on the left side of the heart and/or failure of the left ventricle.[1,2]

Normal Intrapulmonary Vasculature

Normal intrapulmonary vasculature associated with a heart that is normal in size and configuration is compatible with small left-to-right shunts and obstructing lesions that are distal to the ventricles and not associated with ventricular decompensation (Table 1). Any intracardiac defect that results in a left-to-right shunt of less than two to one is not likely to be associated with any change in the size or configuration of the heart or with an alteration of the intrapulmonary vasculature. Thus, it is significant that one cannot make a radiographic diagnosis of a small ventricular septal defect, atrial septal defect, etc. This fact exemplifies the first of the general principles already mentioned, in that the degree of severity of any lesion determines the presence of alterations that can be appreciated radiographically.

Though stenotic lesions such as aortic stenosis, pulmonary stenosis, and coarctation of the aorta may be severe, the heart and intrapulmonary vasculature are normal radiographically as long as the involved ventricle is compensated. Therefore, to make the diagnosis of any one of these stenotic lesions, observations other than the size or shape of the heart and the appearance of the pulmonary vasculature must be used. In aortic stenosis, again depending upon severity, one looks for post-stenotic dilatation of the ascending aorta (Fig. 1). In children, the normal ascending aorta does not project to the right of the spine, and when it does, post-stenotic dilatation should be suspected. Coarctation of the aorta is associated with a small and/or deformed distal arch of the aorta, and at times, the descending aorta may be unusually prominent (Fig. 2). Impressions on the barium-filled esophagus by the small aortic knob above the coarctation and the dilatation of the aorta below the coarctation produce the classic reverse "3-sign." Fluoroscopically, increased pulsations in the left superior mediastinum as a result of the lateral displacement of the left subclavian artery may be appreciated.[3] Notching of the ribs is a valuable clue, and on occasion, the

Table 1. Pulmonary vasculature normal

Minimal or no cardiac enlargement	Cardiac enlargement
Normal	Aortic stenosis
Small shunt <2:1	Coarctation of aorta
Stenosis	Myocardiopathy, e.g., fibroelastosis
Complex lesions, e.g. tetralogy of Fallot	Tumor

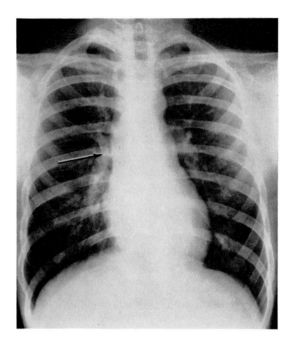

Figure 1. Aortic stenosis, male, 13 years of age. The heart is normal in size and there is no abnormality of the pulmonary vasculature. Post-stenotic dilatation of the ascending aorta is present and visible to the right of the spine (arrow).

dilated and tortuous internal mammary artery may be appreciated anteriorly on the lateral film of the chest. Pulmonary valvular stenosis usually results in post-stenotic dilatation of the trunk of the pulmonary artery (Fig. 3). Fluoroscopically, differential pulsations in the hila may be noted: that is, the right hilum is quiet and there are increased pulsations of the branches of the pulmonary artery on the left side. This observation most likely reflects the anatomic relationship of the left pulmonary artery to the main pulmonary artery.[4]

When the heart is enlarged and the vasculature is normal, the possibilities to be considered should be ventricular decompensation, the primary myocardiopathies, and cardiac or pericardial tumors. Ventricular decompensation secondary to an obstructing lesion on the left side of the heart causes dilatation of the ventricle but may not be associated with demonstrable vascular congestion in the lungs (Fig. 4). The primary myocardiopathies cause cardiac enlargement, usually on the left side, that may not be associated with vascular alterations in the lungs. The lesions usually considered in this group include endocardial fibroelastosis, viral myocarditis, medial necrosis of the coronary arteries, aberrant left coronary artery (arising from the pulmonary artery), and glycogen storage disease of the heart. Cardiac tumors and those of the pericardium present as an enlarged cardiac silhouette with normal intrapulmonary vasculature; the configuration of the heart may be bizarre.

Decreased Intrapulmonary Vasculature

The association of diminished intrapulmonary vasculature with a heart

118

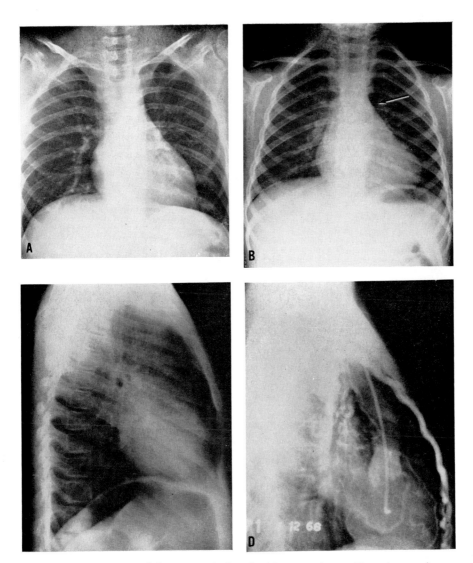

Figure 2. Coarctation of the aorta. A, female, 12 years of age. There is no enlargement of the heart or abnormality of the pulmonary vasculature; the distal arch of the aorta is small and the descending aorta dilated; notching of the ribs is evident. B, male, 5 years of age. A prominent notch just below the distal arch of the aorta is at the site of coarctation. C, a serpiginous soft tissue shadow just behind the sternum represents the enlarged internal mammary arteries and can be compared with the aortogram and subsequent opacification of the same vessels (D).

that is relatively normal in size is indicative of pulmonary obstruction and an intracardiac defect, as may be seen in the tetralogy of Fallot, tricuspid atresia, and at times in transposition of the great vessels (Table 2).[5] The classical radiographic appearance of the tetralogy of Fallot is characterized by an enlarged right atrium, ventricular hypertrophy manifested by round-

119

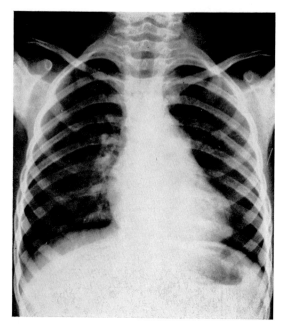

Figure 3. Pulmonary stenosis, valvular. There is slight rounding of the apex of the heart; the pulmonary artery is enlarged; the intrapulmonary vasculature is normal.

ing of the apex of the heart, a small pulmonary artery, diminished intrapulmonary vasculature, and a relatively large aorta (Fig. 5). The aortic arch is on the right in approximately 25 per cent of patients with the tetralogy of Fallot. In the right anterior oblique projection, there may be bulging of the

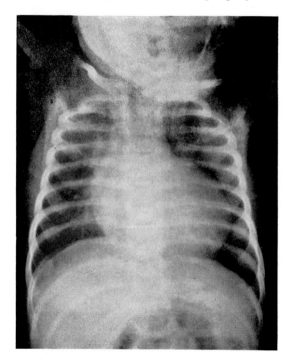

Figure 4. Coarctation of the aorta, male, 3 weeks of age. The heart is enlarged and the apex rounded, but the intrapulmonary vasculature is normal.

Table 2. Pulmonary vasculature decreased

Minimal or no cardiac enlargement	Cardiac enlargement
Tetralogy of Fallot	Pure pulmonary stenosis (infantile)
Tricuspid atresia	Pulmonary atresia
Transposition of great vessels with pulmonary stenosis	Ebstein's anomaly
(Pulmonary atresia— hypoplastic right ventricle)	

outflow tract of the right ventricle, an infundibular chamber (Fig. 6). At times, the prominence of the outflow tract of the right ventricle may be the only alteration that can be appreciated on the roentgenogram. In those instances of tricuspid atresia in which the right ventricle is absent or hypoplastic, one may see deformity of the anterior aspect of the heart in the left anterior oblique projection, i.e., a high bulge reflecting the enlarged right atrium and a concavity below reflecting the hypoplastic right ventricle (Fig. 7). Left atrial enlargement may be present in tricuspid atresia; its enlargement reflects the shunt through the atrial septum and hence the size of the atrial septal defect. In the first weeks or months of life, transposition of the great vessels with pulmonary stenosis may be impossible to differentiate from the others in this group.

Cardiac enlargement associated with diminished pulmonary vasculature suggests the combination of pulmonary obstruction, an intact ventricular septum, and decompensation of the right ventricle, as may occur in isolated pulmonary stenosis (Fig. 8). Similar alterations in the size and appearance

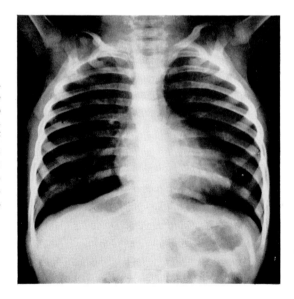

Figure 5. Tetralogy of Fallot, female, 6 months of age. The right atrium is enlarged, the apex is rounded, but the overall size is within the limits of normal. The aorta descends on the right; the superior vena cava is prominent lateral to the right aortic arch. The pulmonary artery is small, as are the intrapulmonary vessels.

121

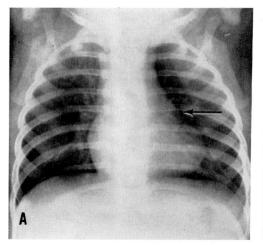
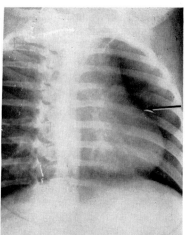

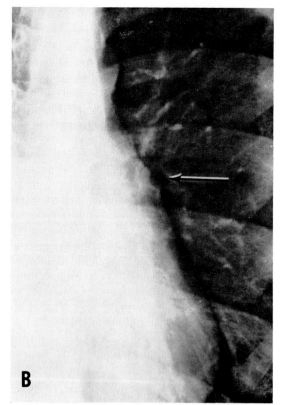

Figure 6. Tetralogy of Fallot. An infundibular chamber is visible as a convexity along the left border of the heart in A, an infant 4 months of age and in B, a male 10 years of age (arrows).

of the pulmonary vasculature may be present in Ebstein's anomaly of the tricuspid valve (Fig. 9). The right atrium is huge in this anomaly, but the total size of the heart reflects the degree to which the right ventricle is "atrialized"; and the degree to which the pulmonary vasculature is dimin-

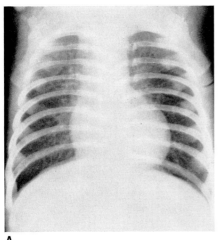 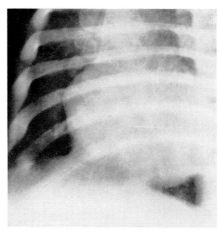

A   B

Figure 7. Tricuspid Atresia. The heart, while little enlarged, is rounded in configuration and associated with a very small pulmonary artery and small, sparse intrapulmonary vessels (A). In the left anterior oblique projection (B), the anterior aspect of the heart is unusual in configuration, the upper bulge reflects the enlarged right atrium, and the lower concavity the absence of a normal right ventricle.

ished depends upon the presence or absence of pulmonary stenosis. In both instances, right-to-left shunting at the atrial level contributes to the diminished vasculature. One expects the intrapulmonary vasculature to be diminished in the presence of pulmonary atresia with an intact ventricular septum; however, the degree of cardiac enlargement depends upon the presence or absence of hypoplasia of the right ventricle.

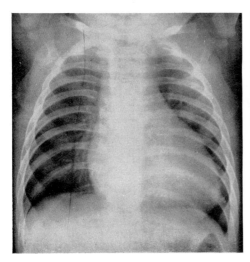 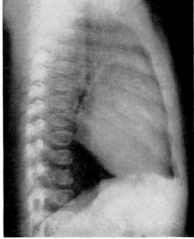

Figure 8. Pure pulmonary stenosis, male, 5 months of age. The heart is enlarged, the intrapulmonary vasculature sparse, and the vessels small.

123

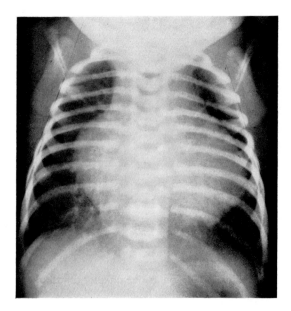

Figure 9. Ebstein's anomaly of the tricuspid valve, infant 1 week of age. The heart is huge, the apex rounded, and the right atrium enlarged. The intrapulmonary vasculature is diminished.

Engorgement of the Intrapulmonary Vasculature

An intracardiac or extracardiac uncomplicated defect resulting in a shunt to the lungs with a flow ratio greater than two to one is associated with both cardiac enlargement and vascular engorgement (Tables 3, 4).[6] In general, the degree of vascular engorgement parallels the size of the heart. In children, it is in this category that one may have the greatest success in evaluating chamber enlargement and localizing the site of the shunt. For example, in a secundum atrial septal defect, the flow, as illustrated in Figure 10, is left-to-right at the atrial level, resulting in an increased load on the right atrium, right ventricle, and pulmonary artery. The left atrium does not enlarge, as there is ready exit of blood from the left atrium to the right

Table 3. Pulmonary vasculature engorged

Cardiac Enlargement
Anomalous pulmonary venous return: not obstructed
Atrial septal defect: secundum
Endocardial cushion defect
Ventricular septal defect
Patent ductus arteriosus
Pulmonary-aortic window
Truncus arteriosus
Transposition (intracardiac-extracardiac shunts)

Table 4. Pulmonary vasculature engorged

Cardiac Enlargement	

Anomalous pulmonary venous return: not obstructed
   No left atrial enlargement
   Wide mediastinum if venous return is to left
      superior vena cava
   Right atrial enlargement
	Patent ductus arteriosus
	   Left atrial enlargement

Atrial septal defect: secundum
   No left atrial enlargement
	Truncus arteriosus
	   Left atrial enlargement
	   Pulmonary trunk not seen
	   Pulmonary branches high

Endocardial cushion defect
   Left atrial enlargement
   Right atrial enlargement
	Transposition great vessels with shunt
	   Left atrial enlargement
	   Pulmonary trunk not seen

Ventricular septal defect Left atrial enlargement	

atrium (Fig. 11). The pathophysiology of partial, unobstructed pulmonary venous return is exactly that of an atrial septal defect, and unless one can visualize the anomalous vein or veins, one cannot recognize this lesion as distinct from that of an atrial septal defect.[7] In total anomalous pulmonary venous return to the left superior vena cava, however, one notes enlargement of the left superior vena cava, the right superior vena cava, and the right

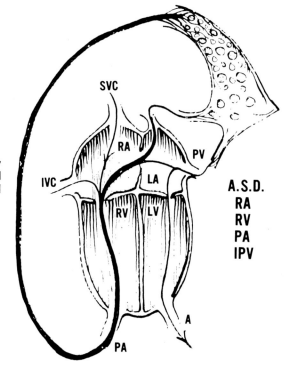

Figure 10. Diagram of flow (heavy black line) associated with a secundum atrial septal defect.

A.S.D.
RA
RV
PA
IPV

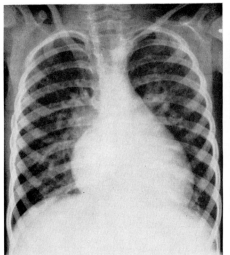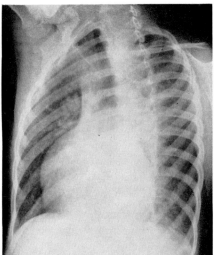

Figure 11. Atrial septal defect (secundum), male, 7 years of age. The heart is enlarged, particularly the right atrium and right ventricle. There is no left atrial enlargement. The pulmonary artery is engorged as is the intrapulmonary vasculature.

side of the heart and the pulmonary artery. The enlargement of the right and left superior venae cavae and enlargement of the right side of the heart may result in a configuration (Fig. 12) that has been termed "figure-8."

Patent ductus arteriosus, Figure 13, results in increased flow through the left side of the heart, the proximal aorta, and the pulmonary artery and its intrapulmonary branches. Fluoroscopically, the aorta shows prominent pulsations (Fig. 14).

In a ventricular septal defect (Fig. 15), the load imposed by the shunt is on the left atrium, the left ventricle, the right ventricle, the pulmonary artery, and the intrapulmonary vasculature (Fig. 16). Frequently, alterations of the right ventricle cannot be appreciated radiographically, and in those

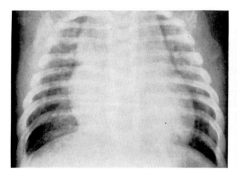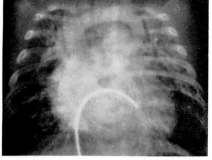

Figure 12. Total anomalous pulmonary venous return to the left superior vena cava. The mediastinum is wide owing to the large cavae; the heart, particularly the right atrium, is enlarged and the intrapulmonary vessels are overfilled.

126

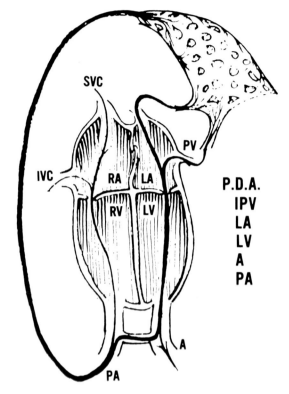

Figure 13. Diagram of flow (heavy black line) associated with a patent ductus arteriosus.

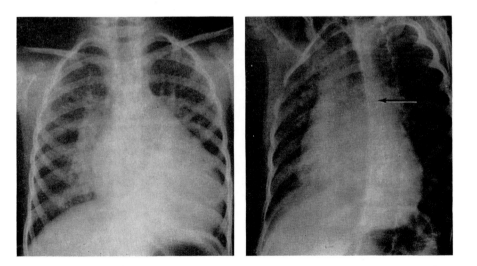

Figure 14. Patent ductus arteriosus. The heart is enlarged. The left ventricle extends laterally, inferiorly, and posteriorly. Enlargement of the left atrium has elevated the left stem bronchus (arrow). The pulmonary artery and its intrapulmonary branches are engorged.

127

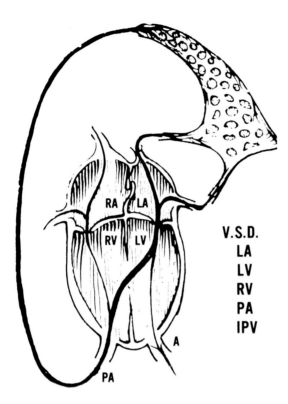

Figure 15. Diagram of flow (heavy black line) associated with ventricular septal defect.

V.S.D.
LA
LV
RV
PA
IPV

instances, it is not possible to differentiate a ventricular septal defect from a patent ductus arteriosus in which the imposed load is on the left atrium, the left ventricle, the pulmonary artery, and the intrapulmonary vasculature.

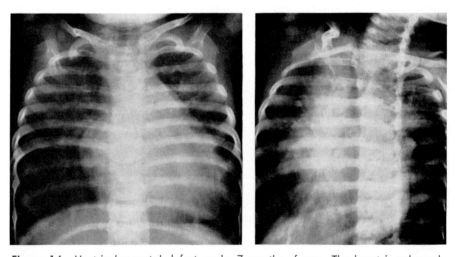

Figure 16. Ventricular septal defect, male, 7 months of age. The heart is enlarged, with biventricular enlargement as well as enlargement of the left atrium. The pulmonary artery is prominent, as are its intrapulmonary branches.

128

It may be very difficult to make the diagnosis of an endocardial cushion defect as distinct from a ventricular septal defect or atrial septal defect. If, in the presence of enlargement of the right atrium and the right ventricle, one notes left atrial enlargement, one should consider the possibility of an endocardial cushion defect (Fig. 17).[8]

The evaluation of the pulmonary artery is most important in the presence of a shunt to the lungs. If the pulmonary artery is not seen as an enlarged, distinct structure when the heart is enlarged and the intrapulmonary vasculature is engorged, two possibilities should be considered; one [9] is that the pulmonary artery is absent, as in a truncus arteriosus (Fig. 18), and the other

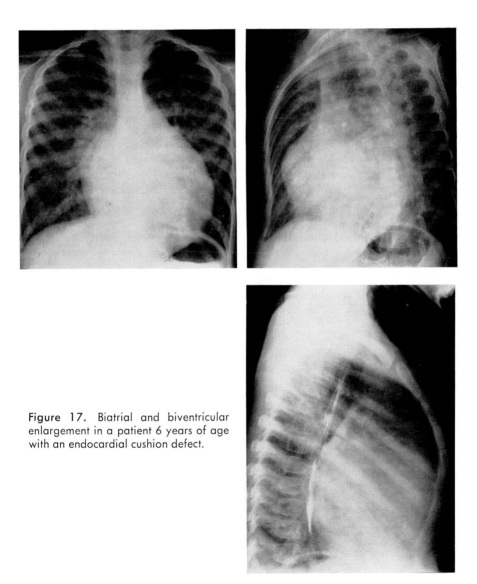

Figure 17. Biatrial and biventricular enlargement in a patient 6 years of age with an endocardial cushion defect.

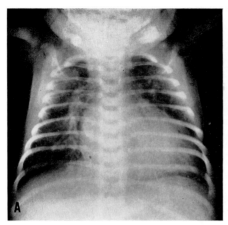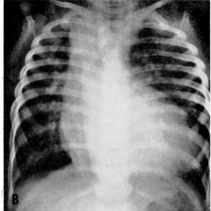

Figure 18. Truncus arteriosus. A, the heart is enlarged and the pulmonary vessels engorged, but the pulmonary trunk is not visible. Note the high position of the right hilum. B, the truncus is on the right.

is that the pulmonary artery is in an abnormal position, as in one of the forms of transposition (Figs. 19, 20).

In left-to-right shunts, it is necessary to evaluate the intrapulmonary vasculature for alterations that reflect increased pulmonary resistance.[10] In general, one suspects high pulmonary resistance when the pulmonary trunk and the hilar vessels are engorged and those vessels in the mid-portion and in the periphery of the lung are small and/or tortuous. In the presence of high pulmonary resistance, flow is altered so that the right side of the heart is dominant no matter what the location of the shunt, and the general rules as given may not be applicable.

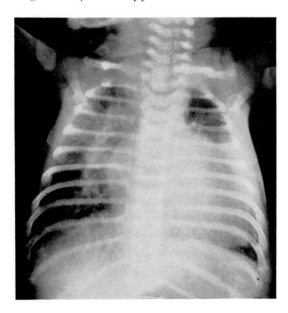

Figure 19. Transposition of the great vessels with associated intracardiac defects, female 1 month of age. The heart is enlarged, the pulmonary vasculature is engorged and congested, the base of the heart is narrow.

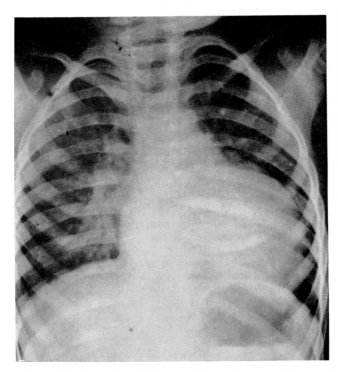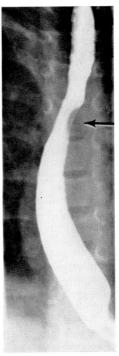

Figure 20. Inversion of the ventricles and ventricular septal defect. The ascending aorta lies laterally along the upper left border of the heart. The enlarged pulmonary artery is located posteriorly and medially and indents the barium-filled esophagus (arrow).

Transposition of the great vessels is a general category. In the usual instance, the aorta arises from the right ventricle and is seen to lie anterior and to the right of the pulmonary artery, which arises from the left ventricle.[11] Cyanosis is to be expected but may not be clinically evident, depending on the size and location of other associated defects. The roentgenographic manifestations also reflect associated defects, that is, there are shunts to the lungs through atrial or ventricular defects or a patent ductus arteriosus. The heart is enlarged, the base narrowed, and the pulmonary vasculature increased in the usual instance (Fig. 19). At times, particularly in the presence of large shunts, it may not be possible to differentiate the roentgen appearance from that of a similar defect in a heart in which the great vessels are normally situated. Transposition of the great vessels may be associated with inversion of the ventricles, wherein the hemodynamics are normal. The anatomic left ventricle lies anterior, receives blood from the right atrium, and empties into the pulmonary artery. The anatomic right ventricle is posterior and lateral, receives blood from the left atrium, and empties into the aorta. Radiographically, the lateral position of the aorta and the posterior position of the pulmonary artery are significant. Associated defects are common (Fig. 20).

Table 5. Pulmonary vasculature congested

Minimal or no cardiac enlargement	Cardiac enlargement
Stenosis of pulmonary veins	Mitral insufficiency Primary

Obstructive anomalous pulmonary
    venous return
	Secondary (left ventricular failure)
	    Aortic stenosis
	    Coarctation of aorta
	    Myocardiopathies

Cor triatriatum	
Mitral stenosis or atresia	
Hypoplastic left heart syndrome	

Congested Intrapulmonary Vasculature

In general, if an obstructing lesion is associated with congestion of the intrapulmonary vasculature, the heart is relatively normal in size when the obstruction is at or proximal to the mitral valve and enlarged when the obstruction is distal to the mitral valve (Table 5, Figs. 21, 22).[12] In the hypoplastic left heart syndrome, pulmonary congestion may be intense and the heart relatively normal in overall size, because the hypoplasia of the ascending aorta and left ventricle act as an obstruction at the mitral valve level.[13] In young infants, it may be impossible to differentiate coarctation of the aorta from aortic stenosis when these anomalies are associated with left heart failure and congestion (Fig. 23).

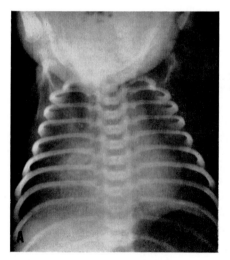 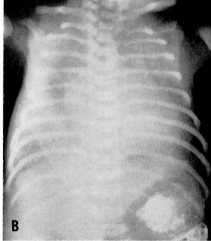

Figure 21. Obstructed anomalous pulmonary venous return to the ductus venosus. At 6 days the pulmonary vessels are indistinct and edema in the right middle lobe is evident (A). 12 hours later there is intense pulmonary edema (B).

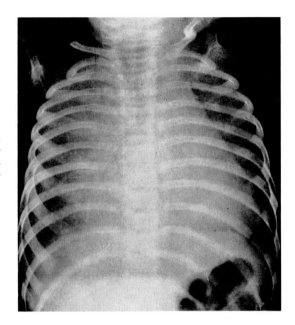

Figure 22. Cor triatriatum. While the heart is not enlarged, the lungs are congested, and there is pulmonary edema.

THE GREAT VESSELS

As has been described, the size and position of the great vessels are significant in diagnosis.[14] The side on which the aorta descends is readily determined by visualization of the distal arch of the aorta or of the descending aorta. If these are not well seen because of the thymus, there is indirect evidence as reflected by the trachea and the barium-filled esophagus. In infants and children, the trachea usually lies to the side opposite the aortic arch, and the barium-filled esophagus is indented by the distal arch on the

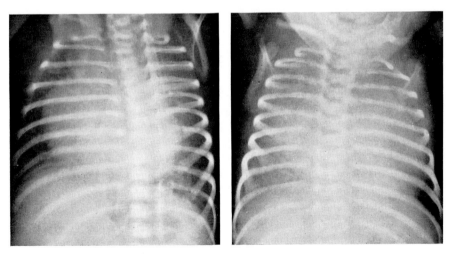

Figure 23. Aortic stenosis, male, 3 months of age. The heart is enlarged and there is intense pulmonary venous and lymphatic congestion.

133

side on which it descends. The mirror-image right aortic arch has been reported to be associated with congenital heart disease in 98 per cent of instances, of which 90 per cent are the tetralogy of Fallot. If there is an anomalous left subclavian artery associated with the right arch, only 12 per cent are associated with congenital heart disease.[15] To determine the above, it is necessary to visualize the barium-filled esophagus in multiple projections, particularly the posteroanterior and the lateral. A careful study of the esophagus and trachea also reveals other anomalies of the aortic arch, such as a double aortic arch (Fig. 24).

The pulmonary artery lies posterior in the usual transposition and, if enlarged, may indent the barium-filled esophagus at a lower level than does the aorta.

THE NEONATE AND YOUNG INFANT

The radiological evaluation of congenital cardiac abnormalities encountered in the neonate and young infant [16, 17] differs from the evaluation of

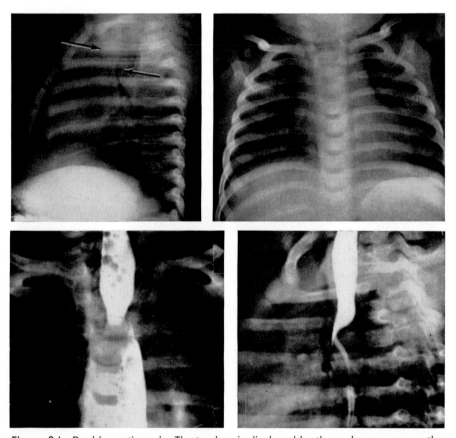

Figure 24. Double aortic arch. The trachea is displaced by the arches as seen on the lateral radiograph (arrows). There are bilateral indentions and a posterior one on the barium-filled esophagus produced by the two arches.

similar lesions encountered in the older infant and child. The usual rules for the recognition of enlargement of the chambers of the heart or of the position of the great vessels and even the size of the heart do not apply because of physiological, anatomical, and clinical factors peculiar to this age group. The neonate or young infant with congenital heart disease commonly presents with either a loud murmur, cyanosis, or cardiac failure—manifestations of either complex lesions, large shunts, or severe stenotic lesions. In addition, the transition from the fetal circulation to the extra-uterine circulation is in progress during this period, with increased pulmonary resistance and dominance of the right side of the heart that may not be a complication of the same lesion or lesions in the older infant or child. The relatively large thymus, the configuration of the chest, and the high position of the diaphragm make evaluation of the size and shape of the heart difficult.

These anatomical and physiological factors, responsible for difficulties in the roentgen evaluation of the heart and great vessels and of the intrapulmonary vasculature, are responsible, too, for the inconstant and atypical murmurs and atypical electrocardiography. For these reasons, many patients in this age group are subjected to special studies in an attempt to separate those anomalies that lend themselves to operative repair or palliation from those for which nothing can be done at this time.

In the newborn period, particularly in the first days of life, it is important to note that the radiographic appearance of the chest may be normal in the presence of even the most complex of cardiac abnormalities (Figs. 25, 26). As a general rule, a lesion or combination of lesions that will sustain intra-uterine life and permit a live birth is not associated with enlargement of the heart and does not result in recognizable alterations in its configuration in the first days of life.[18] This fact is a reflection of fetal circulation, character-

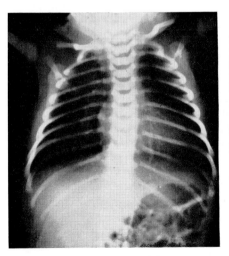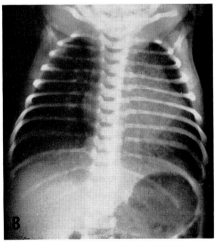

Figure 25. Transposition of the great vessels with intracardiac defects. The heart and great vessels are normal at 22 hours of age (A); there is obvious cardiac enlargement and pulmonary vascular engorgement at 5 days of age (B).

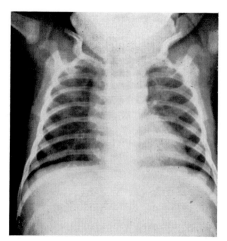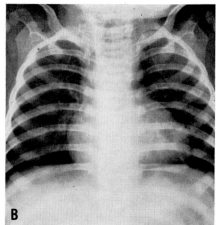

Figure 26. Tetralogy of Fallot. During the first 7 weeks of life, the chest presented no abnormalities (A, 7 weeks of age). By the age of 7 months (B), the heart had become abnormal in configuration and the pulmonary vasculature diminished.

ized by mixing of arterial and venous blood and the dependence of the fetus upon the umbilical circulation rather than the pulmonary circulation. There are exceptions to this rule, and these include abnormalities that interfere with emptying of the ventricles, such as aortic stenosis, severe coarctation of the aorta, and severe pulmonary stenosis, as well as arteriovenous fistulae and myocardial disease. In this context, it is significant that within hours or days of birth, in the presence of severe congenital cardiac defects, the heart enlarges and changes in configuration, as does the intrapulmonary vasculature, depending upon the severity of the defect and/or the complexity of the lesion. The classification given before is, then, equally applicable to this age group. However, the evaluation is apt to result in a differential diagnosis rather than in a more specific one because of the factors noted above.

CONCLUSIONS

Radiological examination of the chest occupies an important position in the diagnosis of congenital heart disease. Its value is increased as the information obtained from the study is correlated with other clinical and laboratory data. The aforementioned classification, which embodies an appreciation of both altered anatomy and pathophysiology, has been found helpful in the roentgen diagnosis of congenital heart disease.

References

1. LESTER, R. G.: *Radiological concepts in the evaluation of heart disease.* Mod. Conc. Cardiov. Dis. 37:113, 1968.
2. LESTER, R. G.: *Radiological concepts in the evaluation of heart disease.* Mod. Conc. Cardiov. Dis. 38:7, 1969.

3. STAUFFER, H. M., AND RIGLER, L. G.: *Dilatation and pulsation of the left subclavian artery in the roentgen ray diagnosis of coarctation of the aorta: Roentgenkymographic studies in 13 cases.* Circulation 1:294, 1950.

4. GAY, B. B., JR., AND FRANCH, R. H.: *Pulsations in the pulmonary arteries as observed with roentgenoscopic image amplification. Observations in patients with isolated pulmonary valvular stenosis.* Amer. J. Roentgen. 83:355, 1960.

5. KLATTE, E. C., AND BURKO, H.: *The differential diagnosis of cyanotic congenital heart disease.* Seminars Roentgen. 3:358, 1968.

6. KAPLAN, S.: *Clinical and hemodynamic bases of the roentgenographic findings in left to right shunts.* Seminars Roentgen. 1:34, 1966.

7. LESTER, R. G., MAUCK, H. P., AND GRUBB, W. L.: *Anomalous pulmonary venous return to the right side of the heart.* Seminars Roentgen. 1:102, 1966.

8. EDWARDS, J. E., CAREY, L. S., NEUFELD, H. N., AND LESTER, R. G.: *Congenital heart disease, correlation of pathologic anatomy and angiocardiography.* W. B. Saunders Co., Philadelphia, 1965.

9. BENTON, C.: *Truncus arteriosus.* Seminars Roentgen. 3:420, 1968.

10. SPITZ, H. B.: *Eisenmenger's syndrome. Seminars Roentgen.* 1:373, 1968.

11. ELLIOTT, L. P., AND SCHIEBLER, G. I.: *X-Ray Diagnosis of Congenital Cardiac Disease.* Charles C Thomas, Springfield, Ill., 1968.

12. LUCAS, R. V., JR., ANDERSON, R. C., AMPLATZ, K., ADAMS, P., JR., AND EDWARDS, J. E.: *Congenital causes of pulmonary venous obstruction.* Pediat. Clin. N. Amer. 10:781, 1963.

13. ROBINSON, A. E., CAPP, P. M., CHEN, J. T. T., AND LESTER, R. G.: *Left-sided obstructive diseases of the heart and great vessels.* Seminars Roentgen. 3:410, 1968.

14. KLATTE, E. C., CAMPBELL, J. A., AND LURIE, P. R.: *Aortic configuration in congenital heart disease.* Radiology 74:555, 1960.

15. STEWART, J. R., KINCAID, O. W., AND TITUS, J. L.: *Right aortic arch: Plain film diagnosis and significance.* Amer. J. Roentgen. 97:377, 1966.

16. ROWE, R. D., AND MEHRIZI, A.: *The Neonate with Congenital Heart Disease. Major Problems in Clinical Pediatrics.* W. B. Saunders Co., Philadelphia, 1968, Vol. 5.

17. KEITH, J. D., ROWE, R. D., AND VLAD, P.: *Heart Disease in Infancy and Childhood,* ed. 2. Macmillan Co., New York, 1967.

18. WITTENBORG, M. H., AND NEUHAUSER, E. B. D.: *Diagnostic roentgenology in congenital heart disease.* Circulation 11:462, 1955.

Natural History of
Ventricular Septal Defect[*]

Arthur J. Moss, M.D., and
Bijan Siassi, M.D.

* Supported in part by USPHS Grants HE05888 and HE5870.

Since the advent of open heart surgery, operative closure of ventricular septal defect has become a relatively common event in most cardiac centers. This lesion, once believed to be relatively benign, was subsequently recognized as a potentially serious abnormality, and its mere presence in the preschool child was, a decade or so ago, generally considered indication for operative intervention. However, accumulating evidence has since established that, although this lesion may indeed result in premature death, it usually pursues a benign course and, in some instances, it may even close spontaneously. In the early years of life, the eventual outcome is often impossible to predict, and so the selection of candidates for operation has currently become a critical and somewhat controversial issue.

Although this lesion was first described some 90 years ago,[1] a definitive answer to the important question of whether or not the asymptomatic child with a *small* defect should be subjected to operation may not be forthcoming for some time. Until more data become available, periodic review of published information pertinent to the natural history of this relatively common lesion seems warranted. This article is, in essence, such a review. It is limited to *isolated* ventricular septal defect, except in those instances where an associated abnormality develops as a complication, i.e., ventricular septal defect with secondary infundibular pulmonic stenosis, with obstructive pulmonary vascular disease, with aortic insufficiency, and with cardiomyopathy. Ventricular septal defect as part of a more complex abnormality, e.g., tetralogy of Fallot, tricuspid atresia, endocardial cushion defect, etc. is not included. Likewise, single or common ventricle is not discussed, since it is quite different anatomically from a large ventricular septal defect.[2]

INCIDENCE

Reported incidence figures for ventricular septal defect at birth range from 1.28 to 3.3 per 1,000 live births (Table 1). The lesion accounts for 27 to 40 per cent of all congenital cardiac defects encountered in live born

Table 1. Incidence of ventricular septal defect at birth

Authors	Location	Total live births	Ventricular septal defect (per 1,000)	Congenital heart lesion (per 1,000)	Ventricular septal defect (% of congenital heart lesions per 1,000)
Carlgren [3]	Gothenberg	58,105	1.70	6.4	27
Richards et al.[4]	New York City	5,628	2.66	7.6	35
Kerrebijn [5]	Leiden	1,817	3.3	8.0	40
Mitchell et al.[6]	USA (Various parts)	50,000	1.28	—	—
Hoffman [7]	New York City	22,957	1.35	—	—

infants. It is the most common congenital cardiac malformation, except at very high altitudes, where the incidence of patent ductus arteriosus apparently exceeds that of ventricular septal defect (Mexico City and the Peruvian Andes).[8]

It is noteworthy that the incidence of ventricular septal defect in school-age children is considerably lower than in the newborn, with a reported occurrence rate of 0.44 to 1.60 per 1.000.[9–13] Very few data are available for adults. Hoffman,[7] quoting from a personal communication with Kannel, indicates that the prevalence rate in an adult population of about 5,000 was only 0.4 per 1.000. Wade and Wright,[14] in a study of pregnant women, found ventricular septal defect to be half as common as isolated pulmonic stenosis and one-sixth as common as atrial septal defect. The declining prevalence rate of ventricular septal defect with age could be a reflection of death during infancy and childhood and of spontaneous closure. The lesion appears to be about equally distributed between the two sexes.[15–17]

ANATOMICAL CLASSIFICATION

Anatomically, defects of the ventricular septum are classified according to their relationship to the crista supraventricularis and the tricuspid valve as follows (Fig. 1).[18]

Type 1. Superior and anterior to the crista supraventricularis
Type 2. Posterior and inferior to the crista supraventricularis

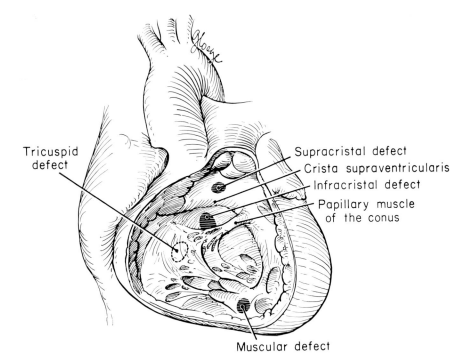

Figure 1. Diagram of the ventricular septum viewed from the right side.

141

Type 3. Under the septal leaflet of the tricuspid valve
Type 4. Single and located in the muscular portion of the septum
Type 5. Multiple and located in the muscular portion of the septum

The size of the shunt, rather than the location of the defect, is the main determinant of the behavior of the cardiovascular system.[19] Thus, muscular defects, generally considered to be relatively benign, may be associated with severe heart disease when multiple.[20,21]

COURSE AND COMPLICATIONS

The clinical course of ventricular septal defect ranges from a benign one with spontaneous closure to a stormy one terminating in death from early heart failure. Some patients eventually develop obstructive pulmonary vascular disease, secondary infundibular pulmonic stenosis, aortic insufficiency due to prolapse of an aortic cusp, cardiomyopathy (?), and bacterial endocarditis. Any of these may be sufficiently severe to lead to premature death during childhood or adulthood.

Heart Failure

The development of congestive heart failure depends on the size of the defect and the resistance of the pulmonary vascular bed. In the fetus, the pulmonary vascular resistance is high because of the unaerated state of the lungs and the thick media of the muscular pulmonary arteries. The thickened media decreases sharply during the first 2 weeks of postnatal life, and a further but more gradual decrease occurs up to 1 or 1½ years of age, when a level similar to that of adults is reached.[22]

In infants with ventricular septal defect, there also is an initial decrease in medial thickness, but from 2 months on, there is an increase; and in some children as young as 3 or 4 months of age, the media may be extremely hypertrophic.[23, 24] The thick muscular pulmonary arteries of the newly born infant are capable of significant vasoconstriction and thus can maintain a higher than normal resistance to pulmonary flow. This mechanism prevents a lethal shunt when lung expansion takes place in the newborn who has a large ventricular septal defect.[25] With involution of the muscular arteries during ensuing weeks or months, however, congestive heart failure may occur. Large defects are associated with systemic pressures in the pulmonary circuit, and if one applies Ohm's law (pressure=flow×resistance), it then becomes clear that these defects must be associated either with high flow or with high pulmonary vascular resistance, or more likely with both.[26]

It is in the early postnatal months that the fall in pulmonary vascular resistance is most critical. It is particularly in this period that patients are apt to die from left ventricular failure due to a large shunt. Congestive heart failure appears almost invariably during the first 6 months of life, mostly within the first 3 months. It practically never occurs during the first week and is rare during the first month. However, premature infants may develop heart failure earlier than do full term infants, presumably because

142

of the lesser development of the media in the pulmonary arteries of prematurely born infants.[15]

A striking decrease in the incidence of heart failure occurs after the age of a year or so, despite the presence of high pulmonary flows and increased pulmonary pressures. In adults, the incidence again increases because of continued pulmonary hypertension or a large left-to-right shunt.[27] According to Vogel et al.,[28] the incidence of congestive heart failure in infants with ventricular septal defect is not as common at the high altitude of Denver as at sea level. These authors attribute this difference to increased pulmonary vascular resistance resulting from hypoxia at the higher altitude. They suggest that the chronic exposure to the lower oxygen tension in Denver results in chronic vasoconstriction, and they refer to the phenomenon as "hypoxic banding."

Overt cardiac decompensation is manifest by tachypnea, tachycardia, hepatomegaly, growth failure, increased sweating, and sometimes by gallop rhythm. Peripheral edema is rare in infants.[29] Associated pulmonary infection is common, and there may be recurrent bouts of pneumonia. Rudolph[30] has pointed out that left ventricular failure may present merely as wheezing and be confused with bronchiolitis, bronchopneumonia, or bronchial asthma.

The exact incidence and mortality of heart failure is not known. However, it seems clear that the mortality of medically treated cases has declined through the years. This decrease, no doubt, is a reflection of earlier diagnosis and more effective decongestive measures. Likewise, the mortality of surgically treated cases appears to be declining. In most centers, banding of the pulmonary artery is currently the operative procedure of choice for infants under 2 years of age. Elective closure of the defect and removal of the band is then carried out at a later age. Direct closure in the infant age group still carries a relatively high risk in most centers, although one group reports a mortality of only 10 per cent in the 6- to 24-month age group.[31]

Pulmonary Vascular Disease

One of the feared complications of ventricular septal defect is the development of obstructive pulmonary vascular disease. It occurs only with the larger defects, not having been reported with defects smaller than 1 cm./m.[2, 26, 32, 33] Clinically, it is manifested by a change from the characteristic holosystolic to a systolic ejection murmur. With increasing obstruction, the intensity lessens and the murmur may even disappear entirely. Coincidentally, the second pulmonic sound becomes accentuated. The electrocardiogram shows evidence of increasing right ventricular hypertrophy, and the cardiac shadow on roentgenogram becomes smaller with a noticeable reduction in the peripheral pulmonary vascular markings. In its most advanced form, progressive cyanosis occurs, heralding Eisenmenger's disease.[34-36] The patient with obstructive pulmonary vascular disease usually survives to early or middle adult life. Common causes of death are heart failure and bacterial endocarditis. Thus, as a result of progressive changes in

143

the medial and intimal layers of the pulmonary arterioles, the noncyanotic infant with a large ventricular septal defect, and perhaps with early heart failure, may become severely cyanotic, polycythemic, and dyspneic as an adult. Other infants, however, maintain a high pulmonary vascular resistance from birth on and characteristically show early and persistent cyanosis. These latter patients presumably fail to achieve normal maturation of the pulmonary vascular bed.[37]

The incidence of pulmonary vascular disease and its course once it occurs remain controversial issues, probably largely because of lack of uniformity in case selection and in methods of assessment.[38-43] The problem obviously has an important bearing on the selection and optimal age for operation. The mortality rate associated with operative repair has a direct relationship to the degree of pulmonary vascular disease as evidenced by pulmonary pressures, pulmonary vascular resistance, and magnitude and direction of shunt. Pulmonary vascular disease sufficiently obstructive to result in a net right-to-left shunt renders the patient inoperable.

Several points appear clearly established. Some infants develop rapidly progressive pulmonary vascular disease. Because of this possibility, it has been recommended by Hoffman and Rudolph [43] that infants under 9 months of age found to have a ventricular septal defect with pulmonary hypertension and moderately elevated pulmonary resistance should be recatheterized about 6 months later. If the pulmonary vascular resistance has not fallen, then, in their view, surgical intervention is indicated. However, the vast majority of children wtih ventricular septal defect do not develop pulmonary vascular disease—at least not up to the age of puberty.[44] Currently available evidence is strong that in the case of the small ventricular septal defect, there is no threat of pulmonary vascular disease, and operative intervention on this basis does not appear justified.

Infundibular Pulmonary Stenosis

In 1957, Gasul et al.[45] published a preliminary report in which they proposed a new concept for the course of some patients with ventricular septal defect, namely that infundibular pulmonic stenosis may develop secondarily and convert the condition into a noncyanotic or cyanotic type of tetralogy of Fallot. This proposal was documented by catheterization studies in three of their patients, one of whom developed the typical findings of tetralogy of Fallot with marked cyanosis and a predominant right-to-left shunt. They suggested the possibility that an infant with isolated large ventricular septal defect may some time later develop hypertrophy of the crista supraventricularis and perhaps of its septal or parietal band, leading to infundibular stenosis. Since this original report, the development of infundibular pulmonic stenosis in patients with isolated ventricular septal defect has been confirmed by a number of investigators.[27, 29, 39, 46, 47]

Its incidence has not been established. Nadas and Fyler [26] estimate that it occurs in about 5 per cent of patients with large ventricular septal defects.

Others [27] indicate that infundibular stenosis may be acquired in 5 to 10 per cent of patients with florid defects.

In their original description, Gasul et al.[45] speculated that the development of infundibular pulmonic stenosis in these patients may be a natural protective mechanism that limits the large pulmonary flow. This certainly seems to be one factor responsible for the general improvement in well-being usually observed after a year or so of age.

Vogel and Blount [48] found that in patients with ventricular septal defect and pulmonary hypertension, the presence of infundibular pulmonic obstruction may be inapparent. They suggest that "masked" infundibular obstruction in these patients may be fairly common. Moreover, they raise the possibility that the obstruction may be present at birth and continue to develop. With maturation of the pulmonary vascular bed and a reduction in pulmonary vascular resistance, it becomes "unmasked."

Aortic Insufficiency

Aortic insufficiency accompanying a large ventricular septal defect is well recognized.[26, 27, 49–53] It is acquired some time after the first year of life, usually toward the end of the first decade. Most commonly, it appears between the ages of 3 and 8 years. In one study of 756 cases of ventricular septal defect, the incidence was slightly less than 5 per cent. However, the true incidence is probably less than 1 per cent. It usually occurs in association with large defects, but it has been reported in at least one patient with a low pressure defect and a small shunt.[50]

The lesion is caused by prolapse of the left coronary cusp and occasionally the noncoronary cusp of the aortic valve into the left ventricle. Rarely, the cusp may prolapse through the defect into the right ventricle or pulmonary artery. In the latter case, the left-to-right shunt may diminish or disappear because of partial or complete plugging of the defect by the pendulous cusp. The defect is generally situated unusually high, just below the pulmonary valve.

The first clinical sign of complicating aortic insufficiency is the characteristic protodiastolic, decrescendo, high-pitched murmur that becomes progressively louder. It is much more serious than the complicating infundibular pulmonic stenosis discussed in the previous section. Indeed, the course may well be one of rapid deterioration. The early detection of complicating aortic insufficiency is probably indication for prompt surgical closure of the ventricular defect to prevent further deformity of the aortic valve cusp.

Van Praagh and McNamara [52] point out that if the ventricular septal defect is subpulmonary, the aortic insufficiency is a problem of herniation, and closure of the ventricular septal defect may be curative. If, however, the defect is subcristal in location, then the basis of the insufficiency may be a defective commissure of the aortic valve, and closure of the ventricular septal defect alone will not cure the aortic insufficiency. In the latter case, repair of the aortic valve is also necessary. In view of the differences in surgical

145

management, we emphasize that the preoperative diagnosis of the anatomic type of ventricular septal defect is of practical importance when associated with aortic insufficiency.

Cardiomyopathy

In 1961, Bloomfield [54] reported nine cases of minor defects of the ventricular septum in which there was evidence of myopathic changes in the left ventricle. Three of the patients were studied during life and six at necropsy. Three of these nine cases had small left-to-right shunts, and in the remaining six, the septal defect was imperforate. In a subsequent report,[33] Bloomfield indicates that four of the patients, all over 50 years of age, were examples of spontaneous closure. All died in cardiac failure, and the inference is made that the defective septum could have been the basis. If this is so, then even a small ventricular septal defect might be the cause of heart failure later in life, even if the defect closes spontaneously. Bloomfield speculates that the ventricular septal defect mechanically interferes with systolic contraction, thereby imposing a strain on the lateral wall of the left ventricle. He further proposes that a defective ventricular septum, whether patent or not, may contribute to the compromise of cardiac function exerted later in life by hypertension or coronary artery disease.

Since these original reports, Goldbarg and Liebman [55] described a 16-year-old boy with a moderate-sized ventricular septal defect who developed evidence of left ventricular cardiomyopathy.

The concept advanced by Bloomfield [33] is an attractive one, but as yet there is no firm evidence to support it. Further observation of patients with ventricular septal defect into and through adult life will be necessary to establish whether or not a relationship exists between ventricular septal defect and left ventricular cardiomyopathy.

Bacterial Endocarditis

The incidence of bacterial endocarditis complicating ventricular septal defect is unknown. The figures recorded in the literature show wide variation, with a range of from 1 to 30 per cent.[27, 33, 47, 50, 51, 56, 57] There is general agreement, however, that this serious complication is a major risk confronting patients with this malformation. It appears to be rare in very young infants and beyond the age of 30 years.[26] In one study of 227,999 children hospitalized over a 10-year period, the disease was encountered only once in every 4,500 admissions.[58]

The most recent estimate of the incidence of bacterial endocarditis during the lifetime of a 5-year-old child with an uncomplicated ventricular septal defect is 13.6 per cent.[57] Since the mortality is about 20 per cent, the *mortal* risk is calculated to be 2.7 per cent. It has not yet been determined whether these figures can be applied to this modern era of antibiotic prophylaxis.

Anatomically, the vegetations of bacterial endocarditis complicating ventricular septal defect are found on the opposing wall of the right ventricle,

146

on the right ventricular rim of the defect, or on the septal leaflet of the tricuspid valve.

Fear of bacterial endocarditis has been advanced by some as an argument in favor of routine operative closure of small ventricular septal defects. In this regard, it should be pointed out that there is no assurance that operative closure eliminates or even reduces the chances of subsequent bacterial endocarditis. In fact, available evidence indicates that when bacterial endocarditis does complicate repair of cardiac lesions, the mortality rate is much higher, ranging from 40 to 100 per cent.[59] It is noteworthy that in the study reported by Zakrzewski and Keith,[58] 12 of the 50 children with bacterial endocarditis were infected following cardiac surgery.

Spontaneous Closure

Spontaneous closure of a ventricular septal defect was first suggested more than half a century ago.[60] However, it was not until 1958 that the first documented case of near closure was reported.[61] Since that time, more than 80 examples of functional or complete closure, documented by catheterization or necropsy studies, have been reported in the literature.[14, 15, 26, 27, 33, 46, 47, 62–71] These include membranous as well as muscular defects, and, in a number of instances, the defect had been large enough to cause congestive heart failure during infancy. Since it is now clearly established that ventricular septal defects may close spontaneously, it is likely that many observations of this phenomenon are no longer being recorded.

This finding was confirmed in a recent survey of 197 board-certified Pediatric Cardiologists.[72] Among this group, the opinion was expressed, largely on the basis of clinical impressions, that more than 3,000 defects had been observed to close spontaneously. The great majority occurred during the first 2 years of life, although a significant number were observed in the 2- to 5-year age group. A declining number of cases were encountered with increasing age, although three instances of closure were believed to have occurred during adulthood.

It is currently estimated that at least 20 per cent[73] and possibly as high as 50 per cent or more of all ventricular septal defects will eventually close spontaneously. This event appears most likely to occur during the first 5 years of life, but may occur even during adulthood. Spontaneous closure of ventricular septal defects during childhood probably explains the marked disparity of incidence of this lesion in children as opposed to adults, since it cannot be explained by autopsy figures. It is possible that careful necropsy examination of the heart may reveal increasing evidence of spontaneous closure (fig. 2).

The mechanism of closure may involve binding of the septal leaflet of the tricuspid valve over the defect, plugging of the defect by vegetations of bacterial endocarditis and, in the case of muscular defects, fusion of the margins. Experimentally, it has been shown that surgically created defects

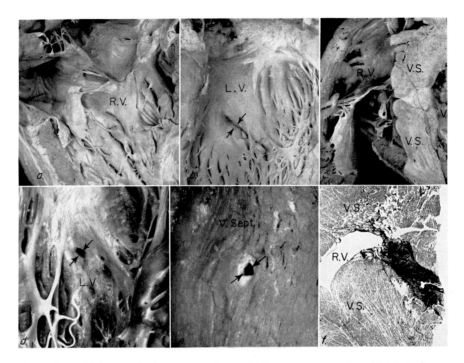

Figure 2. a, Right ventricular aspect of ventricular septum reveals a highly trabeculated ventricular septum. Although suggestive of the presence of a muscular ventricular septal defect, it is within the usual range for the degree of right ventricular trabeculation. b, Interior of left ventricle (L.V.) Between two obliquely oriented muscle bundles within the ventricular septum is a cleft (between arrows) representing the left ventricular aspect of an interventricular communication, now closed. c, Cross section through the ventricular septum (V.S.). From the cavity of the left ventricle (L.V.), an opening (arrow) leads into a fibrous mass that is within the ventricular septum. The fibrous tissue represents the factor closing a preexisting ventricular septal defect of the muscular part of the ventricular septum. R.V., right ventricle. d, e, f, The left ventricular opening of an interventricular communication (point of arrows) is circular in outline. e, A sagittal section has been made through the center of the ventricular septum, showing within it the continuation of the channel seen in e. f, A cross section of the right ventricular side (R.V.) of the ventricular septum (V.S.); the right ventricular side of the channel that began in the left ventricle is closed by the interposition of collagenous plug. (From Simmons et al.,[68] with permission of the American Heart Association.)

in dogs will heal spontaneously if the opening is less than 10 mm. in diameter.[74] The interesting possibility has been raised that aneurysms of the membranous septum may be a residuum of a spontaneously closed defect.[75]

In some instances, it is possible to predict closure of a ventricular septal defect on clinical grounds. The murmur becomes softer and higher pitched and loses its holosystolic quality. This has been termed by some the "puffy" murmur. The typical murmur of a closing defect is decrescendo and occupies early systole, often with extension into the midportion of systole (Fig. 3).

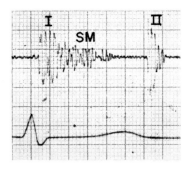

Figure 3. Phonocardiogram of a 13-year-old boy, showing the early decrescendo murmur of a small ventricular septal defect. Tracing was registered at the fourth interspace. I = first heart sound; II = second heart sound; S.M. = systolic murmur.

SURGICAL CONSIDERATIONS

There is general agreement that congestive heart failure due to a large left-to-right shunt that is resistant to medical management is indication for operative intervention. This situation is invariably limited to the infant age group. The operation of choice is banding of the pulmonary artery, although some have advocated corrective surgery even in this young age group.[76] Evidence of progressive pulmonary vascular disease is also indication for operation before the optimal age of 4 or 5 years. The appearance of mild complicating aortic insufficiency may be a further indication for earlier repair of the ventricular septal defect.

Recognition that spontaneous closure may occur has prompted a re-evaluation of the commonly accepted criteria for operation in the asymptomatic uncomplicated case. In the recent survey of Pediatric Cardiologists previously referred to,[72] 95 per cent of those who responded believed that the *small* uncomplicated defect should *not* be closed. The great majority considered a shunt of 1.5:1 or less to represent a small defect. In the authors' opinion, defects of this size should not be closed, in the light of present knowledge. Available evidence suggests that with defects of this size, pulmonary vascular disease is not a threat. The risks of bacterial endocarditis and of aortic insufficiency or the effect on the life-span is not yet sufficiently documented to justify routine closure of *small* uncomplicated defects. However, because of these unknowns, it is important that these patients remain under observation until more data become available.

In considering surgery, one must take into account the long term effects of the ventriculotomy scar, postoperative right bundle branch block, and postoperative heart block, to say nothing about the emotional trauma to the family and the cosmetic disfiguration.

It is disheartening that some 90 years after ventricular septal defect was originally described, we cannot accurately predict its course—which one will close, when it will close, and what will happen if it does not. Still another generation may pass before the answers are forthcoming.

SUMMARY

Ventricular septal defect is the most common congenital heart lesion. It occurs in 1.28 to 3.3 per 1,000 live births. It is encountered with decreasing frequency in older age groups and is relatively uncommon in adults.

The size of the defect, rather than its location, is the main determinant of the behavior of the cardiovascular system. Although the clinical course is usually benign, it may be complicated by heart failure, pulmonary vascular disease, infundibular pulmonic stenosis, aortic insufficiency, bacterial endocarditis, and possibly by cardiomyopathy.

Spontaneous closure of some defects has been clearly established. Closure probably occurs in 20 to 50 per cent of cases and appears to be most prevalent during the first 5 years of life. Spontaneous closure may be predicted in some instances by the characteristic change in auscultatory findings. This change consists essentially of transformation of the holosystolic murmur to a softer early decrescendo systolic murmur of a higher pitch.

Although there is general agreement that the large ventricular septal defect should be closed surgically, preferably at 4 or 5 years of age, management of the *small* uncomplicated defect is not quite so clear. Available evidence indicates that operative intervention is not justified if the left-to-right shunt is 1.5:1 or less.

References

1. ROGER, H.: *Recherches cliniques sur la communication congénitale des deux coeurs, par inocclusion du septum interventriculaire.* Bull. Acad. Nat. Med. Paris, 2nd ser. 8:1074, 1879.

2. VAN PRAAGH, R., ONGLEY, P. A., AND SWAN, H. J.: *Anatomic types of single or common ventricle in man. Morphologic and geometric aspects of 60 necropsied cases.* Amer. J. Cardiol. 13:367, 1964.

3. CARLGREN, L. E.: *The incidence of congenital heart disease in children born in Gothenburg 1941–1950.* Brit. Heart J. 21:40, 1959.

4. RICHARDS, M. R., MERRITT, K. K., SAMUELS, M. H., AND LANGMANN, A. G.: *Congenital malformations of the cardiovascular system in a series of 6,053 infants.* Pediatrics 15:12, 1955.

5. KERREBIJN, K. F.: *Incidence in infants and mortality from congenital malformations of the circulatory system.* Acta Paediat. Scand. 55:316, 1966.

6. MITCHELL, S. C., BERENDES, H. W., AND CLARK, W. M., JR.: *The normal closure of the ventricular septum.* Amer. Heart J. 73:334, 1967.

7. HOFFMAN, J. I.: *Natural history of congenital heart disease. Problems in its assessment with special reference to ventricular septal defects.* Circulation 37:97, 1968.

8. PEÑALOZA, D., ARIAS-STELLA, J., SIME, F., RECAVARREN, S., AND MARTI-CORENA, E.: *The heart and pulmonary circulation in children at high altitudes: physiological, anatomical, and clinical observations.* Pediatrics 34:568, 1964.

9. ROSE, V., AND KEITH, J. D.: *The prevalence of ventricular septal defect in elementary school children in the City of Toronto.* Canad. Med. Ass. J. 95:1132, 1966.

10. ROBINSON, S. J., AGGELER, D. M., AND DANILOFF, G. T.: *Heart disease in San Francisco school children; 1947 registry showing incidence, problems, and supervision techniques.* J. Pediat. 33:49, 1948.

11. MARESH, G. J., DODGE, H. J., AND LICHTY, J. A.: *Incidence of heart disease among Colorado school children; a state-wide study.* J.A.M.A. 149:802, 1952.

12. MORTON, W., BEAVER, M. E., AND ARNOLD, R. C.: *Heart disease screening in elementary school children.* J.A.M.A. 169:1163, 1959.

13. MORTON, W. E., AND HUHN, L. A.: *Epidemiology of congenital heart disease. Observations in 17,366 Denver school children.* J.A.M.A. 195: 1107, 1966.

14. WADE, G., AND WRIGHT, J. P.: *Spontaneous closure of ventricular septal defects.* Lancet 1:737, 1963.

15. HOFFMAN, J. I., AND RUDOLPH, A. M.: *The natural history of ventricular septal defects in infancy.* Amer. J. Cardiol. 16:634, 1965.

16. ASH, R.: *Natural history of ventricular septal defects in childhood lesions with predominant arteriovenous shunts.* J. Pediat. 64:45, 1964.

17. FYLER, D. C., RUDOLPH, A. M., WITTENBORG, M. H., AND NADAS, A. S.: *Ventricular septal defect in infants and children; a correlation of clinical, physiologic, and autopsy data.* Circulation 18:833, 1958.

18. KIRKLIN, J. W., HARSHBARGER, H. G., DONALD, D. E., AND EDWARDS, J. E.: *Surgical correction of ventricular septal defect: anatomic and technical considerations.* J. Thorac. Cardiov. Surg. 33:45, 1957.

19. BECU, L. M., FONTANA, R. S., DUSHANE, J. W., KIRKLIN, J. W., BURCHELL, H. B., AND EDWARDS, J. E.: *Anatomic and pathologic studies in ventricular septal defect.* Circulation 14:349, 1956.

20. SAAB, N. G., BURCHELL, H. B., DUSHANE, J. W., AND TITUS, J. L.: *Muscular ventricular septal defects.* Amer. J. Cardiol. 18:713, 1966.

21. FRIEDMAN, W. F., MEHRIZI, A., AND PUSCH, A. L.: *Multiple muscular ventricular septal defects.* Circulation 32:35, 1965.

22. WAGENVOORT, C. A., NEUFELD, H. N., AND EDWARDS, J. E.: *The structure of the pulmonary arterial tree in fetal and early postnatal life.* Lab. Invest. 10:751, 1961.

23. WAGENVOORT, C. A., NEUFELD, H. N., DUSHANE, J. W., AND EDWARDS, J. E.: *The pulmonary arterial tree in ventricular septal defect. A quantitative study of anatomic features in fetuses, infants, and children.* Circulation 23:740, 1961.

24. NAEYE, R. L.: *The pulmonary arterial bed in ventricular septal defect. Anatomic features in childhood.* Circulation 34:962, 1966.

25. EDWARDS, J. E.: *Functional pathology of the pulmonary vascular tree in congenital cardiac disease.* Circulation 15:164, 1957.

26. NADAS, A. S., AND FYLER, D. C.: *Ventricular septal defect. A review of current thoughts.* Arch. Dis. Child. 43:268, 1968.

27. KAPLAN, S., DAOUD, G. I., BENZING, G., III, DEVINE, F. J., GLASS, I. H., AND MCQUIRE, J.: *Natural history of ventricular septal defect.* Amer. J. Dis. Child. 105:581, 1963.

28. VOGEL, J. H., MCNAMARA, D. G., AND BLOUNT, S. G., JR.: *Role of hypoxia in determining pulmonary vascular resistance in infants with ventricular septal defects.* Amer. J. Cardiol. 20:346, 1967.

29. MORGAN, B. C., GRIFFITHS, S. P., AND BLUMENTHAL, S.: *Ventricular septal defect. I. Congestive heart failure in infancy.* Pediatrics 25:54, 1960.

30. RUDOLPH, A. M.: *Diagnosis and treatment: respiratory distress and cardiac disease in infancy.* Pediatrics 35:999, 1965.

31. CARTMILL, T. B., DUSHANE, J. W., MCGOON, D. C., AND KIRKLIN, J. W.:

Results of repair of ventricular septal defect. J. Thorac. Cardiov. Surg. 52:486, 1966.

32. WOOD, P.: *The Eisenmenger syndrome or pulmonary hypertension with reversed central shunt.* Brit. Med. J. 2:755, 1958.

33. BLOOMFIELD, D. K.: *The natural history of ventricular septal defect in patients surviving infancy.* Circulation 29:914, 1964.

34. SELZER, A., AND LAQUEUR, G. L.: *The Eisenmenger complex and its relation to the uncomplicated defect of the ventricular septum: Review of thirty-five autopsied cases of Eisenmenger's complex, including two new cases.* A.M.A. Arch. Intern. Med. 87:218, 1951.

35. IVERSON, R. E., LINDE, L. M., AND KEGEL, S.: *The diagnosis of progressive pulmonary vascular disease in children with ventricular septal defects.* J. Pediat. 68:594, 1966.

36. WEIDMAN, W. H., DUSHANE, J. W., AND KINCAID, O. W.: *Observations concerning progressive pulmonary vascular obstruction in children with ventricular septal defects.* Amer. Heart J. 65:148, 1963.

37. LUCAS, R. V., JR., ADAMS, P., JR., ANDERSON, R. C., MEYNE, N. G., LILLEHEI, C. W., AND VARCO, R. L.: *The natural history of isolated ventricular septal defect. A serial physiologic study.* Circulation 24:1372, 1961.

38. HOWITT, G., AND WADE, E. G.: *Repeat catheterization in ventricular septal defect and pulmonary hypertension.* Brit. Heart. J. 24:649, 1962.

39. STANTON, R. E., AND FYLER, D. C.: *The natural history of pulmonary hypertension in children with ventricular septal defects assessed by serial right-heart catheterization.* Pediatrics 27:621, 1961.

40. ARCILLA, R. A., AGUSTSSON, M. H., BICOFF, J. P., LYNFIELD, J., WEINBERG, M., JR., FELL, E. H., AND GASUL, B. M.: *Further observations on the natural history of isolated ventricular septal defects in infancy and childhood. Serial cardiac catheterization studies in 75 patients.* Circulation 28:560, 1963.

41. AULD, P. A., JOHNSON, A. L., GIBBONS, J. E., AND McGREGOR, M.: *Changes in pulmonary vascular resistance in infants and children with left-to-right intracardiac shunts.* Circulation 27:257, 1963.

42. ANDERSON, R. A., LEVY, A. M., NAEYE, R. L., AND TABAKIN, B. S.: *Rapidly progressing pulmonary vascular obstructive disease. Association with ventricular septal defects during early childhood.* Amer. J. Cardiol. 19:854, 1967.

43. HOFFMAN, J. I., AND RUDOLPH, A. M.: *Increasing pulmonary vascular resistance during infancy in association with ventricular septal defect.* Pediatrics 38:220, 1966.

44. NADAS, A. S., RUDOLPH, A. M., AND GROSS, R. E.: *Pulmonary arterial hypertension in congenital heart disease.* Circulation 22:1041, 1960.

45. GASUL, B. M., DILLON, R. F., VRLA, V., AND HAIT, G.: *Ventricular septal defects: Their natural transformation into those with infundibular stenosis or into the cyanotic or noncyanotic type of tetralogy of Fallot.* J.A.M.A. 164:847, 1957.

46. LYNFIELD, J., GASUL, B. M., ARCILLA, R., AND LUAN, L. L.: *The natural history of ventricular septal defects in infancy and childhood, based on serial cardiac catheterization studies.* Amer. J. Med. 30:357, 1961.

47. WALKER, W. J., GARCIA-GONZALES, E., HALL, R. J., CZARNECKI, S. W., FRANKLIN, R. B., DAS, S. K., AND CHEITLIN, M. D.: *Interventricular septal*

defect: Analysis of 415 catheterized cases, ninety with serial hemodynamic studies. Circulation 31:54, 1965.

48. VOGEL, J. H., AND BLOUNT, S. G., JR.: *Masked infundibular pulmonary obstruction in ventricular septal defect with pulmonary hypertension.* Circulation 31:876, 1965.

49. EDWARDS, J. E.: *Ventricular septal defect. Unresolved problems.* Amer. J. Cardiol. 19:832, 1967.

50. MUDD, J. G., AYKENT, Y., FAGAN, L., SHIELDS, J. B., DAVIS, M., DONAHOE, J., AND HANLON, C. R.: *Untreated, low-pressure ventricular septal defect. Repeated cardiac catheterization.* Arch. Surg. (Chicago) 89:126, 1964.

51. RITTER, D. G., FELDT, R. H., WEIDMAN, W. H., AND DUSHANE, J. W.: *Ventricular septal defect.* Circulation 32: (Suppl.) 3:42, 1965.

52. VAN PRAAGH, R., AND MCNAMARA, J. J.: *Anatomic types of ventricular septal defect with aortic insufficiency. Diagnostic and surgical considerations.* Amer. Heart J. 75:604, 1968.

53. NADAS, A. S., THILENIUS, O. G., LAFARGE, C. G., AND HAUCK, A. J.: *Ventricular septal defect with aortic regurgitation: Medical and pathologic aspects.* Circulation 29:862, 1964.

54. BLOOMFIELD, D. K.: *Association of left ventricular myopathy with minor congenital defects of the ventricular septum.* (Abstract). Circulation 24:889, 1961.

55. GOLDBARG, A., AND LIEBMAN, J.: *Possible development of cardiomyopathy in a patient with ventricular septal defect.* J. Pediat. 73:411, 1968.

56. STORSTEIN, O., AND SÖRLAND, S.: *Ventricular septal defect. A clinical and hemodynamic study in 100 cases.* Acta Med. Scand. 180:543, 1966.

57. SHAH, P., SINGH, W. S., ROSE, V., AND KEITH, J. D.: *Incidence of bacterial endocarditis in ventricular septal defects.* Circulation 34:127, 1966.

58. ZAKRZEWSKI, T., AND KEITH, J. D.: *Bacterial endocarditis in infants and children.* J. Pediat. 67:1179, 1965.

59. STANTON, R. E., LINDESMITH, G. G., AND MEYER, B. W.: *Escherichia coli endocarditis after repair of ventricular septal defects.* New Eng. J. Med. 279:737, 1968.

60. WEBER, F. P.: *Can the clinical manifestations of congenital heart disease disappear with the general growth and development of the patient?* Brit. J. Dis. Child. 15:113, 1918.

61. AZEVEDO, A. DE C., TOLEDO, A. N., CARVALHO, A. A. DE, ZANIOLO, W., DOHMANN, H., AND ROUBACH, R.: *Ventricular septal defect; an example of its relative diminution.* Acta Card., Brux. 13:513, 1958.

62. CUMMING, G. R.: *Confirmation of closure of ventricular septal defects: value of vasopressor agents.* Amer. J. Cardiol. 15:259, 1965.

63. KAVANAGH-GRAY, D.: *Spontaneous closure of a ventricular septal defect.* Canad. Med. Ass. J. 87:868, 1962.

64. MAJKA, M., RYAN, J., AND BONDY, D. C.: *Spontaneous repair of a ventricular septal defect.* Canad. Med. Ass. J. 82:317, 1960.

65. EDGETT, J. W., JR., NELSON, W. P., HALL, R. J., ET AL.: *Spontaneous closure of a ventricular septal defect after banding of the pulmonary artery.* Amer. J. Cardiol. 22:729, 1968.

66. NADAS, A. S., SCOTT, L. P., HAUCK, A. J., AND RUDOLPH, A. M.: *Spontaneous functional closing of ventricular septal defects.* New Eng. J. Med. 264:309, 1961.

67. GLANCY, D. L., AND ROBERTS, W. C.: *Complete spontaneous closure of ventricular septal defect: necropsy study of five subjects.* Amer. J. Med. 43:846, 1967.

68. SIMMONS, R. L., MOLLER, J. H., AND EDWARDS, J. E.: *Anatomic evidence for spontaneous closure of ventricular septal defect.* Circulation 34:38, 1966.

69. MOORE, D., VLAD, P., AND LAMBERT, E. C.: *Spontaneous closure of ventricular septal defect following cardiac failure in infancy.* J. Pediat. 66:712, 1965.

70. AGUSTSSON, M. H., ARCILLA, R. A., BICOFF, J. P., MONCADA, R., AND GASUL, B. M.: *Spontaneous functional closure of ventricular septal defects in fourteen children demonstrated by serial cardiac catheterizations and angiocardiography.* Pediatrics 31:958, 1963.

71. EVANS, J. R., ROWE, R. D., AND KEITH, J. D.: *Spontaneous closure of ventricular septal defects.* Circulation 22:1044, 1960.

72. MOSS, A. J.: *Conquest of the ventricular septal defect—A period of uncertainty.* Amer. J. Cardiol. (In press).

73. NADAS, A. S.: *Management of infants with ventricular septal defect, a controversy.* Pediatrics 39:1, 1967.

74. GRIFFIN, G. D. J., AND ESSEX, H. E.: *Experimental production of intraventricular septal defects; certain physiologic and pathologic effects.* Surg. Gynec. Obstet. 92:325, 1951.

75. JAIN, A. C., AND ROSENTHAL, R.: *Aneurysm of the membranous ventricular septum.* Brit. Heart J. 29:60, 1967.

76. SIGMANN, J. M., STERN, A. M., AND SLOAN, H. E.: *Early surgical correction of large ventricular septal defects.* Pediatrics 39:4, 1967.

Pulmonary Valvular Stenosis[*]

Russell V. Lucas, Jr., M.D., and James H. Moller, M.D.

[*] Portions of this work were supported by Cardiovascular Project Program Grant HE06314 and the Graduate School, University of Minnesota.

Pulmonary valvular stenosis is the most common form of isolated right ventricular outflow tract obstruction. In this report, pulmonary valvular stenosis will be emphasized and contrasted to less frequently occurring obstructive lesions. Among the latter are dysplasia of the pulmonary valve, stenosis of the ostium infundibuli (infundibular stenosis), anomalous muscle bundles in the right ventricle, and peripheral pulmonary artery stenosis. These uncommon defects will be discussed briefly in the section concerned with differential diagnosis.

Early anatomic description of pulmonary valvular stenosis are found in the works of Morgagne [1] and Corvasiart.[2] In the 1830's, James Hope first presented the clinical findings of pulmonary stenosis and the means to distinguish it from aortic stenosis.[3] Fallot later described seven cases of pulmonary stenosis with intact ventricular septum who were cyanotic because of a right-to-left shunt through a patent foramen ovale. He termed this syndrome "trilogy." [4]

Although it was considered an uncommon form of congenital heart disease until the late 1940's, we now recognize that isolated pulmonary valvular stenosis accounts for perhaps 10 per cent of all congenital cardiac disease, ranking among the six most prevalent cardiac malformations. There is no sex predilection. It presents throughout man's life span, from newborn infants to the eighth decade.

The etiology of pulmonary stenosis in most patients is unknown. Maternal rubella accounts for a small percentage of cases. There is a distinct form that appears to be familial. A few cases are found in patients with the male Turner's syndrome.[5]

Developmentally, the pulmonary value is formed from three bulbous swellings composed of loose embryonic tissue in the distal portion of the bulbus cordis. Through tissue differentiation and growth, the swellings become "scooped out" to form thin valve leaflets and their respective sinuses of Valsalva. If this process is incomplete, the form of stenosis related to valvular dysplasia results. It is difficult to understand the embryological maldevelopment that results in fusion of the commissures of the pulmonary valve.

Abbott,[6] in 1926, suggested that pulmonary valvular stenosis might be secondary to intra-uterine endocarditis. Burch [7] has demonstrated pulmonary valvular (and other valve) changes in animals subjected to Coxsackie B viremia during intra-uterine life. At present, however, the etiology and pathogenesis of pulmonary valvular stenosis are not precisely known.

ANATOMICAL FEATURES

Pulmonary Valve

Viewed from above, the stenotic pulmonary valve has a domed or wind sock appearance with a central orifice that varies in size from patient to patient (Fig. 1, *left*). Three raphae are present at the site of expected commissural development. They extend along the pulmonary arterial surface

156

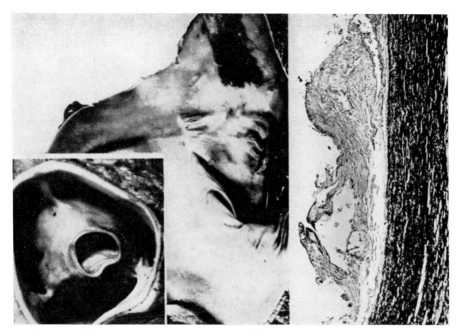

Figure 1. Anatomic features in pulmonary valvular stenosis. *Left:* Domed pulmonary valve viewed from above. The commissures are fused. Three raphae can be seen extending from the base of the pulmonary valve to the pulmonary arterial wall at the base of the sinus of Valsalva. The free edge of the pulmonary valve is thickened. *Center:* The opened pulmonary trunk just distal to the pulmonary valve orifice. A corrugated patch (upper) represents a "jet lesion." *Right:* Photomicrograph of the jet lesion (ELVG, × 30). (From Edwards, J. E., and Burchell H. B., Endocardial and intimal jet lesions (jet impact) as possible sites of origin of murmurs.[8])

of the domed valve to insert in the pulmonary arterial wall in the sinus of Valsalva. In rare cases, there is a fourth raphae. Isolated bicuspid pulmonary valves have been described that are not stenotic, but it is conceivable that with time, these valves might result in obstruction of pulmonary outflow. The edge of the domed valve often is thickened and occasionally exhibits evidence for preceding endocarditis in the form of multiple small nodules.

Pulmonary Artery

The pulmonary trunk originates normally from the right ventricle and is in normal relationship to the aorta, which in turn has a normal origin from the left ventricle. This latter relationship forms the basis for the synonym "pulmonary stenosis with normal aortic root."

Some degree of post-stenotic dilatation of the pulmonary trunk and left pulmonary artery occurs in most patients with pulmonary valvular stenosis. The involvement of the left pulmonary artery, which is a direct extension of the pulmonary trunk, and the absence of post-stenotic dilatation of the right pulmonary artery, which exits from the pulmonary trunk at a right

157

angle, support the concept that the post-stenotic dilatation is due to turbulence of flow distal to the stenotic valve. The magnitude of post-stenotic dilatation is not, however, directly related to the severity of the pulmonary valvular stenosis. Occurrence of significant post-stenotic dilatation in patients with minimal pulmonary valvular stenosis suggests that a congenital defect in the wall of the pulmonary artery may play a contributory role.

Raised patches, rugiform in appearance and composed of nonvascular fibrous tissue, frequently are present on the wall of the main pulmonary artery or the proximal left pulmonary artery (Fig. 1, center and right). These are felt to be "jet lesions" representing an endothelial response to the stress of turbulent flow. Edwards suggested that these jet lesions may be a site for bacterial endocarditis.[8]

Right Ventricle

The ventricular septum is normally formed and intact. The right ventricular infundibulum may be hypertrophied and its lumen encroached upon. In patients with severe pulmonary valvular stenosis, infundibular hypertrophy may be significant and may form the basis for temporary, residual pulmonary outflow obstruction following pulmonary valvotomy. The hypertrophy of the right ventricular myocardium has been termed concentric hypertrophy.[9] In fact, however, the hypertrophy is asymmetrical, particularly in those patients who develop systemic pressure within the right ventricular cavity. Muscular hypertrophy and increased trabeculation occur predominantly at the right ventricular apex and along the lateral portion of the free wall. Asymmetrical right ventricular hypertrophy alters the shape of the right ventricular cavity from crescentric to conical, thus converting the right ventricle to a more efficient pressure pump (Fig. 2).

On microscopic examination, there appears to be a gross increase in myocardial fiber size. In addition, diffuse, patchy fibrosis has been noted in the subendocardial and subpericardial areas of the myocardium. When fibrosis of the right ventricular myocardium occurs, the papillary muscles seem to be most severely affected.[10, 11]

Tricuspid Valve

The tricuspid valve often is normal. Both the chordae tendineae and the valve leaflets, however, may be thickened, and evidence of significant tricuspid insufficiency may be present.

Atrial Septum

Usually the atrial septum is intact, but it may possess a valve-competent foramen ovale or may have a true atrial septal defect with the potential for bidirectional flow. Selzer and associates[12] reported 52 patients with pulmonary valvular stenosis and found a patent foramen ovale in 29 and an intact atrial septum in the remaining 23. Of 69 patients reported by Abrahams and Wood,[13] 15 had an interatrial shunt. In seven, the shunt was

Figure 2. Right ventricular form and function in pulmonary valvular stenosis. *Upper:* Right ventriculogram (during systole) in a child with mild pulmonary valvular stenosis (right ventricular systolic pressure 72 mm. Hg). The right ventricular cavity retains its normal crescentric or wedge shape. *Lower:* Right ventriculogram (during systole) in a child with severe pulmonary stenosis (right ventricular systolic pressure 250 mm. Hg). Asymmetric hypertrophy of the right ventricle has occurred. The right ventricular cavity assumes a conical shape, geometrically a more efficient pressure pump.

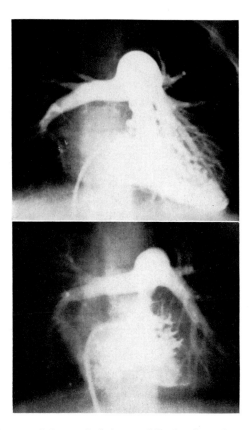

left-to-right, implying presence of an atrial septal defect; while in the other eight patients, the shunt was right-to-left, an occurrence compatible with either atrial septal defect or patent foramen ovale.

Pulmonary Vasculature

The pulmonary arterial vessels in pulmonary stenosis have not been extensively studied.

In an anatomic study of 26 patients with pulmonary stenosis and intact ventricular septum, Thomas [14] found 13 with "adequate" bronchial arteries and 13 with "minimal" bronchial artery development. Development of adequate bronchial arteries tended to be positively correlated with increasing age and increasing severity of stenosis; nonetheless, several older patients with severe stenosis had minimal bronchial collaterals.

Thomas also described pulmonary arteriolar changes in the 26 patients. In the majority of the infants, the pulmonary arterioles were normal. In those infants with severe pulmonary valvular stenosis and inadequate bronchial collaterals, however, there was delayed evolution of the pulmonary vasculature from the thick-walled, small-lumened fetal pattern. On the other hand, in those patients with severe stenosis and adequate bronchial collaterals, evolution of the pulmonary arterioles proceeded normally.

Associated Cardiac Defects

Associated cardiac defects are unusual in patients with pulmonary valvular stenosis. A small ventricular septal defect is rarely associated with pulmonary valvular stenosis.[15] Unlike tetralogy of Fallot, this disorder is associated with a normal aortic root. The hemodynamics and symptoms are dominated by the pulmonary obstructive lesion. Patent ductus arteriosus is seen occasionally.[16] Other rare associated cardiac anomalies include right aortic arch, bicuspid aortic valve, aortic valvular stenosis, subaortic stenosis, and partial anomalous pulmonary venous connection.[17, 18]

Pulmonary valvular stenosis may coexist with other right-sided obstructive lesions, such as peripheral pulmonary artery stenosis, infundibular stenosis, and anomalous muscle bundles of the right ventricle.

NATURAL HISTORY

The relatively recent clinical recognition of pulmonary stenosis and the early surgical success in the treatment of this condition have prevented the accumulation of precise data regarding its natural history. General autopsy studies uncover few patients over 40 years of age with this condition. An occasional, unusual patient with pulmonary valvular stenosis has survived until the sixth or seventh decade. Clinical observation of patients with pulmonary stenosis defines two distinct patterns.

Cyanotic Infant

Infants with severe pulmonary valvular stenosis and right ventricular dysfunction are cyanotic at birth or shortly thereafter. Life expectancy is a few weeks or months, and the infants succumb to the combination of right heart failure and hypoxia. Many infants respond dramatically to early operation. Others, however, even when valvular obstruction is recognized early and relieved operatively, continue to demonstrate signs of right ventricular dysfunction in the absence of a postoperative pressure difference across the pulmonary valve function. Right ventricular myocardial fibrosis, papillary muscle dysfunction with resultant tricuspid insufficiency, and relative hypoplasia of the right ventricle may singly or in combination be responsible for this poor postoperative prognosis.

Asymptomatic Patient

Most patients follow a quite different natural history. They present a period of well-being with absence of symptoms and with normal growth and development. When the stenosis is mild (right ventricular pressure (RVP) < 40 mm. Hg), life expectancy is normal. When the stenosis is moderate or severe, symptoms may develop at any age, but usually in the second decade of life. Increased fatigability on exercise occurs first. In the ensuing years, first cyanosis and then congestive heart failure appear. Three factors have been proposed to explain the progressive course of this group of patients.

Fixed Pulmonary Valve Area

If the orifice of the stenotic pulmonary valve remained of fixed dimensions as the child grew, one could explain deterioration with increasing age by the fact that the normal increase in cardiac output would be accompanied by increasing right ventricular pressure. Thus, the right ventricular pressure and the right ventricular work must increase to provide the increased cardiac output, and ultimately the physiological capabilities of the right ventricle are exceeded. Serial cardiac catheterizations in patients with pulmonary valvular stenosis do not support this concept. In our study of children with pulmonary stenosis,[19] the right ventricular pressure remained constant despite significant increase in body size and cardiac output. Similar findings have been reported by others in patients with mild to moderate pulmonary valvular stenosis.[20, 21] Such studies strongly suggest that the orifice of the stenotic pulmonary valve increases with growth of the patient with mild to moderate pulmonary valvular stenosis. Unfortunately, comparable data are not available in patients with severe pulmonary stenosis, since in these patients, operation is invariably performed following the initial cardiac catheterization.

Myocardial Fibrosis

Increasing evidence is accumulating to suggest that development of right ventricular myocardial fibrosis may be an important determinant of the natural history of pulmonary stenosis. This idea was stressed by Brock.[18] He said, "We do not attribute enough importance to the state of myocardium in our own management of cases of congenital heart disease, and especially of pulmonary stenosis." The inability of some patients to increase their cardiac output following complete surgical relief of pulmonary valvular stenosis has been reported by McIntosh and Cohen [22] and by Johnson.[23] Studies done in our laboratory indicate that the right ventricular myocardium of patients with pulmonary stenosis has significantly more fibrosis than the right ventricular myocardium in normal individuals of the same age or in patients with tetralogy of Fallot.[24] The right ventricular papillary muscles show the greatest degree of fibrosis, and this may be the basis of the tricuspid insufficiency that is occasionally seen in patients with severe pulmonary stenosis and that may persist following successful valvotomy. It is our belief that the state of the right ventricular myocardium is the dominant factor governing the natural history of the disease and is the limiting factor in successful surgical handling of pulmonary valvular stenosis.

Infundibular Hypertrophy

In studies of patients with pulmonary valvular stenosis, the severity of infundibular hypertrophy increases with each decade.[25] This finding suggests that infundibular stenosis may develop and lead to a secondary and, at times, major site of right ventricular outflow obstruction. To date, no serial cardiac catheterization studies have proved this point. Moreover, the postoperative findings of Engle and associates [26] indicate that following

161

successful valvotomy, residual obstruction secondary to infundibular hyper-trophy regresses within one year following operation. If infundibular hypertrophy and consequent obstruction is an important determinant in the natural history of pulmonary stenosis, it is, nonetheless, a factor that appears to be completely reversible following surgical correction.

CLINICAL RECOGNITION

Symptoms in pulmonary valvular stenosis depend on (1) the severity of the obstruction, (2) the presence or absence of a patent foramen ovale that will allow a right-to-left atrial shunt, and (3) the functional competence of the right ventricle. The last is altered by myocardial fibrosis, papillary muscle dysfunction and resultant tricuspid valve insufficiency, and encroach-ment upon the right ventricular cavity by muscular hypertrophy.

Clinical Features

The majority of children with pulmonary valvular stenosis are asympto-matic and show normal growth and development. Easy fatigability is present in an occasional child with severe stenosis and in many adults with moderate or severe stenosis. Cyanosis is uncommon, and when present, is a consequence of a right-to-left shunt at the atrial level and accompanies severe or long-standing valvular stenosis. It thus may be present at birth or develop in adult life. Squatting is rare.

Physical Examination

The prominent clinical finding is a systolic ejection murmur that is maximally heard in the second left intercostal space and radiates well to the left upper back. The murmur usually is loud and is associated with a thrill in both the pulmonic area and in the suprasternal notch. The characteristics of the murmur vary with the severity of the stenosis; with more significant stenosis, the murmur becomes longer, and its peak intensity occurs later in systole. The murmur is usually initiated by a systolic ejection click, but in severe stenosis, this finding may be absent. The intensity of the second heart sound may be normal or diminished. Although there is normal respiratory variation of the second heart sound, the degree of splitting varies directly with severity of stenosis.

In severe stenosis, particularly when accompanied by congestive cardiac failure, the systolic ejection murmur is softer, and a pansystolic murmur of tricuspid insufficiency may be heard along the lower left sternal border. In such patients, a prominent fourth heart sound may be present and a large jugular A wave found. These patients frequently show mild cyanosis.

Electrocardiographic Findings

The electrocardiogram may be used to predict right ventricular systolic pressure roughly. Cayler and associates [27] compared the height of the R wave

162

of lead V_1 in patients with pulmonary stenosis with the right ventricular systolic pressure and found fair correlation, although there was considerable overlap. Other authors found better correlation of the electrocardiogram and cross sectional area of the pulmonary valve orifice.[28] The electrocardiogram is, at best, a fair guide of severity.

In mild pulmonary stenosis, although the electrocardiogram may be normal, mild right ventricular hypertrophy is observed in many. In these patients, lead V_1 usually reveals an rSR' pattern and lead V_6 a qRs, the S wave being deeper than normal.

Among patients with moderate stenosis, the electrocardiogram is almost always abnormal (Fig. 3). There is slight right axis deviation. Lead V_1 reveals either an rR' or Rs pattern. The T waves may be positive or negative.

When pulmonary stenosis is severe, the QRS is between $+110$ and $+150$ degrees. Lead V_1 reveals either an R or a qR pattern. Although the T waves may be either positive or negative in V_1, in severe pulmonary stenosis there may be discordance between the QRS complex and the T wave and, in addition, ST-segment depression.

Gamboa and associates[29] studied the vectorcardiogram of patients with pulmonary stenosis and found good correlation between right ventricular pressure and the sum of the maximum QRS vectors. In patients with pulmonary stenosis, the QRS vector loop is nearly always clockwise in the

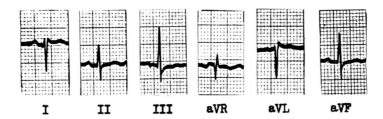

I   II   III   aVR   aVL   aVF

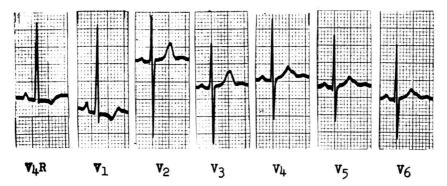

V_4R V_1 V_2 V_3 V_4 V_5 V_6

Figure 3. Electrocardiogram in a 4-year-old female with pulmonary valvular stenosis (right ventricular systolic pressure 105 mm. Hg). QRS axis $+135°$. Precordial leads reveal pattern of right ventricular hypertrophy with tall R waves in leads V_4R and V_1. Leads V_5 and V_6 show a qRS pattern with S waves significantly greater than normal.

163

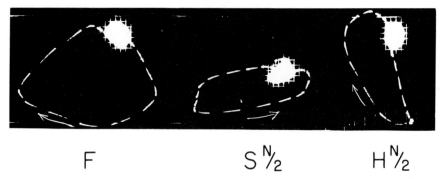

F $S^{N/2}$ $H^{N/2}$

Figure 4. Vectocardiogram of patient in Fig. 3. Sagittal and horizontal planes recorded at half-standardization (N/2). Major QRS forces are directed anteriorly and rightward. The horizontal vector loop is inscribed in a clockwise direction, which is markedly abnormal for a 4-year-old patient, and indicates significant right ventricular hypertrophy.

frontal plane. The most significant changes are observed in the horizontal plane. Among mild cases, the loop frequently is of the figure-8 contour, the terminal portion being directed posteriorly and rightward. As the severity increases, the initial anterior and leftward forces are foreshortened and the terminal forces are increased. In moderate stenosis, the loop is entirely clockwise and shows normal initial rightward and anteriorly directed forces (Fig. 4). With severe stenosis, the loop retains its clockwise rotation, but the initial forces are directed anteriorly and to the left. Marked discrepancy of the T loop is observed in these patients.

Radiographic Features

In the majority of patients with dome-shaped pulmonary valvular stenosis, both the cardiac size and the pulmonary vasculature are normal (Fig. 5).

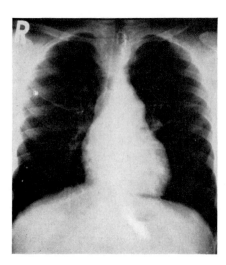

Figure 5. Thoracic roentgenogram of a 10-year-old boy with valvular pulmonary stenosis. Cardiac size and pulmonary vasculature are normal. Pulmonary trunk and left pulmonary artery are prominent.

The characteristic finding is enlargement of the main and left pulmonary arteries. Lateral and oblique views reveal evidence of enlargement of the right ventricle.

The patient with severe pulmonary valvular stenosis, right ventricular dysfunction, and right-to-left atrial shunt presents a different roentgen picture (Fig. 6). The cardiac silhouette may be moderately to markedly enlarged as a consequence of right ventricular and right atrial dilatation. The pulmonary vasculature is characteristically decreased.

HEMODYNAMIC FEATURES AND CARDIAC CATHETERIZATION

Isolated pulmonary valvular stenosis generally can be diagnosed from clinical examination supported by electrocardiographic and roentgenographic findings. Cardiac catheterization and selective angiography are helpful in defining the precise type and site of right ventricular obstruction and in excluding associated lesions such as atrial septal defect. In addition, quantitation of the right ventricular pressure and cardiac output are helpful in reaching a decision as to the advisability of surgical intervention and in providing information of prognostic value to the patient.

Pressure Measurement

In the normal subject, a systolic gradient across the pulmonary valve does not exceed 5 mm. Hg. In patients with increased pulmonary blood flow as a consequence of left-to-right shunts, the pressure difference across the pulmonary valve may reach 20 mm. Hg, but it seldom exceeds this value. In patients with isolated pulmonary valvular stenosis, we have observed right ventricular systolic pressure values from 40 to above 250 mm. Hg in the resting state, and as high as 300 mm. Hg during exercise.

In pulmonary valvular stenosis, the right ventricular pressure pulse is abnormal in form.[30] The normally present ejection plateau is absent, and instead, the pressure pulse rises to a peak late in systole and then declines

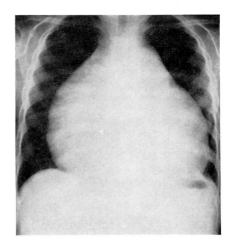

Figure 6. Thoracic roentgenogram of 4-year-old boy with severe pulmonary valvular stenosis and tricuspid insufficiency. Greatly enlarged heart. The prominent right cardiac shadow represents right atrial enlargement. The pulmonary vasculature is diminished.

rapidly to the baseline. When pulmonary stenosis is severe, the pressure pulse in the pulmonary arteries is damped and the mean pressure low. When the cardiac catheter lies just distal to the stenotic pulmonary valve, negative deflections, synchronous with maximal systolic ejection, are noted in the pulmonary pressure pulse and are due to Venturi effect of high velocity flow in the pulmonary artery. Withdrawal of the catheter across the pulmonary valve results in a sudden increase in systolic pressure. If the catheter is withdrawn slowly, the withdrawal tracing may allow definition of infundibular stenosis or anomalous muscle bundles in the right ventricle. In both these subvalvular obstructions, however, the catheter frequently recoils from the pulmonary artery directly into the proximal portion of the right ventricle and does not record the intermediate pressure.

The right atrial pressure is often normal, but in severe pulmonary valvular stenosis, a prominent A wave is present. When right ventricle failure and tricuspid regurgitation are present, a prominent V wave in the atrial pressure pulse occurs.

In the patient with pulmonary valvular stenosis, the right ventricular pressure must always be measured before directing the catheter into the pulmonary artery. Right heart failure, syncope, and sudden death have occurred when the cardiac catheter has been positioned within the critically small pulmonary valve orifice.[31] If the right ventricular pressure is over 200 mm. Hg, it is advisable not to attempt passage of the catheter tip into the pulmonary artery; or if passage is accomplished, the catheter should not remain in the pulmonary artery for more than a few seconds.

The level of right ventricular pressure or the systolic gradient across the pulmonary valve have been used as primary indications for operation in patients with pulmonary valvular stenosis. Right ventricular pressure is dependent on the cross-sectional area of the pulmonary valve orifice as well as on the cardiac output. The rather significant variation in cardiac output depending on the patient's state of sedation or anxiety is well known.

For a given pulmonary valve area, the anxious patient may have a high cardiac output and a comparably high right ventricular pressure and be considered a candidate for operation. The same patient, well sedated, will have a low cardiac output, and thus a lower right ventricular pressure. Consideration of right ventricular pressure alone would place him in a nonoperative category. The fallacy of using only right ventricular pressure as a criterion for operation is thus apparent.

Pulmonary Valve Area

Calculation of pulmonary valve area is a practical means of relating cardiac output and right ventricular pressure in patients with pulmonary valvular stenosis.

The formulae of Gorlin [32,33] for calculation of pulmonary valve area (PVA) are

$$PVA \ (cm.^2) = \frac{\text{systolic flow}}{\text{velocity through valve}}$$

166

$$PVA = \dfrac{\dfrac{CO \times 1{,}000}{SEP \times HR}}{44.5\sqrt{RV_{sm} - PA_m}}$$

where CO=cardiac output, SEP=systolic ejection period, HR=heart rate, RV_{sm}=mean right ventricular systolic ejection pressure, and PA_m=mean pulmonary artery pressure.

Moller and Adams [34] derived the following simplified, clinically useful method of calculation of pulmonary valve area.

To determine the pulmonary valvular area, the formula for pulmonary valvular resistance is utilized:

$$PVR = \dfrac{RV_{sm} - PA_m}{CO} \times \dfrac{1{,}332 \times 60}{1{,}000}$$

A substitution of 0.66 peak right ventricular systolic pressure is made for the mean right ventricular systolic ejection pressure, and the pulmonary valvular resistance is calculated:

$$PVR = \dfrac{0.66\,RV - PA_m}{CO} \times 80$$

This value for resistance is located on the abscissa of Fig. 7, and the corresponding pulmonary valvular area is found on the ordinate.

Exercise Hemodynamics

Measurement of hemodynamics in a resting child may not accurately reflect his status during everyday activities, and thus may provide less than optimal means of determining his prognosis or need for operation. For this reason, we now routinely measure pressures and cardiac output both at rest and during supine exercise. A bicycle ergometer is used for these studies. Data obtained during moderate exercise allow estimation of right ventricular pressure and work during everyday activities and provide a means of estimating, by extrapolation, the right ventricular stress imposed during severe exercise. Moreover, the state of the right ventricular myocardium can be appreciated by noting the level and change of right ventricular end-diastolic pressure, the increase in cardiac output, and the relationship of oxygen consumption to cardiac output (exercise factor).

Exercise studies have also provided insight into the natural history of patients with pulmonary valvular stenosis. Lewis and associates [35] reported results of exercise in 13 adults (ages 19 to 61) with pulmonary valvular stenosis. Their patients fell into two groups. In group I patients (right ventricular systolic pressures below 80 mm. Hg), cardiac output and right ventricular end-diastolic pressures were normal at rest. Heart rate and cardiac output increased normally with exercise. In group II patients (right ventricular systolic pressures above 80 mm. Hg), the resting cardiac output was less than normal. With exercise, there was a subnormal increase in

167

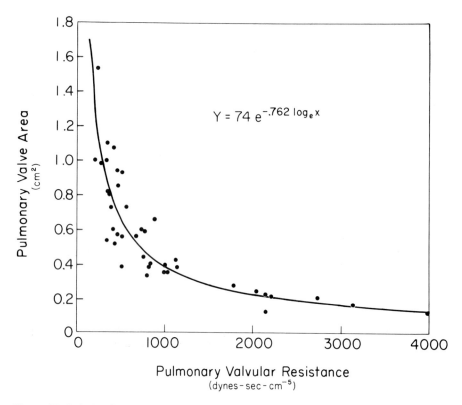

Figure 7. Relationship between pulmonary valve area and pulmonary valvular resistance calculated from data in 40 children with pulmonary valvular stenosis. (From Moller, J. E., and Adams, P., Jr., A simplified method for calculating the pulmonary valve area.[34])

cardiac output, despite a normal increase in heart rate. Exercise increased the right ventricular end-diastolic pressure in all their patients.

We have studied 42 children (ages 5 to 16) with pulmonary valvular stenosis during rest and exercise.[36]

In 29 of these 42 children, the resting right ventricular systolic pressure was less than 80 mm. Hg and the resting cardiac output was normal. In these patients, the heart rate and cardiac output increased normally during exercise. Exercise did not result in an increased right ventricular end-diastolic pressure; indeed, the end-diastolic pressure decreased during exercise in some of them.

In 13 children, the resting right ventricular systolic pressure was above 80 mm. Hg. Eleven had normal resting cardiac output and end-diastolic pressure. Exercise resulted in a normal increase in cardiac output and heart rate in these 11 patients, and the end-diastolic pressure increased modestly or not at all.

Two children, by contrast, showed impaired right ventricular function at rest (elevated end-diastolic pressure or low cardiac output) and responded to exercise by subnormal increase in cardiac output and by increase in end-diastolic pressure.

These studies indicate that at comparable levels of pulmonary valvular obstruction, the majority of children have normal or near-normal right ventricular function, while adults demonstrate significant impairment of right ventricular function. These data support the concept that the natural history of pulmonary valvular stenosis is related to impairment of right ventricular myocardial function.

ANGIOGRAPHY

Clinical features almost always allow a diagnosis of pulmonary outflow obstruction, and cardiac catheterization establishes the severity of the obstruction and the level of right ventricular function.

Angiography illustrates the precise anatomic site and nature of the obstructive lesion and allows definition of coexisting obstructions. Thus, the usefulness of angiography lies in the anatomic differential diagnosis of pulmonary valvular stenosis. We believe right ventriculography is a prerequisite to surgical management of the patient with pulmonary valvular stenosis.

The characteristic features described below may be contrasted to the angiographic findings in other types of pulmonary outflow obstruction illustrated in the section on differential diagnosis.

The form or shape of the right ventricular cavity is normal in mild stenosis (Fig. 2, left). When the right ventricular pressure exceeds 100 mm. Hg, asymmetrical hypertrophy of the right ventricle occurs, and the resultant conical shape of the right ventricular cavity is well illustrated by angiography (Fig. 2, right). The infundibulum may be hypertrophied and may appear obstructive in late systole. The infundibular cavity opens to adequate size during diastole and early systole, however.

The valve appears thickened and is domed during systole (Fig. 8). The sinuses of Valsalva are dilated and clearly defined. A jet of opaque enters the pulmonary trunk during systole and may allow an estimate of the orifice size. A "negative jet" of unpacified blood in the pulmonary artery may be observed late in the study.

Poststenotic dilatation of the pulmonary trunk and left pulmonary artery are typically present. The right pulmonary artery is of normal size.

DIFFERENTIAL DIAGNOSIS

The conditions that must be considered in the differential diagnosis of pulmonary valvular stenosis depend upon the severity of the obstruction and the presence or absence of cyanosis.

Mild Pulmonary Valvular Stenosis

In the asymptomatic patient with mild pulmonary stenosis, one must also consider atrial septal defect, idiopathic dilatation of the pulmonary artery,

169

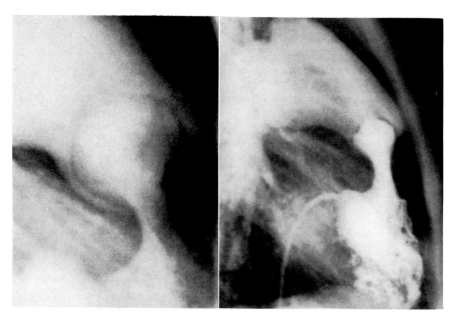

Figure 8. *Left:* Close-up of pulmonary valve in the lateral projection of a right ventriculogram. The pulmonary valve domes and the valve cusps are thin. The sinuses of Valsalva are distinctly seen and well opacified. The infundibulum is narrowed during this systolic phase. Poststenotic dilatation of the pulmonary trunk is present. *Right:* Lateral view, right ventriculogram in patient with pulmonary valvular stenosis. Doming of the pulmonary valve is evident. A jet of contrast is seen passing through the stenotic pulmonary valve. The pulmonary trunk shows significant post-stenotic dilatation. The infundibular area of the right ventricle is narrowed during this systolic phase.

and the innocent pulmonary flow murmur. Atrial septal defect can be distinguished on the basis of fixed splitting of the second heart sound, increased pulmonary vascular markings, and the incomplete right bundle branch block on the electrocardiogram. The differentiation among mild pulmonary stenosis, idiopathic dilatation of the pulmonary artery, and functional pulmonary flow murmur may at times be difficult. However, this is an academic consideration, since each of the conditions results in a normal, asymptomatic life span.

Cyanotic Infant

The infant with pulmonic stenosis and cyanosis is characterized by a large heart, decreased pulmonary vasculature, and evidence of congestive cardiac failure. Included in the differential diagnosis are all the causes of cyanotic congenital heart disease in infancy. In particular, the following must be differentiated.

Pulmonary Atresia, Tricuspid Atresia, and Hypoplastic Right Ventricle

These conditions result in decreased pulmonary vascular markings but may have a small cardiac silhouette. Precise diagnosis usually requires the use of the catheterization laboratory.

Ebstein's Malformation of the Tricuspid Valve

Physical findings and roentgen features of Ebstein's anomaly in infancy may mimic precisely those of severe pulmonary stenosis. The major clue lies in electrocardiographic evidence of right ventricular hypertrophy in patients with pulmonary valve stenosis and absence of normal right ventricular forces in patients with Ebstein's anomaly. However, we have observed patients in whom clinical differentiation was impossible. Since pulmonary valvular stenosis in infancy necessitates surgery on a semiemergency basis and Ebstein's malformation of the tricuspid valve is best treated medically, confirmation in the cardiac catherization laboratory is necessary.

Tetralogy of Fallot

The patient with tetralogy of Fallot can be differentiated on the basis of a small heart and the absence of congestive cardiac failure. However, the so-called tetrad variants, which include transposition of the great vessels with pulmonic stenosis and single ventricle with pulmonic stenosis, may be difficult to differentiate from pulmonary valvular stenosis with intact ventricular septum. As a consequence of the urgency demanded in the surgical care of the patient with severe pulmonary valvular stenosis, definitive diagnosis in the catheterization laboratory is necessary.

Moderate to Severe Pulmonary Stenosis in the Child or Young Adult

Differentiation of pulmonary valvular stenosis from aortic stenosis, ventricular septal defect, and acyanotic tetralogy of Fallot is not difficult. The major diagnostic problem in these patients is the anatomic definition and location of the pulmonary outflow obstruction. Lesions that must be considered include dysplastic pulmonary valve, infundibular stenosis, anomalous muscle bundle of the right ventricle, and peripheral pulmonary artery stenosis. Since recognition of these lesions is important to appropriate surgical management, they will be considered in some detail.

Infundibular Stenosis

Stenosis of the ostium infundibulum usually is associated with ventricular septal defect (tetralogy of Fallot). When infundibular stenosis occurs in the presence of an intact ventricular septum, it may be secondary to pulmonary valvular stenosis. In this situation, the infundibulum is diffusely hypertrophied and may produce additional obstruction to right ventricular outflow before or after surgical elimination of valvular obstruction.

When infundibular stenosis occurs as an isolated lesion, it is more localized and seen typically at the inlet to the infundibulum. Of 215 operated cases of pulmonary outflow obstruction, Brock found 17 cases of pure infundibular stenosis, an incidence of 8 per cent.[18]

The hemodynamic alterations and symptoms are comparable to those

171

in pulmonary valvular stenosis and depend on the severity of the obstruction. Pure infundibular stenosis may be indistinguishable clinically from pulmonary valvular stenosis. At times, the murmur is located slightly lower on the left sternal border. The systolic ejection click usually present in pulmonary valvular stenosis is not heard in isolated infundibular stenosis. Electrocardiography has not been helpful in our hands in differentiating these two lesions. Roentgen evidence of post-stenotic dilatation of the main pulmonary artery and left pulmonary artery may not be present in infundibular stenosis, while these features are typically seen in pulmonary valvular stenosis.

Identification of infundibular stenosis is possible in the catheterization laboratory. Careful pressure withdrawal tracings from pulmonary artery to right ventricle may show an intermediate pressure with systolic pressure equal to pulmonary artery systolic and diastolic pressure equal to right ventricular diastolic, followed by high pressure right ventricular tracing. However, the catheter not infrequently traverses the intermediate chamber so rapidly that no intermediate pressure is recorded. Right ventriculography provides a definite diagnosis.

Anomalous Right Ventricular Muscle Bundles

In 1962, attention was directed to the fact that significant right ventricular outflow obstruction may be caused by large muscle bundles traversing the right ventricular cavity proximal to the infundibulum.[37] Subsequent reports have confirmed that the occurrence of this cause of pulmonary outflow obstruction is not uncommon.[38-40] In the majority of cases, the muscle bundles are associated with ventricular septal defect and the physiology is comparable to that seen in tetralogy of Fallot. Anomalous muscle bundles may occur in association with pulmonary valvular stenosis or may be the sole site of right ventricular outflow obstruction.

Anatomically, these muscle bundles are found within the sinus portion of the right ventricle, below and distinct from the infundibular tract. They arise from the central portion of the crista supraventricularis or the subjacent ventricular septum. After traversing the ventricular cavity, the bundles attach broadly to the parietal ventricular wall. A portion of the muscle bundle mass has its attachment at the base of the anterior papillary muscle. The muscle bundles form an imperfect partition between the proximal and distal right ventricular cavity (Fig. 9).

In addition to anatomic outflow obstruction, the muscle bundles result in inflow obstruction and functional outflow obstruction.

Physical examination, electrocardiogram, and chest X ray have failed to provide a clue to differentiate obstruction secondary to anomalous muscle bundles from that associated with pulmonary valvular stenosis.

In five of nine patients reported by Warden and associates,[39] a pressure gradient was noted between the proximal and distal portions of the right ventricle. In the other four patients, however, the pressure tracing was comparable to pressure tracings seen in pulmonary valvular stenosis. In

172

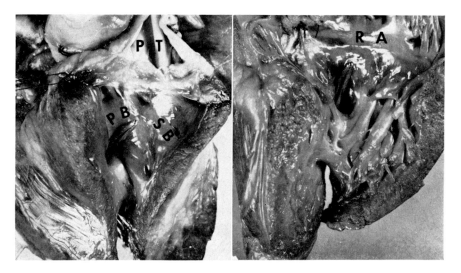

Figure 9. Autopsy specimen from 3½-year-old patient with anomalous muscle bundles of the right ventricle. *Left:* The hypertrophied parietal and septal bands of the crista supraventricularis are clearly distinguished from the junction of the septal and parietal bands of anomalous muscle bundle that originates from the crista to insert on the anterior wall of the right ventricle. The tip of the hemostat protrudes through the major communication between the proximal and distal right ventricular chambers. The pulmonary valve is stenotic. PT = pulmonary trunk. (From Lucas et al., anomalous muscle bundles of the right ventricle. Hemodynamic consequences and surgical consideration.[37]) *Right:* The anomalous muscle bundles seen from the right atrium and proximal right ventricular cavity. The relationship of the anomalous muscle mass to the anterior papillary muscle is shown. The hemostat lies in the major channel between proximal and distal right ventricle.

these patients, the catheter apparently snapped rapidly from the pulmonary artery into the proximal right ventricular cavity.

Angiography, on the other hand, has proved to be a consistently accurate diagnostic tool. Right ventriculography demonstrates characteristic filling defects within the body of the right ventricle (Fig. 10).

The natural history of this lesion is not clearly defined. In four patients, nonobstructive muscle bundles were demonstrated in infancy and became obstructive with time.[40]

With preoperative diagnosis, the surgeon's task in relieving this type of obstruction is not difficult.[39] Appropriate surgical approach necessitates cardiopulmonary bypass and a longitudinal cardiotomy placed so as to enter the largest of the channels from proximal to distal right ventricle. The muscle bundles are then resected after their relationship to the anterior papillary muscle is clearly defined. Valvotomy for associated pulmonary valvular stenosis, when it is present, is best done via a separate transverse pulmonary arteriotomy.

On the other hand, failure to recognize this type of right ventricular outflow obstruction before operation or at the time of surgery results in a

173

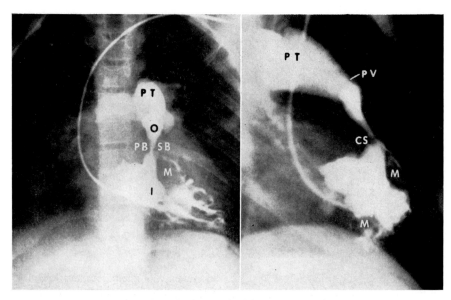

Figure 10. Selective right ventriculogram in a patient with pulmonary valvular stenosis and anomalous muscle bundles of the right ventricle. *Left:* Anteroposterior view during systole. The septal band (SB) and parietal band (PB) of the crista supraventricularis are hypertrophied. The anomalous muscle mass (M) clearly separates the right ventricle into inflow (I) and outflow (O) portions. *Right:* In the lateral view, the filling defects (M) represent the attachment of the muscle mass to the anterior right ventricular wall and to the anterior papillary muscle. The pulmonary valve is domed. (Pt, pulmonary trunk.) (From Warden, H. E., et al., Right ventricle obstruction resulting from anomalous muscle bundles.[39])

significant residual obstruction and a possible fatal issue from the operative procedure.[37]

Stenosis Due to Valvular Dysplasia

Recently we have described a distinct anatomic type of pulmonary valvular stenosis associated with rather specific clinical and laboratory findings.[41] In this form, the pulmonary valve shows three distinct cusps without commissural fusion, but the cusps are greatly thickened and redundant (Fig. 11). The obstruction results from the bulk of valvular tissue in the right ventricular outflow tract. These patients present with a pulmonary ejection murmur but without the pulmonary systolic ejection click usually observed in typical valvular stenosis. There is a familial tendency for this form of pulmonary stenosis. Many children present with triangular-shaped face, ptosis, hypertelorism, and low-set ears.

We have recognized this anatomic form of pulmonary stenosis in patients with the rubella syndrome and in children with a syndrome of multiple lentigines, hearing defect, hypogenitalism, and the facies described above.[42] This type of pulmonary valve is present also in patients with the male Turner's syndrome (Noonan syndrome).

174

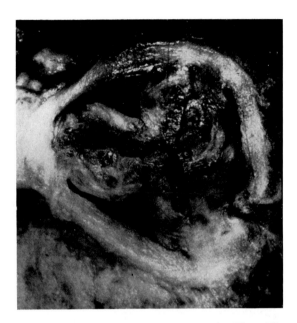

Figure 11. Dysplastic pulmonary valve, transected and viewed from above. Three distinct pulmonary valvular cusps are present. There is no commissural fusion. The valvular cusps are greatly thickened. The sinus of Valsalva, at the right, is obliterated by tissue proliferation.

The electrocardiogram and vectorcardiogram are unusual (Fig. 12). Generally, the QRS axis is located between +210 and +270 degrees, and the major QRS electrical forces are directed posteriorly in the horizontal plane. Thoracic roentgenograms usually fail to show an enlarged pulmonary artery. Cardiac catheterization reveals a gradient at the level of the pulmonary valve. In our patients, the level of right ventricular systolic pressure has ranged between 100 and 200 mm. Hg.

The angiographic features of this valve are characteristic; the valve fails to dome, there is rarely a jet, the thickened valve leaflets are evident, and the sinuses of Valsalva are not well visualized (Fig. 13).

The clinical recognition of this distinct form of pulmonary stenosis is important, for before we were aware of its nature, operative repair was accompanied by 40 per cent mortality and significant residual stenosis in patients who survived operation. Pulmonary valvotomy is not beneficial, since commissural fusion is minimal or absent.

At operation, an outflow patch must be placed across the pulmonary annulus, one or more valve cusps must be resected, or both procedures must be carried out. Operative results in two patients in whom this condition was recognized before operation have been good; a third, a 7-day-old infant, died in the immediate postoperative period.

Peripheral Pulmonary Arterial Stenosis (Pulmonary Artery Coarctation)

Stenosis of the pulmonary arteries may occur either as an isolated lesion or in association with other congenital cardiac abnormalities, particularly tetralogy of Fallot and pulmonary valvular stenosis. The stenotic lesions in the pulmonary artery may occur as single, localized constrictions or as multiple, diffuse narrowings throughout both lung fields. The lesions may

175

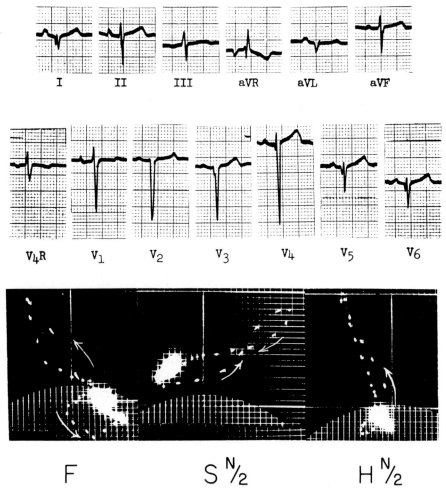

I   II   III   aVR   aVL   aVF

V₄R   V₁   V₂   V₃   V₄   V₅   V₆

F   S ᴺ/₂   H ᴺ/₂

Figure 12. Electrocardiogram and vectorcardiogram in 10-year-old patient with pulmonary valvular dysplasia. Right ventricular systolic pressure was 175 mm. Hg. The QRS axis is +210 degrees. The precordial leads reveal the predominant QRS electrical forces to be directed posteriorly, and no pattern of right ventricular hypertrophy. The sagittal and horizontal planes of the vectorcardiogram are recorded at half standardization (N/2). The major forces are directed posteriorly and to the right and the initial forces are normal. The frontal plane reveals a predominantly counterclockwise rotation. In the horizontal plane, the QRS vector loop also is predominantly counterclockwise in inscription. In each plane, the QRS vector loop is narrow. Contrast these to the electrocardiogram of typical pulmonary valvular stenosis (Figs. 3 and 4).

be represented anatomically by a diaphragm across a pulmonary artery or its branch, or, more commonly, as a hypoplastic segment of an artery. The etiology is more frequently discernable in this condition than in pulmonary valvular stenosis. It often is present in the rubella syndrome of infancy[43] and occurs in the male Turner's syndrome.

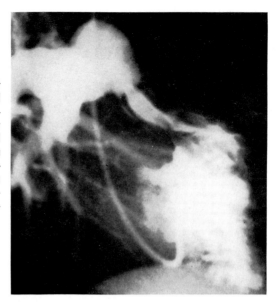

Figure 13. Lateral view, right ventriculogram in a 6-year-old patient with dysplastic pulmonary valve. The pulmonary valvular cusps are thickened and the sinuses of Valsalva narrowed. Doming of the pulmonary valve is absent and a jet is not present. The pulmonary annulus and the subpulmonary area are narrowed.

Hemodynamic alterations include elevation of right ventricular systolic pressure and elevation of pressure in the pulmonary artery proximal to the obstruction. Single or multiple pressure gradients may be recorded in the pulmonary arteries. The pulmonary arterial pressure pulse proximal to the obstruction characteristically shows a wide pulse pressure with a low dicrotic notch. In most patients, obstruction is of mild to moderate severity; right ventricular systolic pressure rarely exceeds 100 mm. Hg.

Generally, the children are asymptomatic. If obstruction is severe, easy fatigability is present. Cyanosis is rare. Growth may be slow in the patients in whom the cardiac condition is a portion of a specific syndrome. The prominent physical finding is a systolic ejection murmur along the upper left sternal border, which is also well heard throughout both lung fields, anteriorly and posteriorly. Continuous murmurs are uncommon, since there is rarely a diastolic gradient across the stenotic lesion. Pulmonary systolic ejection clicks are rare, and the pulmonic second heart sound is of normal loudness (low dicrotic notch) as in valvular pulmonary stenosis.

The electrocardiogram varies from normal to a pattern of right axis deviation, right atrial enlargement, and right ventricular hypertrophy in more severe cases. In patients with rubella syndrome, the QRS axis is frequently superiorly oriented in the frontal plane. Thoracic roentgenograms are usually normal or reveal mild cardiac enlargement. The pulmonary arterial segment is not dilated, and the pulmonary vasculature is normal.

Stenotic pulmonary arterial lesions can be recognized by pulmonary arteriography (Fig. 14). One study of the natural history revealed that the condition is not progressive over a 5-year period, although the long-term consequences are unknown.[44] The majority of patients either require no operative therapy or are inoperable because the stenotic areas are multiple

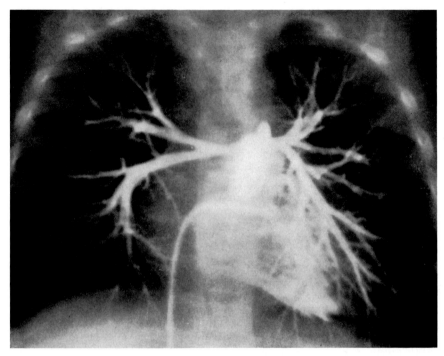

Figure 14. Anteroposterior view of right ventriculogram in 14-month-old child with peripheral pulmonary artery stenosis. Stenotic lesions are present at the bifurcation of the pulmonary trunk. The proximal right pulmonary artery appears hypoplastic. The caliber of the distal right pulmonary artery is greater than that of the proximal right pulmonary artery. The pulmonary trunk is of normal size.

and peripherally located. If the stenotic areas are isolated and proximally located and if the condition severe, excision may be performed.

THERAPY

Indication for Operation

Significant obstruction at the pulmonary valve necessitates increased right ventricular work and ultimately results in impaired right ventricular function and associated symptoms. Optimal treatment consists of timely relief of the obstruction, before right ventricular function is irreversibly impaired.

Thus, we are faced with two questions:

1. Is the pulmonary valvular obstruction significant? Will it ultimately impair right ventricular function?

2. If obstruction is significant, when should operative relief of the obstruction be performed?

These questions will be considered in the following types of patients.

The Cyanotic Infant

Infants with severe pulmonary valvular stenosis, right ventricular failure, and right-to-left atrial shunt have severely impaired right ventricular func-

178

tion. They represent medical and surgical emergencies. Such an infant requires immediate and intensive anticongestive treatment and emergency pulmonary valvotomy.

The Patient with Right Heart Failure

Right heart failure may occur in the infant, child, or adult. Pulmonary valvotomy should be carried out promptly, as soon as heart failure has been treated and diagnosis confirmed. Unfortunately, many of these patients, and particularly the older ones, have irreparable right ventricular damage, and operation may result in minimal improvement.

The Asymptomatic Patient

This group embraces patients with insignificant obstruction and normal life expectancy, patients with severe stenosis, and patients with mild and moderate pulmonary valvular stenosis.

Careful assessment of physical findings, ECG, VCG, and X rays allows identification of the patient with insignificant pulmonary valvular stenosis.

The clinical signs we utilize to identify the patient with severe stenosis often are dependent on impairment of right ventricular function. Use of these indicators may delay operative intervention beyond the optimal time. For this reason, we feel that cardiac catheterization is indicated at about age 6 years in any child thought to have significant pulmonary valvular stenosis. We recommend early elective operation in all those children with significant obstruction.

What is significant obstruction? A simple, definitive sign is always comforting, and a right ventricular pressure above 70 mm. Hg has been so utilized. We have discussed the drawback of using right ventricular pressure in the absence of knowledge of cardiac output as an indication for operation. In general, we perform valvotomy in patients with a pulmonary valve area of less than 0.5 cm.^{2}/m.^{2} The patient's hemodynamic response to exercise has been of help in borderline cases. We can thereby estimate the right ventricular pressure during everyday activity. Should this value exceed 100 to 120 mm. Hg, we would favor operation. Moreover, exercise stress allows assessment of right ventricular function. Failure of right ventricular end-diastolic pressure to decrease with exercise, suboptimal increase in cardiac output, and abnormal exercise factor all favor a decision for operation.

Operation

Three operative approaches have been used.

Brock Valvotomy

This operation is of historical interest but is rarely used today. A cutting valvulotome and then dilators are inserted through a right ventriculotomy and passed blindly through the stenotic pulmonary valve orifice. Brock performed the operation in 114 patients, with an operative mortality of

12 per cent.[18] In a followup of 57 patients operated upon in this way by Brock, Campbell found 61 per cent to have excellent relief of the obstruction, while the remaining 39 per cent had significant residual pulmonary stenosis.[45]

Open Pulmonary Valvotomy Under Conditions of Cardiopulmonary Bypass

The patient is placed on bypass, a pulmonary arteriotomy is performed, and the surgeon inspects and incises the commissural fusions without haste. This approach also allows the surgeon to define other sites of obstruction (infundibular stenosis, anomalous muscle bundles of the right ventricle) and correct these when necessary. While the risk of cardiopulmonary bypass is low, it is significant, and in the majority of patients with pulmonary valvular stenosis, use of cardiopulmonary bypass is not required.

Open Pulmonary Valvotomy Under Conditions of Inflow Stasis

In this method, introduced by Varco in 1951,[46] blood flow to the right heart is temporarily interrupted by occluding the venae cavae. Under normothermic conditions, occlusion for 1.5 to 2 minutes is well tolerated. This time is adequate for inspection and incision of the fused commissures.

The addition of hypothermia to this procedure allows occlusion for periods of 8 to 10 minutes. In our opinion, this amount of time is not needed for the routine valvotomy and may be insufficient should additional obstructive sites be identified.

At present, we use inflow stasis under normothermic conditions for pulmonary valvotomy. Cardiopulmonary standby is maintained for every operation.

Prophylaxis Against Bacterial Endocarditis

Patients with pulmonary valvular stenosis (postoperative state also) should receive appropriate antibiotic prophylaxis for dental procedures, genitourinary manipulation, and bowel surgery, following the recommendation of the American Heart Association.[47]

Results of Therapy

Operative Risk

We have operated on 73 patients with pulmonary valvular stenosis, using cardiopulmonary bypass. At the time of operation, only a pulmonary valvotomy was performed. Of these 73 patients, 10 died (14 per cent) either at the time of operation or shortly thereafter. Two of the ten were less than 1 year or age and tolerated the procedure well, but died of infection following operation. In six other patients, each a child, the right ventricular systolic pressure was greater than 175 mm. Hg. The other deaths occurred in a 21-month-old child and a 33-year-old woman who previously had undergone Blalock-Taussig anastomosis at another institution.

In the last eighty-one patients operated upon for pulmonary stenosis using

180

inflow occlusion under normothermic conditions, five died (6 per cent). Of these five, three were less than 2 weeks of age at the time of operation. One of the other two patients represents an instance of pulmonary valvular dysplasia unrecognized at operation. In the remaining patient, the right ventricular systolic pressure was 175 mm. Hg.

Because of this experience, we feel that in the older patient with mild to moderate pulmonary valvular stenosis, pulmonary valvotomy performed under conditions of inflow occlusion can be carried out with extremely low risk.

Clinical Postoperative Status

Since many patients are asymptomatic before operation, there is no change following operation. Successful operation in more severe cases results in improvement of the patient's condition in the majority of patients. Easy fatigability and cyanosis disappear, but not invariably. In a few children and in some adults these persist, despite near-normal right ventricular pressure. This is the result of altered right ventricular compliance, undoubtedly due to myocardial fibrosis.

Cardiac examination following operation invariably reveals a pulmonary systolic ejection murmur, which is, however, less loud than it had been before operation. Many patients reveal a murmur of pulmonary insufficiency, which probably exists in all patients following valvotomy.

The electrocardiogram returns toward normal, frequently revealing an rSR' pattern in lead V_1. The enlarged pulmonary artery, seen on X rays, persists.

Hemodynamic Postoperative Status

The results of postoperative cardiac catheterization have shown good results. In only two of our fifty-three patients undergoing postoperative cardiac catheterization has the right ventricular systolic pressure exceeded 70 mm. Hg; most patients had pressures less than 40 mm. Hg. Ten patients had preoperative systemic arterial oxygen desaturation; seven of these had normal postoperative arterial saturations, while three were mildly desaturated (88, 88, and 84 per cent). Despite normal systemic saturations, two additional patients had small right-to-left shunts at rest, by indicator dilution studies.

Postoperative cardiac catheterization invariably reveals findings of pulmonary valvular insufficiency. Although this has been considered benign, its long term effects are unknown. Our postoperative exercise studies in eighteen children have shown a normal response to this work stress in fifteen and a less than normal increase in the cardiac output in the remaining three. Reports of similar studies in adults frequently reveal an inability to increase the cardiac output normally with exercise, indicating impaired right ventricular myocardial response.

181

SUMMARY

Isolated pulmonary valvular stenosis accounts for about 10 per cent of all congenital cardiac defects.

Clinical recognition, using physical findings, electrocardiogram, and thoracic roentgenograms, is not difficult.

We recommend cardiac catheterization in all patients with pulmonary valvular stenosis to (1) define the need for operation and (2) demonstrate the precise anatomical site of obstruction.

The natural history of pulmonary valvular stenosis depends primarily on the function of right ventricular myocardium, which is in turn dependent on the degree of myocardial fibrosis. The amount of myocardial fibrosis correlates with severity of obstruction and its duration.

Utilizing inflow occlusion under normothermic conditions, operative results are excellent and operative mortality is exceedingly low.

References

1. WILLIUS, F. A., AND DRY, T. J.: *A History of the Heart and the Circulation.* W. B. Saunders Co., Philadelphia, 1948, p. 85.

2. WILLIUS, F. A., AND DRY, T. J.: *A History of the Heart and the Circulation.* W. B. Saunders Co., Philadelphia, 1948, p. 108.

3. WILLIUS, F. A., AND DRY, T. J.: *A History of the Heart and the Circulation.* W. B. Saunders Co., Philadelphia, 1948, p. 121.

4. FALLOT, A.: *Contribution à l'anatomie pathologique de la maladie bleue (cyanose cardiaque).* Marsielle Med. 25:77, 1888.

5. NOONAN, J. A.: *Hypertelorism with Turner phenotype. A new syndrome with associated congenital heart disease.* Amer. J. Dis. Child. 116:373, 1968.

6. ABBOTT, M. E., LEWIS, D. S., AND BEATTIE, W. W.: *Differential study of a case of pulmonary stenosis of inflammatory origin (ventricular septum closed).* Amer. J. Med. Sci. 165:636, 1926.

7. BURCH, G. E., SUN, S. C., COLCOLOUGH, H. L., SOHAL, R. S., AND DE PASQUALE, N. P.: *Coxsackie B viral myocarditis and valvulitis identified in routine autopsy specimens by immunofluorescent techniques.* Amer. Heart J. 74:13, 1967.

8. EDWARDS, J. E., and BURCHELL, H. B.: *Endocardial and intimal lesions (jet impact) as possible sites of origin of murmurs.* Circulation 18:946, 1958.

9. EDWARDS, J. E.: *Congenital malformations of the heart and great vessels,* in Gould, S. E. (ed.): *Pathology of the Heart.* Charles C Thomas, Springfield, Ill., 1960.

10. ALLANBY, K. D., AND CAMPBELL, M.: *Congenital pulmonary stenosis with closed ventricular septum.* Guy Hosp. Rep. 98:18, 1949.

11. MOLLER, J. H.: Unpublished observations.

12. SELZER, A., CARNES, W. H., NOBLE, C. A., JR., HIGGINS, W. H., JR., AND HOLMES, R. O.: *The syndrome of pulmonary stenosis with patent foramen ovale.* Amer. J. Med. 6:3, 1949.

13. ABRAHAMS, D. G., AND WOOD, P.: *Pulmonary stenosis with normal aortic root.* Brit. Heart J. 13:519, 1951.

182

14. THOMAS, M. A.: *Pulmonary vascular changes in pulmonary stenosis with and without ventricular septal defect.* Brit. Heart J. 26:655, 1964.

15. HOFFMAN, J. I. E., RUDOLPH, A. M., NADAS, A. S., AND GROSS, R. E.: *Pulmonic stenosis, ventricular septal defect, and right ventricular pressure above systemic level.* Circulation 22:405, 1960.

16. HEINER, D. C., AND NADAS, A. S.: *Patent ductus arteriosus in association with pulmonic stenosis. A report of six cases with additional non-cardiac anomalies.* Circulation 17:232, 1958.

17. EDWARDS, J. E.: *Congenital malformation of the heart and great vessels,* in Gould, S. E. (ed.): *Pathology of the Heart.* Charles C Thomas, Springfield, Ill., 1960, p. 344.

18. BROCK, R.: *The surgical treatment of pulmonary stenosis.* Brit. Heart J. 23:337, 1961.

19. MOLLER, J. E., AND ADAMS, P., JR.: *The natural history of pulmonary valvular stenosis. Serial cardiac catheterizations in 21 children.* Amer. J. Cardiol. 16:654, 1965.

20. TINKER, J., HOWITT, G., MARKMAN, P., AND WADE, E. G.: *The natural history of isolated pulmonary stenosis.* Brit. Heart J. 27:151, 1965.

21. FABRICUS, J.: *Isolated pulmonary stenosis.* Munksgaard, Copenhagen, 1959, pp. 131–145.

22. MCINTOSH, H. D., AND COHEN, A. I.: *Pulmonary stenosis: The importance of the myocardial factor in determining the clinical course and surgical results.* Amer. Heart J. 65:715, 1963.

23. JOHNSON, A. M.: *Impaired exercise response and other residua of pulmonary stenosis after valvotomy.* Brit. Heart J. 24:375, 1962.

24. MOLLER, J. H.: Unpublished observations.

25. JOHNSON, A. M.: *Hypertrophic infundibular stenosis complicating simple pulmonary valve stenosis.* Brit. Heart J. 21:429, 1959.

26. ENGLE, M. A., HOLSWADE, G. R., GOLDBERG, H. P., LUKAS, D. S., AND GLENN, F.: *Regression after open valvotomy of infundibular stenosis accompanying severe valvular pulmonary stenosis.* Circulation 17:862, 1958.

27. CAYLER, G. G., ONGLEY, P. A., AND NADAS, A. S.: *Relation of systolic pressure in the right ventricle to the electrocardiogram. A study of patients with pulmonary stenosis and intact ventricular septum.* New Eng. J. Med. 258:979, 1958.

28. BASSINGTHWAIGHTE, J. B., PARKIN, T. W., DUSHANE, J. W., WOOD, E. H., AND BURCHELL, H. B.: *The electrocardiogram and hemodynamic findings in pulmonary stenosis with intact ventricular septum.* Circulation 28:893, 1963.

29. GAMBOA, R., HUGENHOLTZ, P. G., AND NADAS, A. S.: *Right ventricular forces in right ventricular hypertension.* Brit. Heart J. 28:62, 1966.

30. HARRIS, P.: *Some variations in the shape of the pressure curve in the human right ventricle.* Brit. Heart J. 17:173, 1955.

31. PAUL, M. H., AND RUDOLPH, A. M.: *Pulmonary valve obstruction during cardiac catheterization.* Circulation 18:53, 1958.

32. GORLIN, R., AND GORLIN, S. G.: *Hydraulic formula for calculation of the area of the stenotic mitral valve, other cardiac valves, and central circulatory shunts.* Amer. Heart J. 41:1, 1951.

33. GORLIN, R., HAYNES, F. W., GOODALE, W. T., SAWYER, C. G., DOW, J. W., AND DEXTER, L.: *Studies of circulatory dynamics in mitral stenosis. II. Altered dynamics at rest.* Amer. Heart J. 41:30, 1951.

34. MOLLER, J. E., AND ADAMS, P., JR.: *A simplified method for calculating the pulmonary valve area.* Amer. Heart J. 72:463, 1966.

35. LEWIS, J. M., MONTERO, A. C., KINARD, S. A., JR., DENNIS, E. W., AND ALEXANDER, J. K.: *Hemodynamic response to exercise in isolated pulmonic stenosis.* Circulation 29: 1964.

36. MOLLER, J. M., AND LUCUS, R. V., JR.: Unpublished observations.

37. LUCAS, R. V., JR., VARCO, R. L., LILLEHEI, C. W., ADAMS, P., JR., ANDERSON, R. C., AND EDWARDS, J. E.: *Anomalous muscle bundles of the right ventricle. Hemodynamic consequences and surgical consideration.* Circulation 25:443, 1962.

38. HARTMANN, A. F., TSIFUTIS, A. A., ARVIDSSON, H., AND GOLDRING, D.: *The two chambered right ventricle.* Circulation 26:279, 1962.

39. WARDEN, H. E., LUCAS, R. V., JR., AND VARCO, R. L.: *Right ventricle obstruction resulting from anomalous muscle bundles.* J. Thorac. Cardiov. Surg. 51:53, 1966.

40. HARTMANN, A. F., JR., GOLDRING, D., AND CARLSSON, E.: *Development of right ventricular obstruction by aberrant muscular bands.* Circulation 30:679, 1964.

41. KORETZKY, E. D., MOLLER, J. H., KORNS, M. E., SCHWARTZ, C. J., AND EDWARDS, J. E.: *Congenital pulmonary stenosis resulting from dysplasia of valve.* Circulation 40:43, 1969.

42. GORLIN, R. J., ANDERSON, R. C., AND BLAW, M.: *Multiple lentigenes syndrome.* Amer. J. Dis. Child. 117:652, 1969.

43. ROWE, R. D.: *Maternal rubella and pulmonary artery stenosis.* Pediatrics 32:180, 1963.

44. HARTMANN, A. F., JR., ELLIOTT, L. P., AND GOLDRING, D.: *The course of peripheral pulmonary artery stenosis in children.* J. Pediat. 73:212, 1968.

45. CAMPBELL, M.: *Valvotomy as a curative operation for simple pulmonary stenosis.* Brit. Heart J. 21:415, 1959.

46. VARCO, R.: *Discussion of a paper by Merlin, W. H., and Longmire, W. F.* Surgery 30:41, 1951.

47. COMMITTEE REPORTS: PREVENTION OF BACTERIAL ENDOCARDITIS. Amer. Heart Association. Circulation 31:948, 1965.

Congenital Aortic Valve Stenosis

Daniel F. Downing, M.D., and
Vladir Maranhão, M.D.

Congenital aortic stenosis has gained increasing attention during the past two decades. Not many years ago, it was thought to be a relatively uncommon anomaly. The growing, but not as yet mature, awareness on the part of physicians of the importance of complete examination of the heart in infants and children has resulted in the recognition that this type of obstruction is not as infrequent in incidence as once was believed. Relatively large series of patients have been presented and there has been a gratifying addition to our knowledge of the natural history of the various forms of the defect. However, there is much yet to be learned. The present study was undertaken with the hope of contributing to our knowledge and of confirming observations of others.

Although the ultimate significance of the different types of aortic stenosis—subvalvular, valvular, and supravalvular—may be the same, there are gross differences that make it unwise to lump them together in considering natural history. For this reason, the current presentation has been confined to valvular obstruction.

Three hundred patients were analyzed. The diagnosis was established in 265 by retrograde left ventricular catheterization, by simultaneous aortic catheterization and left ventricular puncture, by simultaneous brachial artery and left ventricular puncture, by surgery, by autopsy, or by a combination of means. In 35, the left ventricle was not entered because it was impossible to do so or was not attempted. Right heart catheterization was accomplished in 33 of these individuals, as it was in all but a half dozen of the entire series. Sixteen of the thirty-five were operated upon and the diagnosis thus determined. Angiocardiography was diagnostic in one, and autopsy in three. In 15 patients, the diagnosis was decided by clinical means only: murmur, thrill, and dilated ascending aorta.

Excluded were all patients with coexisting anomalies of the right or left heart or great vessels. The presence of aortic insufficiency was allowed if it was felt to be of little or no dynamic importance or if it became significant during the course of continuing observation, increasing regurgitation in this instance being considered part of the natural history of the obstruction.

We believe that any difference in pressure between the left ventricle and ascending aorta, constant on multiple withdrawals of the catheter, is indicative of a degree of aortic stenosis. The range of difference in the present series was 5 to 155 mm. Hg.

CHARACTERISTICS

There were 216 males and 84 females, a ratio of 2.57:1. The age at the time of first examination ranged from 1 month to 54 years. Of the subjects, 153 were under 10 years of age, 88 were 10 to 15 years old, and 30 were between 15 and 20. Birth month and parental age were not significant. There were no unusual pregnancy complications. Eleven patients had been born prematurely and one was a twin. Twenty-three individuals had anomalies of other organ systems, none major; the most frequent were inguinal hernia (4), hemangioma (3), and pectus excavatum (2).

186

Diabetes was present in the immediate families of 31 per cent of the victims. In 20 families, multiple instances of congenital cardiovascular defects were documented. The most common anomaly was aortic stenosis (16 patients).

The initial indication of a cardiac anomaly in almost every patient was the discovery of a murmur. The age of discovery ranged from birth to 39 years: neonatal period in 49, remainder of first year in 37, first to fifth year in 110, fifth to tenth year in 38, tenth to fifteenth year in 31, over fifteen in 7, and unknown in 28.

Weight gain and motor development were almost invariably normal. One child did not sit up unaided until 1 year and did not walk until 2 years. His obstruction was of little physiological significance. Ambulation was delayed to 15 to 19 months in seven others.

A history of pneumonia was elicited in 17 patients. No attempt at verification of the diagnosis was made because only a few had been hospitalized. Significant illness other than this had existed in five, each with a separate entity.

At the time of the initial visit, inquiry was made in regard to undue fatigue (embracing activity from taking formula to participation in sports); shortness of breath; rapid, noisy breathing in infancy, increased perspiration (a wet skin even in cool weather); chest pain; dizziness; faintness; syncope; headache; cough; epistaxis; palpitation; convulsions; edema; and cardiac failure.

All signs and symptoms were denied by parent or patient in 87 instances. Among the remaining 213, single complaints were fatigue in nine, shortness of breath in six, increased perspiration in twenty-three, chest pain in twelve, syncope in six, dizziness in seven, and convulsions in six. The total number with fatigue was 113; with shortness of breath, 81; with increased perspiration, 75; with chest pain, 54; with syncope, 39; with dizziness, 7; and with convulsions, 15. Thirteen patients had experienced cardiac failure.

Only 14 could be considered physically underdeveloped. The rest were normal or, indeed, superior. Twelve were definitely obese. It was striking that many were athletes.

Brown, flat nevi were present on the chest or neck in 72 per cent. In the dermatology literature, these are referred to as junction nevi. Their association with other cardiac defects has been, in our experience, uncommon.

Cardiac enlargement was appreciable in only five patients. The apical impulse was judged to be more vigorous than normal in 40 per cent. A systolic thrill was present in 68 per cent. The thrill was felt in the second and third right interspaces, in the suprasternal notch, over the right carotid artery, or in all three areas, except in four children, in whom it was present at the upper left sternal border. The rate was below 100 beats per minute in 53 per cent, and rapid rates were much less frequent than in any other common cardiac defect. The second sound in the aortic area was faint in twenty-two patients, accentuated in three, and judged normal in the rest.

A systolic murmur was present in all patients. At the time of initial examination, the murmur was more prominent in the second and third right interspaces near the sternal border in 225 (75 per cent). In 16, it was heard equally well in the second and third right and left interspaces. The suprasternal notch was the site in fourteen, the right carotid artery in seven, the second and third left interspaces in thirteen. Commonly, the murmur was harsh, crescendo, and moderately loud. Twenty-five patients initially had their murmurs at the lower left sternal border, with superior radiation. A soft, early diastolic blow was present in 32 patients, most commonly along the left sternal border.

The blood pressure determined by cuff was, in general, low normal in patients who were proved to have the higher degrees of obstruction. In a few of these, however, there was a degree of systolic hypertension.

On X-ray study, there was slight cardiac enlargement in 26 per cent. In 4 per cent, enlargement was graded 2 to 3 plus. The ascending aorta was dilated in 91 per cent. In 28 per cent, the main pulmonary artery was unduly prominent, probably displaced to the left by the dilated aorta. Almost invariably, the left cardiac border was lengthened and rounded. Calcification of the aortic valve was visible in four.

Review of the electrocardiograms revealed seven types of tracings: normal, 82; left axis deviation in children with otherwise normal complexes, 5; left ventricular preponderance (small R, deep S in V_3R–V_1 and R, qR, or Rs in V_6 in children), 101; the same, with left axis deviation, 9; rsr' or variant in V_3R–V_1, 19; left ventricular hypertrophy by voltage criterion (SV_1 plus RV_6 45 mm. or more), 19; and left ventricular strain (ST depression and T-wave inversion in V_5 and V_5), 65.

CORRELATIONS

The significance of the aforementioned characteristics can be related to the severity of the obstruction. This severity was determined in 265 by measurement of pressure, in 16 by operation alone, and in 1 by angiocardiography and autopsy.

Those in whom pressure was measured were divided into six groups on the basis of difference in pressure between left ventricle and ascending aorta or brachial artery (Table 1). Although brachial artery pressure is higher than central aortic, no correction was attempted for this fact. Therefore, the actual difference across the valve in some patients was greater than represented. Without exception, those whose study involved brachial artery puncture fell into the groups with differences above 50 mm. Hg.

When symptoms are analyzed according to pressure, it can be appreciated that there is an increase in affected patients from group to group. It is noteworthy, however, that a significant number in group 1, those with the mildest obstructions, also were symptomatic. Fatigue, shortness of breath, and increased perspiration were the most common complaints.

Thirty-five of the thirty-nine patients with a history of syncope were among those catheterized. They were distributed among all pressure groups. Frequency of episode was no more marked in one group than in another. The

Table 1.

Group	Pressure difference LV–AA or BA (mm. Hg)	Number	Symptoms (%)	Syncope	Chest pain	Congestive failure	Thrill (%)	Diastolic murmur	Electrocardiogram	No.	Per cent
1	5–24	166	52	15	24	0	44	8	N	54	32.0
									LAD	3	1.8
									LVP	68	40.0
									LAD–LVP	7	4.2
									LVH (v)	7	4.2
									LVS	9	5.4
									rsr'	18	10.0
2	24–49	41	68	5	8	1	85	6	N	11	26.0
									LVP	19	46.0
									LAD–LVP	1	
									LVH (v)	5	12.0
									LVS	4	9.7
									rsr'	1	
3	50–74	26	61	7	7	5	100	4	N	4	15.0
									LVP	11	42.0
									LVH (v)	2	7.6
									LVS	9	34.0
4	75–99	13	84	3	4	2	100	1	N	2	15.0
									LVP	1	7.6
									LVH (v)	1	7.6
									LVS	9	69.0
5	100–150	17	76	3	4	1	100	6	N	1	5.8
									LVP	6	35.0
									LVH (v)	1	5.8
									LVS	9	52.0
6	>150	2	100	2	2	0	50	0	LVS	2	100

LV   Left ventricle
AA   Ascending aorta
BA   Brachial artery
N   Normal

LAD   Left axis deviation
LVP   Left ventricular preponderance
LVH (v)   Left ventricular hypertrophy, voltage
LVS   Left ventricular strain

same observations held for the 49 of 54 patients with chest pain who were catheterized.

Fourteen of the fifteen patients who had history of one or more convulsions were catheterized. Ten of these were in group 1, two in group 2, and two in group 5.

Pressures are known for nine of the thirteen patients who had experienced congestive heart failure. The pressure difference was 50 mm. Hg or greater in all but one, in whom it was 30 mm. Hg.

A thrill was present in all patients with a difference across the valve of 34 mm. Hg or greater. Under 25 mm., it was most often felt over the carotid artery or in the suprasternal notch; over 25 mm., in the second and third right interspaces.

At least one normal electrocardiogram was found in all pressure groups but one, that being the highest. 31 per cent of those with differences below 50 mm. Hg showed no abnormality. A left ventricular strain pattern was found in at least some patients in all groups. However, the incidence of this pattern was clearly greatest in those with high pressure. The most common (48 per cent) abnormal pattern involved voltage of R and S in V_3R and V_6 (left ventricular preponderance) and was absent only in group 6.

Four of the patients with two to three-plus cardiac enlargement on X rays had pressure differences of 90 mm. Hg or more. However, in the other two who were catheterized, the figures were 14 and 30 mm. Calcification of the aortic valve occurred in one patient in group 3, two in group 4, and one in group 5. The last was a 3-year-old female.

OBSERVATIONS ON NATURAL HISTORY

Unfortunately, repetitive examination was available to us in only 107 patients. Of these, 60 were followed for more than 5 years, 18 longer than 10 years. The longest period was 20 years. The remaining 47 were seen from one to four times during the 4 years after the initial study.

Of those followed more than 5 years, 13 who were initially asymptomatic developed complaints including fatigue, shortness of breath, chest pain, dizziness, weakness (pressure difference 5 to 110 mm. Hg). A thrill appeared in five (p.d. 10 to 110 mm. Hg), nevi in nine (p.d. 5 to 80 mm. Hg), an early diastolic murmur at the left border in six (p.d. 10 to 103 mm. Hg). In four patients who initially had an early diastolic blow, the murmur became louder and harsher with the passage of time, and the pulse pressure widened as much as 10 mm. Hg. The systolic murmur migrated from the left sternal border to the aortic area in three.

Of those followed under 5 years, symptoms appeared in 11: fatigue, shortness of breath, perspiration, chest pain, syncope (p.d. 5 to 100 mm. Hg). A thrill appeared in one (p.d. 6 mm. Hg), nevi in six (p.d. 6 to 50 mm. Hg), an early diastolic murmur in five (p.d. 11 to 152 mm. Hg). In four patients, the murmur shifted from the left sternal border to the aortic area (p.d. 5 to 102 mm. Hg).

190

Significant electrocardiographic changes occurred in two patients in group 1. In one there was a transition from normality at age 4 to left ventricular hypertrophy (voltage) (LVH(v)) at age 15 (p.d. 10 mm. Hg); in the other, from normality at age 5, when the p.d. was 5 mm. Hg, to an rsr' pattern in $V_3R–V_1$ at age 14, when the p.d. was 24 mm. Hg. In group 2, one patient who showed LVH(v) at 8 years had a strain pattern at age 12 (p.d. 25 mm. Hg). Another changed from normality at age 4 to LVH(v) at age 12 (p.d. 40 mm. Hg), and a third from left ventricular preponderance (LVP) at 6 months to LVH(v) at 3 years (p.d. 42 mm. Hg). In group 3, one individual whose tracing was not remarkable at 4 years showed LVH(v) at 9 years and a strain pattern at 13 (p.d. 65 mm. Hg). The one patient in group 5 whose tracing was normal initially at 10 months of age had LVH(v) at 4 years (p.d. 110 mm. Hg). Another showed transition from LVP at 4 years to LV strain at 10 years (p.d. 110 mm. Hg).

Recatheterization was accomplished in only 10 of the unoperated patients. Eight studies were performed 5 to 12 years after the first, the others at intervals of 3 and 4 years. Four were in group 1 initially, four in group 2, and one each in groups 3 and 4. Pressures remained stable in all but two. These showed an increase in pressure difference of 19 and 11 mm. Hg, respectively, the first being in group 1, the second in group 2. The former was the child whose electrocardiogram changed from normality at age 5 to an rsr' pattern at age 14. One, whose pressure did not change between 7 months and 3 years, showed a change in the electrocardiogram from LVP to LVH(v).

To five patients in the series, death came at ages 10 weeks and 6, 8, 9, and 17 years, respectively (Table 2). In none was left ventricular catheterization accomplished. The infant's obstruction was delineated by angiocardiography, and he was autopsied. In the others, valvular stenosis was diagnosed on the basis of murmur, thrill, and dilated ascending aorta.

R.W. was first seen at 5 weeks, and study was urged. Parents and pediatrician temporized. At 6 weeks, there was an episode of syncope, and at 7 weeks, he became decompensated. At 8 weeks, following digitalization, he was studied and surgery was suggested. At 10 weeks he expired suddenly.

C.R. and W.R. were among the first patients studied. At the time, the available operation appeared inadequate and was not recommended. Both died suddenly some months later while engaged in quiet pursuits.

Table 2. Medical deaths *

Subject	Age	Sex	Syncope	CHF
R. W.	10 wk.	M	+	+
C. R.	6 yr.	M	0	0
W. R.	8 yr.	M	0	0
B. P.	9 yr.	F	+	+
D. S.	17 yr.	F	0	+

* All ECG's showed left ventricular strain.

Surgery was recommended for B.P. when she was studied at age 6 years. Other opinions prevailed, however. At 9 years of age, she died suddenly while at play.

D.S. was studied at 12 years of age and, as with C.R. and W.R., operation was not recommended. Several attempts were made to have her return, but these were unsuccessful. At age 17, she was hospitalized elsewhere with evidence of congestive failure. She appeared to be responding satisfactorily but developed ventricular fibrillation and expired.

DISCUSSION

Rheumatic fever as the cause of aortic stenosis in this series was dismissed because of the age of discovery of the first sign in the majority, because of absence of any evidence of rheumatic involvement historically and lack of involvement of the mitral valve and, in those operated upon, the configuration of the valve.

The lack of symptoms in patients with aortic stenosis is stressed in most publications. In this series, symptoms were not uncommon. Adding to the 213 patients who were symptomatic when first seen the 24 who developed a complaint during the followup period, 79 per cent had manifestations that might be referable to the cardiovascular system. It is true, however, that disability was rare and most victims were significantly less handicapped than those with other defects of comparable importance. Perhaps one reason for the discrepancy between this and other series is the fact that the history was obtained by the same individual in almost all instances.

It must be admitted that it is difficult to ascribe certain symptoms in some patients to the defect. For example, did syncope occur in 15 patients as a result of obstruction that produced a pressure difference across the valve of only 5 to 14 mm. Hg? Did the chest pain in 24 of the same group or the convulsions in 10 result from the mild stenosis? Probably not, yet they may have.

The frequent association of aortic stenosis and brown, flat nevi on the chest or neck has intrigued us for many years. Apparently this correlation has not been noteworthy to others. They were present in 72 per cent on initial examination and appeared subsequently in an additional 15 patients.

Subacute bacterial endocarditis was diagnosed on only one patient. She was first examined at age 12 and had classic signs of valvular stenosis. Two years later, a faint, early diastolic murmur appeared along the left sternal border. At age 17, she developed endocarditis caused by Streptococcus viridans. During the subsequent 6 years, the diastolic murmur became harsh and very prominent, but her peripheral diastolic pressure remained relatively stable.

Calcification of the valve was demonstrable in four patients by X ray. In an additional 10, it was discovered at operation. The youngest patient and only child was a female, age 3, whose pressure difference across the valve was 100 mm. Hg. At operation, calcium was present diffusely in the substance of both the right and left coronary cusps. The noncoronary cusp was diminutive but free of visible calcium. The striking finding was a bulbous calcific

192

mass projecting cephalad from the edge of the valve and measuring about 4 mm. in greatest diameter.

Congestive failure occurred in one infant, three children, and two adolescents. The others with cardiac failure ranged in age from 28 to 59 years. The electrocardiograms of ten showed left ventricular strain; that of one child showed LVH(v), of another, LVP, and of a third, an rSr' pattern in V_3R. The infant and a 6-year-old child died. Operation interrupted the natural history in eight, of whom two died. The remaining three patients are well compensated from 3 to 6 years following the initial episode. That congestive failure does not necessarily mean a very poor prognosis was indicated by two patients who first decompensated 7 and 10 years before surgery.

The value of the electrocardiogram in the assessment of valvular aortic stenosis lies in its reflection of the importance of the burden to the individual at the time the tracing is made. The instrument is not a transducer that measures left ventricular pressure. Rather, it is a method that, in an imperfect way, allows a judgment of the quality of the left ventricular myocardium. A normal electrocardiogram in a patient who has marked left ventricular hypertension has the same clinical value as the finding of left ventricular strain pattern in a patient who has a relatively modest pressure differential across the valve. One may judge that the first individual has an excellent myocardium and that the second has not been so blessed.

The area in which we continue to be relatively ignorant of the natural history of this defect embraces the young patient who has mild to moderate obstruction when first studied. Will the stenosis become relatively more severe over the years? If not, will the existing degree of stenosis have a deleterious effect on the myocardium and shorten life span? It seems clear that the answers will be available only when a large number of patients have been studied and restudied over a period of years. This study will involve a much more liberal use of left ventricular catheterization, extending the procedure to all children who have an aortic systolic murmur and thrill, with repetition at intervals whether or not there has been an observable change in symptoms, signs, X ray, or electrocardiogram.

SUMMARY

The data of 300 patients with congenital aortic valve stenosis were examined with particular attention to the natural history of the condition.

Two thirds of the patients had mild obstruction, but a significant number of these had symptoms and abnormal electrocardiograms. Of those with moderate or severe obstruction, a number were asymptomatic and had normal electrocardiograms.

Repetitive examinations were possible in only 107 patients, and of these only 10 were recatheterized. The changes observed suggest that in some patients with mild original obstruction, there may be a relative increase in severity, but the data were too few to be significant.

We reached the conclusion that only the more liberal use of cardiac catheterization and recatheterization in children with aortic stenosis will allow satisfactory elucidation of the natural history.

Tetralogy of Fallot: Natural Course, Indications for Surgery, and Results of Surgical Treatment

Barbara J. Bourland, M.D.,[*] and
Dan G. McNamara, M.D.

* Supported by NIH Grant IT12HE5756-04.

Distinct differences among patients with tetralogy of Fallot (TF) call for hemodynamic classification [1] so that natural course, indications for surgery, and results of surgical treatment may be discussed. Unlike anomalies such as ventricular septal defect or ductus arteriosus, which, if small, are benign, TF is never benign. A few patients with TF may not have obvious subjective symptoms until fairly late in childhood or even in young adult life, so their early course may resemble that of patients with benign congenital cardiac defects.

To understand the several anatomical, clinical, and hemodynamic differences in TF, it is helpful to know the elements of this anomaly shared by each case.

ANATOMICAL SIMILARITIES AND DIFFERENCES

RIGHT VENTRICULAR OUTFLOW TRACT STENOSIS. The rotated septal limb of the crista supraventricularis narrows the outflow tract in TF with varying severity. Fusion of the pulmonary valve commissures or stenosis of the pulmonary valve annulus or both may be present and may produce more important obstruction than the infundibular stenosis. This infundibular narrowing may be short and located close to the valve, so that on pressure withdrawal of the cardiac catheter, the abrupt change in pressure may create the false impression that the obstruction is entirely valvular. A normal right ventricular outflow tract, as occurs in pulmonary valve stenosis with normal aortic root, is not found in TF. Right ventricular angiocardiography identifies the infundibular stenosis much better than does the pressure tracing (Fig. 1).

ROTATION OF THE OUTFLOW TRACT. The septal limb of the crista supraventricularis in this anomaly has rotated into a superior and leftward direction from the normal location and produces the infundibular narrowing that gives the distinctive angiographic appearance of TF seen in both mild and severe forms (Fig. 2).

LARGE VENTRICULAR SEPTAL DEFECT. Both the mild and the severe forms of tetralogy have a ventricular septal defect (VSD) large enough to allow equalization of pressure between right and left ventricle. Direct relationship of the VSD to the septal limb of the crista occurs in the common form of VSD as it does in TF, but in TF, the septal limb of the crista is rotated leftward and superior. The ventricular communication in TF occasionally may be partially covered by the septal leaflet of the tricuspid valve. Thus, the effective size of the large VSD may be reduced, preventing equalization of pressure between the two ventricles.

DIRECT RELATIONSHIP BETWEEN DEGREE OF OVERRIDING OF AORTA AND SEVERITY OF THE PULMONARY STENOSIS. This feature of TF causes an inverse relationship between the size of the aorta and the size of the pulmonary artery. A small pulmonary artery and a large aorta, while "typical," are not common to every heart with TF; the two vessels may be of nearly equal size

196

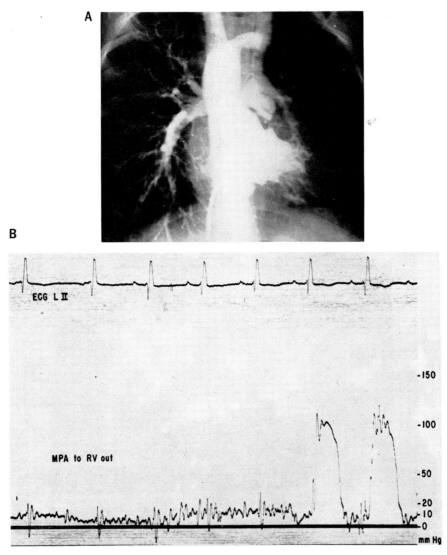

Figure 1. A, right ventricular angiocardiogram demonstrating infundibular stenosis and lateral displacement of the outflow tract in a patient with TF. B, pressure withdrawal tracing in the same patient, demonstrating an abrupt change.

when the two circulations are balanced, or the pulmonary artery may be larger than the aorta in cases with excessive pulmonary blood flow.

HEMODYNAMIC SIMILARITIES AND DIFFERENCES

PRESSURE GRADIENT BETWEEN BODY OF RIGHT VENTRICLE AND PULMONARY ARTERY. The gradient determined at cardiac catheterization may be abrupt, seemingly at the valve (Fig. 1B); more often, it is abrupt but lower than the

197

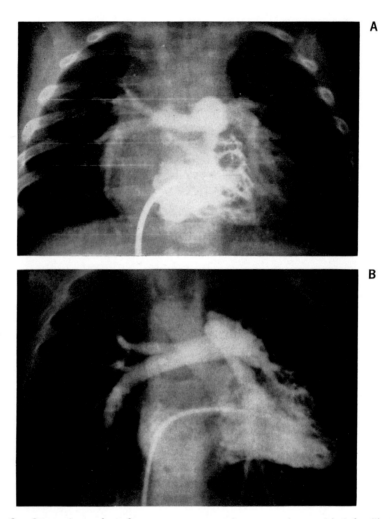

Figure 2. Comparison of outflow tract anatomy in two patients with infundibular stenosis and VSD. In A, a patient without TF and with normal aortic root, the outflow tract is in its normal medial position. In B, a patient with TF, the outflow tract is rotated to the left and lies lateral to the left pulmonary artery.

fluoroscopically estimated position of the valve. Less frequently, two distinct pressure gradients are observed when an infundibular chamber is present and of sufficient dimension to permit the development of a distinct pressure curve (Fig. 3).

PEAK PRESSURE IN THE RIGHT VENTRICLE AT SYSTEMIC LEVEL. Equalization of pressure between right and left ventricles occurs in nearly every instance of tetralogy of Fallot, but even here, there are occasional exceptions. The septal leaflet of the tricuspid valve may partially close the large VSD and prevent the obligatory equalization of pressures. If the infundibular stenosis under this circumstance is mild, then the right ventricular pressure can be

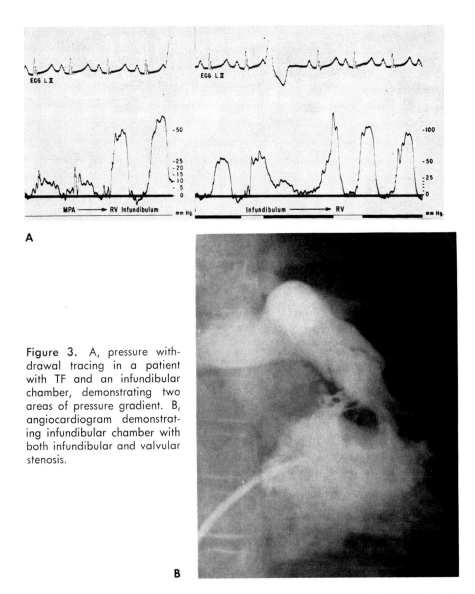

Figure 3. A, pressure withdrawal tracing in a patient with TF and an infundibular chamber, demonstrating two areas of pressure gradient. B, angiocardiogram demonstrating infundibular chamber with both infundibular and valvular stenosis.

less than the systemic, or if the stenosis is quite severe, right ventricular pressure may exceed systemic pressure.

SHUNTING. In the majority of patients with tetralogy of Fallot, the VSD is both anatomically and hemodynamically large, and peak pressure is equal in the right ventricle and left ventricle (or aorta). The size and direction of the shunt then depends upon the relationship between the resistance produced by the infundibular, valvular, or annular stenosis and the resistance offered by the systemic circulation: neither is this relationship constant. The shunting varies in degree with different conditions. Right-to-left shunting through the VSD usually increases with exercise, anxiety, fever,

199

or infection and increases in some patients in a paroxysmal manner. Considering that the patient usually undergoes cardiac catheterization at rest and sedated, the direction and quantity of the ventricular shunt fails to represent the hemodynamic conditions under stress. This lability of shunting appears to be more characteristic of TF than of any other malformation. A careful history obtained from an observant parent often confirms this observation.

CLINICAL CONSIDERATIONS

Variable Cyanosis

The preceding material indicates that both the direction and the quantity of the ventricular shunt differ from one patient to the next. The increase in cyanosis with exercise is unsurprising, but the abrupt increase in cyanosis without obvious precipitation remains baffling. This paroxysmal change could result from either a decrease in systemic arterial resistance or a spasmodic increase in resistance offered by the right ventricular outflow tract stenosis. Drugs such as neo-synephrine can temporarily relieve the spell, presumably by raising systemic resistance; but beta-adrenergic drugs such as propranolol can relieve right ventricular infundibular spasm.[2,3] Morphine has been shown to stop the spell, evidently by its central nervous system action.

Patients with TF may range from those with severe cyanosis through those with mild cyanosis to others with normal color of lips and nail beds. Among those with a normal color, some are found to have a decreased level of arterial oxygen saturation—too slight to be clinically evident—while in others, the saturation is entirely normal. Many children, only faintly cyanotic or not cyanotic at all, have a pronounced intolerance to exercise—a paradox likely to delay proper surgical treatment. This discussion points out that neither a single observation of the patient nor a single determination of the arterial oxygen saturation necessarily reflects the severity of the malformation, unless the observation is made at a time of stress for the patient.

Variable Degree of Polycythemia and Clubbing

A significant and persistently low level of systemic arterial oxygen saturation must be present for polycythemia and clubbing to be present; however, some significantly desaturated patients in early infancy have not had time to develop polycythemia and clubbing. Further, the patient may lack sufficient iron stores in the body to develop polycythemia.

Variable Exercise Tolerance

Exercise intolerance cannot be judged by the hemoglobin level, the degree of clubbing, the visible cyanosis, or a determination of the resting arterial oxygen saturation.[4] This limitation varies considerably with different times of the day and from one day to the next. Extremes of temperature appear to affect the patient's ability to exercise. In the young infant, this limitation is likely to delay motor development, such as walking, and sometimes is mistaken for mental retardation.

Right Ventricular Hypertrophy

Right ventricular hypertrophy is a measurable feature common to all cases of TF. Hypertrophy results from the elevated right ventricular pressure, the one compensatory part of the four elements of the so-called tetralogy. The hypertrophy evidently regresses with successful surgical correction.

Murmur

The murmur in TF with left-to-right shunting is long and plateau ("regurgitant") like that of isolated VSD. However, in typical TF with only right-to-left shunt, the murmur is ejection and results not from the VSD but from the pulmonary stenosis. The more severe the stenosis, the less prominent the murmur. The murmur is absent when there is complete obstruction of the right ventricular outflow tract. Right-to-left shunting through the VSD evidently produces no murmur.

Clinical Types

Patients with TF as seen by the clinician present in one of at least five categories.

Atypical Acyanotic with Left-to-Right Ventricular Shunt

The patient has clinical features of ventricular septal defect with left-to-right shunt. Symptoms in the infant are those of a large left-to-right shunt: tachypnea, sweating, irritability, feeding problems, and growth failure. Radiography shows that both right and left ventricles are dilated (Fig. 4A). The pulmonary vascular markings are increased. The electrocardiogram is interpreted as combined right and left ventricular hypertrophy. Pulmonary stenosis is suspected only by reduced intensity of the second heart sound in the pulmonary area in a patient who, by the other features mentioned, might be suspected of having pulmonary hypertension.

Cardiac catheterization provides the diagnosis by demonstration of pressure gradient between right ventricle and pulmonary artery. If the left-to-right shunt is large, the increased pulmonary flow may elevate pulmonary artery pressure to a level higher than ordinarily expected in pulmonary stenosis. For example, assuming that right ventricular peak systolic pressure is 90 mm. Hg, the pulmonary artery peak systolic pressure might measure 40 mm. Hg in this type of patient. By angiography, the atypical form of tetralogy of Fallot should be suspected by the rotation of the right ventricular outflow tract to the left. The pulmonary artery has a larger caliber than in the cyanotic form of tetralogy of Fallot. During the first few years of

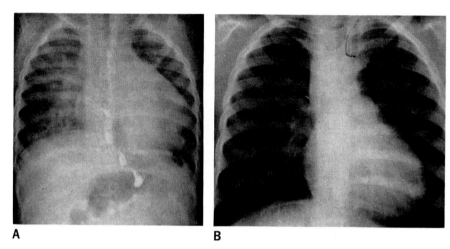

A   B

Figure 4. A, chest roentgenogram of a 10-month-old girl, demonstrating cardiac enlargement and increased size of pulmonary vessels. Right ventricular pressure was at systemic level and there was a left-to-right ventricular shunt. B, at 5 years of age, radiography of chest revealed decrease in heart size and smaller pulmonary vessels. Patient had become cyanotic at rest and developed hypoxemic spells. Hemodynamics at cardiac catheterization were consistent with severe typical TF.

life, patients in this category develop increasing severity of pulmonary (infundibular) stenosis, which reduces the volume of left-to-right shunt and eventually leads to a right-to-left shunt.[5] Along with these changes, the electrocardiogram and radiographic signs of left ventricular enlargement subside, and the heart is no longer dilated (Fig. 4B). It might appear initially that the child is spontaneously recovering from heart disease as he loses the tachypnea and other signs of left-to-right shunt.

Acyanotic Mild Tetralogy of Fallot

Patients in this group may have no symptoms during infancy and early childhood and grow normally. Heart disease is suspected by the loud ejection murmur and by the reduced single second sound. The X ray could be interpreted as normal, so far as heart size and lung vascular markings are concerned, but right ventricular hypertrophy by cardiac contour might be suspected (Fig. 5). The electrocardiogram would be helpful in suspecting tetralogy of Fallot by the presence of right ventricular hypertrophy.

Cardiac catheterization will confirm the diagnosis, provided that the right ventricular and pulmonary artery pressure gradient can be shown and that one can demonstrate ventricular septal defect by passage of catheter from right ventricle to aorta, by angiography from right ventricle, or by indicator dye curves (injecting into the right ventricle and sampling from a systemic artery). Otherwise, ventricular septal defect in this group may not be suspected, since neither left-to-right nor right-to-left shunt is always shown by sampling of blood for oxygen saturation.

Patients with this mild (or subjectively asymptomatic) form of tetralogy

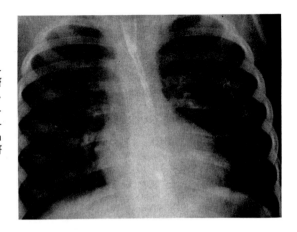

Figure 5. Chest roentgenogram showing normal size of heart and pulmonary vessels— but the cardiac contour suggests RV hypertrophy. The patient, 2 years old, was an acyanotic TF who had spells of paroxysmal hypoxemia.

of Fallot eventually develop symptoms of exercise intolerance, though they may reach adult life without the appearance of resting *visible* cyanosis.

Acyanotic: Severe

This form of tetralogy of Fallot is one of the most difficult anomalies to recognize, much less to understand fully. The patient grows normally and seems well at rest. Frequently spells of paroxysmal dyspnea are mistaken for CNS seizures. These spells occur most commonly in the early morning on awakening, when the physician does not have the opportunity to observe them. By means of a careful history or direct observation of the patient at different times of the day, the nature of the attacks becomes clear.

Physical signs with the patient at rest or between attacks are identical with those of the acyanotic, mild tetralogy of Fallot. During the spell, the systolic ejection murmur disappears. The patient usually has a normal level of hemoglobin; thus, a slight or moderately severe level of arterial oxygen desaturation may go unnoticed. When laboratory measurement is possible, a normal resting oxygen saturation usually is followed by desaturation with exercise or effort (such as crying).

The electrocardiogram and radiographic findings are no different from those in the mild acyanotic case, nor from those of the typical cyanotic patient, for that matter. Likewise, cardiac catheterization and angiocardiography demonstrate similar features. The major difference between the mild and the severe acyanotic TF is their response to exercise.

Typical Cyanotic Form

Characteristically, the "typical" tetralogy of Fallot patient appears cyanotic at birth and for the first week or two, then improves in color to the point that only the trained observer recognizes the abnormal color of the infant's lips and nailbeds. Late in the first year of life, the infant usually begins to show very obvious cyanosis. His activity is fairly limited, so that exercise intolerance is not noticed much and may not be observed until he starts walking.

This infant may or may not have spells of paroxysmal increase in hypoxemia. Spells are difficult to recognize when the observer lacks familiarity with them. They have been misinterpreted as "colic," temper tantrums, "constipation," mild allergy, CNS seizures, and so forth. The patient is always tachypneic and usually seems to be in some discomfort. He may lose consciousness and lie limp for a time; some individuals develop a clonic seizure. Spells are ominous when they occur several times a day, when the spell lasts for 20 or 30 minutes, when the patient has no murmur or a very faint murmur between attacks, and when spells occur in the first 3 months of life and after about 3 years of age.

Severe Cyanotic Tetralogy of Fallot Associated with Main Pulmonary Artery Atresia

Some refer to this anomaly (Fig. 6) simply as "pulmonary atresia," though this term might lead to confusion with pulmonary *valve* atresia with intact ventricular septum or with atresia of both right and left pulmonary artery branches as well as main pulmonary artery (type IV truncus). Some refer to the anomaly as "pseudotruncus," which is convenient for conversation, if not very acceptable semantically. In any event, the anomaly produces symptoms and signs of a very severe tetralogy of Fallot. The natural course of the anomaly is like that of the typical cyanotic tetralogy of Fallot, except that symptoms appear earlier and are more severe. Spells of paroxysmal increase in hypoxemia occur almost invariably. Bronchial artery collaterals form between aorta and right and left pulmonary arteries, but as the ductus

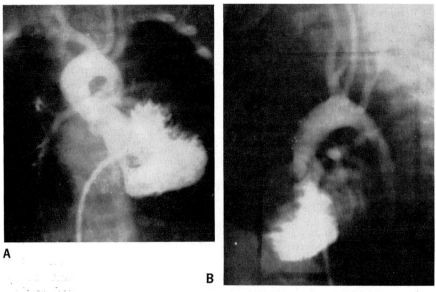

A

B

Figure 6. A, anteroposterior angiocardiogram of a patient with severe cyanotic TF associated with main pulmonary artery atresia, showing the right and left pulmonary arteries filling from a ductus arteriosus. B, simultaneous lateral projection.

closes, spells occur and frequently (though not invariably) end fatally. At times, this malformation is seen in school-age children who have survived the spells in infancy and have gradually improved. The ductus remains open into childhood in a few of these patients. Collateral circulation increases and might produce in some patients a continuous murmur, louder in the axillae and back of the chest than over the heart. Since patients with *only* bronchial artery supply to the lung (type IV truncus) also may develop continuous murmurs, this physical sign does not aid in making this difficult differential diagnosis.

INDICATIONS FOR SURGERY

With a knowledge of what operations are available for treatment of TF and an understanding of the potential variations in this malformation, it is not quite so necessary (and perhaps not even so desirable) to compile a list of what operation to do and when (assuming that such a guide could be devised successfully).

Palliative Operations

Palliative AO-PA shunt surgery generally is performed for the significantly symptomatic infant who is too small to survive total correction necessitating cardiopulmonary bypass. Shunting procedures, however, have problems of their own, including a certain mortality. While successful shunting operations relieve spells of paroxysmal dyspnea and improve exercise tolerance, some of the sequelae and complications of TF are unaffected by a successful shunt. One example is subacute bacterial endocarditis. Another is brain abscess or cerebral emboli, thrombosis, or hemorrhage. Furthermore, a systemic-pulmonary shunt procedure must be occluded when the patient subsequently undergoes intracardiac surgery. The shunt might, in some cases, produce pulmonary hypertension, adding to the morbidity and mortality of the eventual total correction. The shunt operation occasionally leads to irreversible pulmonary vascular obstructive disease, possibly rendering the patient inoperable.

On the other hand, a shunt procedure performed on the cyanotic, polycythemic child can serve to dilate the pulmonary arteries and favorably enlarge the often small left atrium and left ventricle, as well as sustain life. Reduction in polycythemia by a successful shunt carries the added advantage of minimizing bleeding problems, incident to profound polycythemia, at the time of total correction.

Each of the shunt operations has its own particular advantages and disadvantages.

Subclavian Artery-to-Pulmonary Artery Anastomosis (Blalock-Taussig)[6, 7]

ADVANTAGES. The size of the anastomosis is determined by the diameter of the severed end of the artery. In very cyanotic TF, the subclavian artery is found to be of propitiously large size. Heart failure from an excessively

205

large subclavian artery has not occurred in our experience in uncomplicated TF. Heart failure following a subclavian anastomosis usually indicates that the patient has some defect other than TF or some additional defect.

Cardiovascular surgeons generally agree that surgical obliteration of the subclavian-pulmonary artery shunt presents little technical problem at the time of intracardiac repair. The exception is the rarely performed end-to-end rather than the usual end-to-side subclavian-to-pulmonary anastomosis. In end-to-end, the anastomosis must be left undisturbed when the patient undergoes corrective operation.

DISADVANTAGES. In the young infant, the operation reputedly is difficult, and a nonfunctioning shunt has forced many surgeons to use the side of a segment of aorta for the shunt.

Some cardiologists and surgeons object to the sacrifice of subclavian supply to the arm. It is true that the arm so deprived may measure a few millimeters smaller than the opposite arm several years later, but no dysfunction appears to result. Parents must be notified that the arm will lack a pulse following a Blalock-Taussig operation and that auscultatory blood pressure will be unobtainable. The Horner's syndrome so commonly seen in early postoperative period subsides completely. Even those who retain anisocoria have no functional visual disturbance as a result.

Descending Thoracic Aortic-to-Left Pulmonary Artery Anastomosis (Potts) [8]

ADVANTAGES. This operation, once mastered by the surgeon, reputedly is easier and faster to perform than is the subclavian shunt. Even though external inspection of the heart is no more possible than with the approach provided by the subclavian shunt, neither is it necessary to enter the pericardial space.

DISADVANTAGES. The operation cannot easily be done on the right side when there is a right aortic arch unless there should be left pulmonary isomerism, a fortuitous arrangement too rare to count on. The Potts anastomosis cannot be done on the left in a left arch if there is right pulmonary isomerism.

The size of the anastomosis must be carefully controlled—not too large, not too small. Here the built-in control offered by the subclavian anastomosis is lacking. The sometimes unavoidably large shunt may lead to excessive pulmonary flow and heart failure and for those who tolerate and survive an excessive shunt, pulmonary hypertension may occur.

However, these theoretical problems seldom occur, and the only universal objection to the Potts anastomosis is the difficulty in obliterating it surgically at the time of the intracardiac repair.

Ascending Aorta-to-Right Pulmonary Artery Side-to-Side Intrapericardial Anastomosis

Despite the long descriptive title for this operation, there appears to be some difficulty in assigning a suitable eponym.[9, 10, 11, 12]

ADVANTAGES. The operation was devised to simplify surgical obliteration of the shunt at the time of open-heart repair. It has the added advantage of availability whether there is a right or a left aortic arch. In one patient with L-transposition, VSD, and subpulmonary stenosis, this shunt was performed from ascending aorta to left pulmonary artery through a left thoracotomy.

DISADVANTAGES. This shunt unfortunately requires opening into the pericardial space, sometimes resulting in a bothersome pericarditis.

The clinician may be disturbed by the fact that this shunt does not produce the loud, continuous murmur characteristic of the Potts or Blalock-Taussig anastomosis.

"Total Correction" (Intracardiac Repair)[13, 14]

Currently, total correction is recommended for the patient with disabling symptoms who is about 3 years of age or more and for any patient with TF who is about 8 to 10 years of age or older.

For the patient who is less than 18 months old with severe symptoms, a shunt procedure is performed. For the patient between 18 months and 3 years of age, every effort would be made to avoid operation of either type. This happens to be an age at which delay of surgery usually may be safely recommended.

Total correction might better be termed intracardiac repair of TF. Patients are usually greatly improved symptomatically by the operation, and a few have virtually normal dynamics, but many with good clinical result have persistent though mild pulmonary stenosis, and a few patients with a spectacular symptomatic result have a persistent ventricular communication.

Discussion

This paper does not propose to present a statistical analysis of results of operations based on postoperative cardiac catheterization. While it is our intention to recatheterize all patients with TF following intracardiac repair, this recommendation is a difficult thing for the parent and the patient to accept when the progress is good. The studies unfortunately more often are performed in the patient who may not have a good result.

It may be difficult to assess clinically the result of intracardiac repair of TF, because a systolic murmur often persists in the patient with a good result. This murmur may be the result of mild pulmonary stenosis, some deformity of the tricuspid valve, or even a small persistent ventricular communication. It could result from an additional unrecognized defect, such as stenosis of a branch of the pulmonary artery or a deformity of the mitral valve. Thus, a persistent murmur following the operation frequently is heard and may or may not represent an important lesion. A pulmonary insufficiency murmur, common following the repair in which pulmonary annulotomy is necessary, does not imply a poor result.

The ECG is not too helpful in evaluating the postoperative result, since

207

right branch bundle block incident to the surgery renders the QRS voltage and R:S ratio invalid as criteria for ventricular hypertrophy.

Radiographic appearance of heart size and contour does not provide reliable information about the hemodynamic result, since a moderate increase in heart size follows successful repair. Great cardiac enlargement, of course, would be an ominous sign following operation. It appears that pulmonary insufficiency, while perhaps not life-threatening, does lead to right ventricular and right atrial dilatation. If the postoperative pulmonary artery pressure is elevated, for whatever reason, then pulmonary insufficiency becomes functionally more important.

In the normal heart, the maximal peak right ventricular (RV) pressure in the resting state is 30 mm. Hg. In patients with congenital pulmonary stenosis and intact ventricular septum, a peak pressure in RV of 50 mm. Hg or less is considered mild.

Among 53 patients who are doing well objectively and subjectively following corrective surgery and on whom postoperative catheterization data are available, 10 have a normal RV peak systolic pressure of 30 mm. Hg or less. Thirteen patients have a peak RV pressure between 30 mm. Hg and 40 mm. Hg and thirty patients between 40 and 50 mm. Hg.

It would appear from the benign course of patients with mild pulmonary stenosis and an RV peak systolic pressure of 50 mm. Hg or less that this degree of RV pressure is acceptable in predicting a relatively normal existence for them.

A few preliminary studies indicate that the exercise ability may be reduced in the patient with corrected TF despite a good resting hemodynamic result. However, since the operation is done sometimes as a life-saving procedure or to relieve disabling symptoms, it becomes relatively unimportant that it may not enable the patient to become an unrestricted athlete. In our enthusiasm to secure patient and parent approval for operation, we should not promise future gridiron glory; but we can anticipate a remarkable relief of symptoms, sufficient for the patient to plan an education, a gainful occupation, and a family life.

References

1. McCord, M. C., Van Elk, J., and Blount, S. G., Jr.: *Tetralogy of Fallot. Clinical and hemodynamic spectrum of combined pulmonary stenosis and ventricular septal defect.* Circulation 16:736, 1957.

2. Cumming, G. R., and Carr, W.: *Relief of dyspnoeic attacks in Fallot's tetralogy with propranolol.* Lancet 1:519, 1966.

3. Eriksson, B. O., Thoren, C., and Zettergvist, P.: *Long-term treatment with propranolol in selected cases of Fallot's tetralogy.* Brit. Heart J. 31:37, 1969.

4. Gold, W. M., Mattioli, L. F., and Price, A. C.: *Response to exercise in patients with tetralogy of Fallot with systemic-pulmonary anastomoses.* Pediatrics 43:781, 1969.

5. Gasul, B. M., Dillon, R. F., Vrla, V., and Hait, G.: *Ventricular septal defects: Their natural transformation into those with infundibular stenosis or into the cyanotic or noncyanotic type of tetralogy of Fallot.* J.A.M.A. 164:847, 1957.

208

6. BLALOCK, A., AND TAUSSIG, H. B.: *The surgical treatment of malformations of the heart in which there is pulmonary stenosis or pulmonary atresia.* J.A.M.A. 128:189, 1945.

7. TAUSSIG, H. B., CRAWFORD, H., PELARGNIO, S., AND ZACHARIOUDAKIS, S.: *Ten to thirteen year follow-up on patients after a Blalock-Taussig operation.* Circulation 25:630, 1962.

8. POTTS, W. J., SMITH, S., AND GIBSON, S.: *Anastomosis of the aorta to a pulmonary artery.* J.A.M.A. 132:627, 1946.

9. COOLEY, D. A., AND HALLMAN, G. L.: *Intrapericardial aorto-right pulmonary artery anastomosis.* Surg. Gynec. Obstet. 122:1084, 1966.

10. WATERSON, D. J.: *The treatment of Fallot's tetralogy in infants under the age of one year.* Rozhl Chir. 41:183, 1962.

11. FULLER, D.: *Aorta-right pulmonary artery anastomosis.* S. Afr. J. Surg. 3:117, 1965.

12. EDWARDS, W. S., MOHTASHEMI, M., AND HOLDEFER, W. F., JR.: *Ascending aorta to right pulmonary artery shunt for infants with tetralogy of Fallot.* Surgery 59:316, 1966.

13. KIRKLIN, J. W., ELLIS, F. H., JR., McGOON, D. C., DuSHANE, J. W., AND SWAN, H. J. C.: *Surgical treatment of the tetralogy of Fallot by open intracardiac repair.* J. Thorac. Cardiov. Surg. 37:22, 1959.

14. KIRKLIN, J. W., WALLACE, R. B., McGOON, D. C., AND DuSHANE, J. W.: *Early and late results after intracardiac repair of tetralogy of Fallot: Five-year review of 337 patients.* Amer. Surg. 162:578, 1965.

Transposition of the Great Arteries: Recognition and Management

Elizabeth Fisher, M.D., and
Milton H. Paul, M.D.

Transposition of the great arteries (TGA) is a common and lethal congenital cardiac malformation.[1, 2] In recent years, the prognosis has been altered dramatically and extensively with the development of a succession of palliative and corrective procedures. TGA has been estimated to occur in 1 per 2,000 live births, causes 15 to 20 per cent of all infant deaths from heart disease in the first month of life, and is responsible for about 15 per cent of all deaths resulting from congenital heart disease. Without treatment, about 50 per cent of these infants die within the first month of life, 70 per cent within 6 months and 90 per cent within the first year. Early diagnosis and prompt palliative treatment are essential for the survival of these critically ill infants to an older age, when surgical correction becomes feasible.

ANATOMY

Defined literally, TGA means that the great arteries are abnormally placed across the interventricular septum, and consequently, the aorta and pulmonary artery arise from the wrong ventricle. Thus, the aortic root is abnormally anterior and arises from the right ventricle; the main pulmonary artery is abnormally posterior and arises from the left ventricle (Fig. 1). This discussion will be restricted to the common form of TGA, also termed complete (simple) dextro (D-) transposition of the great arteries.[3] The modifying term "dextro-" implies that the abnormal anteroposterior positioning of the great arteries is associated with normal or usual right-left disposition of atria, ventricles, and great arteries, and is derived from the normal embryological right (dextro) looping of the cardiac tube. In contrast, levo (L-) TGA, a consequence of abnormal left (levo) looping of the cardiac tube, manifests inversion (right-left reversal) of the great arteries as well as transposition (anteroposterior reversal). In L-TGA, the ventricular chambers also are inverted, making the morphologically right ventricle left-sided relative to the morphologically left ventricle. Additional useful morphological landmarks in complete D-TGA (Fig. 2) relate to the abnormal presence of subaortic conus musculature (parietal band) and the absence of normal subpulmonary conus.

The term "complete" (simple) implies the usual anatomical D-transposition of the great arteries malformation, as contrasted with other types of abnormalities with malpositioned aorta or so-called partial transpositions, such as double outlet right ventricle, Taussig-Bing anomaly, and transposition complexes with single-ventricle pathology.

The modifying term "complete" is also understood to refer physiologically to an uncorrected transposition; i.e., systemic venous blood going to the aorta and pulmonary venous blood to the pulmonary artery, as opposed to the modifying term "corrected," which indicates that despite the presence of anatomic transposition, systemic venous blood is directed to the pulmonary artery and pulmonary venous blood to the aorta (Fig. 1); i.e., physiologically corrected transposition.[3]

Complete D-TGA commonly occurs as an isolated abnormality with an

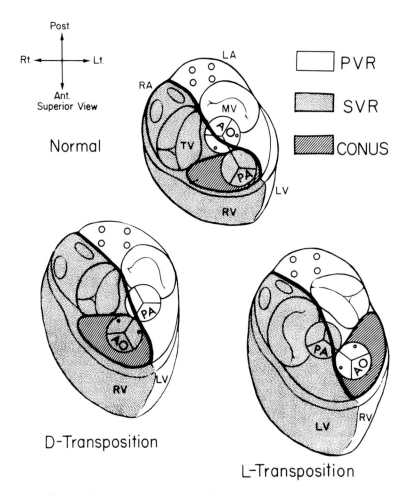

Figure 1. Abnormal anatomical and physiological relationships in D- and L-TGA. In the normal, note: (1) the *right posterior* position of the aorta (AO) arising from the left-sided morphologically left ventricle (LV), (2) the *subpulmonary conus* of normally related great arteries, and (3) the desaturated systemic venous return (SVR) being directed to the pulmonary circulation (RA→RV→PA) and the oxygenated pulmonary venous return (PVR) being directed to the systemic circulation (LA→LV→AO). In D-TGA, note: (1) the *right anterior* position of the aorta arising from the right-sided morphologically right ventricle (RV), (2) the *right-sided subaortic conus* of typical D-TGA, and (3) the desaturated systemic venous return being redirected to the systemic circulation (RA→RV→AO) and the oxygenated pulmonary venous return to the pulmonary circulation (LA→LV→PA). In L-TGA (usual type of "corrected" transposition), note: (1) the *left anterior* position of aorta arising from the left-sided morphologically right ventricle (= bulboventricular inversion); (2) the *left-sided subaortic conus* of typical L-TGA; and (3) despite transposition of the great arteries, a normal *physiological* pathway for SVR (RA→LV→PA) and PVR (LA→RV→AO).

213

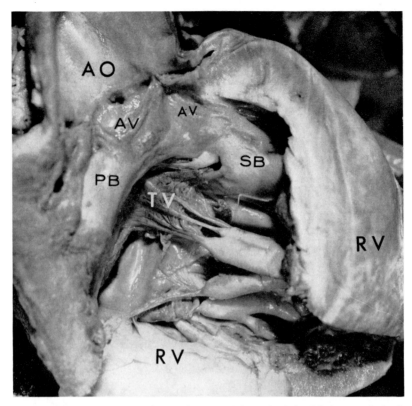

Figure 2. Typical anatomy of complete D-TGA. RV, right-sided, morphologically right ventricle; PB, subaortic conus, i.e., parietal band; SB, septal band joins with the PB to form arch, crista supraventricularis; AO, transposed aorta with subaortic conus resulting in aortic valve (AV)-tricuspid valve (TV) fibrous discontinuity.

intact ventricular septum (IVS), but may be associated with ventricular septal defect (VSD), patent ductus arteriosus (PDA), or various forms of left ventricular outflow tract or pulmonary valve stenosis (PS). TGA may be associated with other major malformations, such as tricuspid atresia, single ventricle, severe coarctation, common atrioventricular canal, pulmonary atresia, and dextrocardia, but this presentation will exclude all such complicated forms.

PHYSIOLOGY

The dominant physiological abnormalities in TGA are hypoxemia and congestive heart failure. Hypoxemia results from large quantities of systemic venous return re-entering the aorta directly without traversing the pulmonary circulation. Congestive heart failure results from excessive cardiac pressure and flow work.

In the normal infant, the systemic and pulmonary circulations function as a series circuit, with desaturated systemic venous return traversing the right heart, being oxygenated in the pulmonary circulation, and returning to the left ventricle for ejection into the systemic circulation (Fig. 3).

In the infant with TGA, the systemic and pulmonary circulations function as parallel circuits. The systemic venous return to the right heart is re-ejected directly into the aorta and systemic circulation, only to return again to the right heart. The oxygenated pulmonary venous return to the left heart is ejected from the left ventricle back into the pulmonary circulation, with resulting purposeless recirculation through the lungs.

The independent, parallel circulation pathways imposed by the transposition anatomy preclude survival unless there is an adequate exchange of oxygenated and unoxygenated blood between the pulmonary (left heart) and systemic (right heart) circulations. Intracardiac shunting may occur at both the atrial or ventricular levels, and extracardiac shunting may occur through a patent ductus arteriosus or pulmonary collateral vessels.[4]

The volume of these life-sustaining, cross-circulation shunts may be estimated from the effective pulmonary blood flow (EPF), since this is a measure of the amount of systemic venous return that ultimately traverses and is oxygenated in the pulmonary circulation. There must be an equal and opposite (pulmonary to systemic) shunt to maintain volume equilibrium within the pulmonary and systemic vascular beds. This shunt is a measure of the effective systemic blood flow in TGA; i.e., that volume of pulmonary venous return that eventually traverses the systemic circulation and delivers oxygen to the body.

In infants with TGA and an intact ventricular septum (TGA with IVS), bidirectional shunting (pulmonary ⇆ systemic) occurs at the patent foramen ovale opening. This shunt volume often is quite small and is determined by the size of this opening. In most infants with TGA, the pulmonary blood flow is quite increased, representing a rapidly recirculating blood volume, with resulting increased left heart volumes and elevated left atrial pressures. Resting systemic blood flow also is commonly increased in the more cyanotic infants, and significantly narrowed arteriovenous oxygen-saturation differ-

Figure 3. Normal and D-TGA circulation pathways. Black solid line and arrows represent pathway of unsaturated mixed venous return; open line and arrows, pathway of oxygenated pulmonary venous blood; broken-line arrows, cross-circulation shunts.

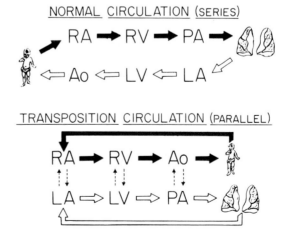

215

ences and peripheral vasodilation are observed. The ductus arteriosus is patent in about half the infant patients, but the lumen usually is small and of little clinical consequence.

When TGA is associated with a large VSD, a second site for bidirectional shunting is present. Cyanosis is less notable in these infants because, proportionately, a larger volume of pulmonary venous return enters the aorta.

When TGA with VSD is associated with significant pulmonary stenosis (PS) such as to restrict pulmonary blood flow, cyanosis again is intense because of the reduced volume of blood oxygenated in the lung.

The pulmonary vascular bed resistance is of prime importance in considering compensatory shunt mechanisms, clinical prognosis, and surgical management. TGA infants with IVS or a small VSD, and also TGA with a large VSD with significant PS or surgical pulmonary artery banding will maintain a favorably low pulmonary artery to aorta peak systolic pressure ratio (PA:AO), and these patients usually do not demonstrate progressive pulmonary vascular obstruction in infancy or early childhood (Fig. 4). In contrast, infants with persisting large VSD manifest pulmonary hypertension

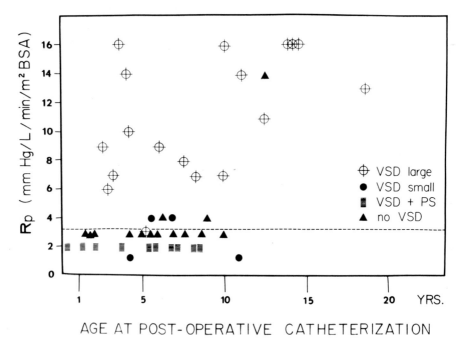

AGE AT POST-OPERATIVE CATHETERIZATION

Figure 4. Estimated pulmonary vascular resistance (Rp) in TGA patients 1 to 9 years after palliative surgery (partial venous correction). The pulmonary artery was entered in 35 of 46 patients studied by cardiac catheterization. Note that all TGA patients with a large VSD (by angiocardiographic criteria) had a significantly elevated Rp, with one exception in a child with previous palliative pulmonary artery banding. In contrast, patients with TGA with IVS, TGA with small VSD, or TGA with large VSD and PS did not manifest physiological pulmonary vascular obstructive changes and had normal Rp, with one exception in a child with TGA and IVS who had a systemic-pulmonary anastomosis performed in infancy.

216

of systemic level, and by about 12 months of age, most have a significantly elevated pulmonary vascular resistance. The wide extent of histological pulmonary vascular obstructive changes observed even in young infants [5] suggests that TGA is associated with an accelerated, more malignant pulmonary vascular obstructive process than that in infants with normal great artery relationships and large VSD.

The various anatomical and physiological subgroups of TGA can be integrated into a useful clinical classification.[6]

I. TGA (IVS): with increased pulmonary blood flow and intact ventricular septum

II. TGA (VSD): with increased pulmonary blood flow and significant ventricular septal defect

III. TGA (VSD & PVO): with restricted pulmonary blood flow, ventricular septal defect and pulmonary vascular obstruction

IV. TGA (VSD & PS): with restricted pulmonary blood flow, ventricular septal defect and pulmonary stenosis

CLINICAL FEATURES

Cyanosis, congestive heart failure, hypoxemic deterioration, and early death characterize the clinical course of TGA without palliative intervention. Infants with TGA with IVS (group I) have obvious clinical difficulties early in the first days or weeks of life (Fig. 5) and manifest intense and increasing cyanosis accompanied by signs of severe hypoxemia, such as tachypnea, tachycardia, weakness, and hypothermia.

Infants with large VSD (group II) usually manifest symptoms somewhat later in the first weeks or months of life, and have less intense cyanosis than do group I infants, but more prominent signs of congestive heart failure, such as tachypnea, tachycardia, weakness, anorexia, hepatomegaly, and cardiomegaly.

Anoxic spells, characterized by prolonged labored breathing with increasing cyanosis but without unconsciousness or convulsion, may occur particularly in group I infants. These anoxic spells are a consequence of inadequate intracardiac shunting with resultant hypoxemic metabolic acidosis and herald clinical deterioration and early death.

Infants having TGA with VSD and PS (group IV) with significantly diminished pulmonary blood flow present many clinical features similar to severe tetralogy of Fallot and indeed require similar surgical palliative procedures to increase the pulmonary blood flow with a systemic-to-pulmonary shunt.

Generally, patients with TGA and VSD do not present with advanced pulmonary vascular obstruction (group III) early in infancy but rather demonstrate progressive pulmonary vascular obstructive physiology toward the end of the first year of life and later. Again, because of more adequate intracardiac pulmonary-to-systemic mixing at the VSD level, cyanosis is less intense than in group I children until late deterioration.

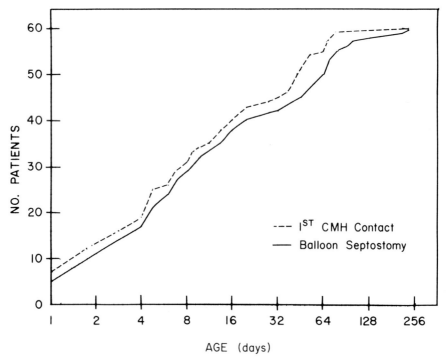

Figure 5. Age (days) of 60 infants with D-TGA at time of admission to Children's Memorial Hospital (first CMH contact) and time of cardiac catheterization (balloon septostomy). TGA with IVS, 32 infants; TGA with VSD, 28 infants. Note that about half the infants had hospital admission and balloon atrial septostomy by 8 days of age.

AUSCULTATION

Auscultation is not particularly helpful in recognizing infants with TGA and is of only limited value in diagnosing the associated lesions.

The aortic and pulmonary components of the second heart sound have maximum intensity at the upper left sternal border. Although frequently closely split, the two components often are interpreted as a single loud aortic valve closure sound.

Infants with TGA and IVS may have a low-intensity systolic ejection murmur along the left sternal border, probably resulting from the increased blood flow across the left ventricular outflow tract. A low-frequency mid-diastolic rumble also may be heard at the apex. In many group I infants, no significant systolic or diastolic murmurs are present.

Infants with TGA and VSD usually have more significant auscultatory findings. After the first weeks of life, harsh, loud, almost pansystolic murmurs are heard, sometimes associated with a precordial thrill. These infants with VSD more commonly also present an apical mid-diastolic rumble and gallop third heart sound.

Infants with TGA, VSD, and significant PS have an ejection systolic murmur of moderate intensity along the mid left sternal border, often characterized by transmission to the right upper sternal border.

218

Development of pulmonary vascular obstruction eventually modifies the auscultatory findings in TGA with large VSD. An attenuated intensity and shortened duration of the systolic murmur is noted, and eventually the murmurs of pulmonary and mitral valve insufficiency result from massive cardiac dilatation.

ELECTROCARDIOGRAM (ECG)

In TGA, there should be expected ECG evidence for abnormal right ventricular hypertrophy, since the right ventricle is systemic in function. Since the normal newborn heart has significant right ventricular myocardial mass as a consequence of the intra-uterine circulation, it may not be possible, by ECG criteria, to establish the presence of abnormal right ventricular hypertrophy in the newborn infant with TGA during the first week of life.[3] After the first week, however, persistence of upright (anteriorly oriented) T waves over the right precordium can signify the persistence of an abnormal right ventricular load despite the absence of QRS axis and voltage criteria of abnormality (Fig. 6).

In general, infants with TGA with IVS, TGA with small VSD, and TGA

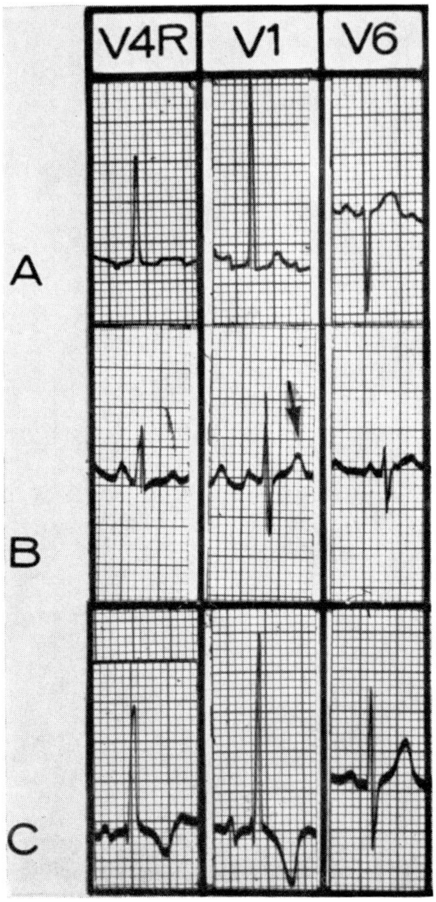

Figure 6. Electrocardiograms (precordial leads V₄R, V₁, V₆). A, TGA with IVS, 2 days old, with evident abnormal right ventricular hypertrophy. B, TGA with IVS, 5 days old, with persistent upright T waves (arrow) over right precordium suggesting persistent abnormal right ventricular load. C, TGA with large VSD, 2 years old, with combined ventricular hypertrophy.

with VSD and PS show right atrial hypertrophy, right axis deviation, and right ventricular hypertrophy by 1 or 2 months of age. Most infants with a large VSD have normal or right axis deviation and combined ventricular hypertrophy.[7]

ROENTGENOGRAMS

In a cyanotic infant, the chest X ray is the single most helpful clinical item in suggesting the diagnosis of TGA (Figs. 7, 8). The important findings of diagnostic value are: (1) cardiac enlargement, often progressing from a normal heart size at birth; (2) oval or egg-shaped cardiac configuration; (3) narrow superior mediastinum (vascular pedicle); and (4) increased pulmonary vascular markings, except when PS is advanced.

Characteristically (and treacherously), the heart may be nearly normal in size during the first week or two of life (Fig. 8A), but thereafter, enlargement is usual. Cardiac enlargement may be minimal in the rare older child with IVS and a large interatrial communication or in those who have maximally

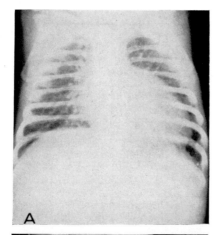
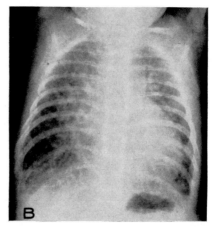
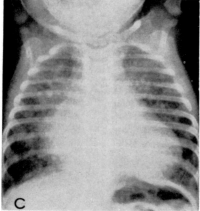

Figure 7. Frontal chest roentgenograms. A, TGA with IVS, 4 weeks old, with classical oval heart configuration (egg on side), narrow vascular pedicle, and increased pulmonary vascular markings. B, TGA with VSD, 8 weeks old, with wider vascular pedicle but typical oval heart. C, TGA with VSD and mild PS, 12 weeks old, with increased pulmonary vascular markings.

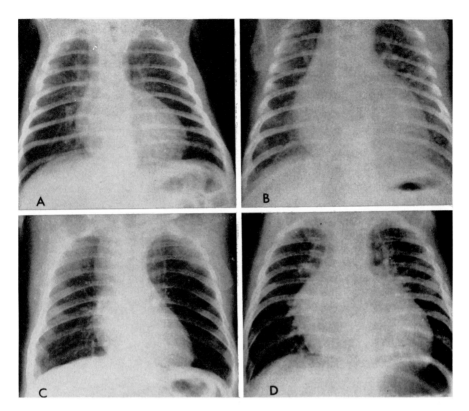

Figure 8. Frontal chest roentgenograms. A, TGA with IVS, 2 weeks old, oval heart configuration, increased pulmonary vascular markings, but minimal cardiac enlargement. B, TGA with IVS, 6 weeks old, marked cardiac enlargement following clinically unsuccessful balloon atrial septostomy. C, TGA with VSD and fibromuscular tunnel subpulmonary stenosis (PS), 4 months old, without cardiac enlargement and diminished pulmonary vascular markings. D, TGA with large VSD, 8 months old, with marked cardiomegaly and increased pulmonary vascular markings.

benefited from palliative surgery and, also, in patients with TGA, VSD, and significant PS.

The characteristic oval cardiac configuration and narrow vascular pedicle are observed in only about half the TGA infants, primarily those with IVS. Right aortic arch is rare in TGA, in contrast to a 25 to 30 per cent incidence in the other common cyanotic congenital cardiac malformation, tetralogy of Fallot.

The assessment of the pulmonary vascular markings during the first week of life is difficult, and in TGA with IVS, the pulmonary vasculature may appear normal at first, just as the heart size often appears near normal at first. The fact that the vascular markings are not diminished in the first week of life helps to exclude severe tetralogy or pulmonary atresia and to implicate TGA as the cause of cyanosis.

DEFINITIVE DIAGNOSIS:
CARDIAC CATHETERIZATION-ANGIOCARDIOGRAPHY

Newborn infants with significant persistent cyanosis should have evaluation by a team experienced in the diagnosis and management of infants with congenital heart disease.

Successful management of infants with TGA requires: (1) prompt initiation of supportive medical therapy, such as oxygen, digoxin, diuretics, acid-base correction, and antibiotics; (2) early establishment of the correct diagnosis; and (3) appropriate palliative treatment with the least possible delay.

The diagnosis of TGA is established by cardiac catheterization and angiocardiography. The catheterization should be viewed as an emergency procedure because of the critical condition of many of these infants and because balloon catheter septostomy during the catheterization procedure is a very effective initial palliative therapy.

In the newborn and very young infant, the hazards of catheterization are minimized by: (1) a staff skilled and experienced with infant cardiac patients, (2) maintaining optimum body temperature with external thermal regulating devices, (3) avoiding cardiopulmonary depression from sedation, (4) providing humidified 100 per cent oxygen during the preparatory and angiocardiographic phases of the procedure, (5) treating metabolic acidosis with appropriate intravenous sodium bicarbonate or amine buffer therapy, (6) restricting angiocardiographic media dosage to the essential minimum, (7) replacing significant procedural blood losses, and (8) instituting endotracheal intubation and artificial ventilation if cardiorespiratory depression is extreme because of hypoxemic acidosis.

The diagnosis of TGA is most directly confirmed by selective ventricular angiocardiography (Fig. 9). In the critical newborn infant, particularly with IVS, it is our policy to restrict initial angiocardiography to a single confirming injection into the left ventricle. Then, after proceeding directly with palliative balloon septostomy, additional right and left ventricular and ascending aortic injections are performed to establish whether VSD, PS, or patent ductus arteriosus is present.

With the diagnosis confirmed, nonsurgical enlargement or creation of an atrial septal defect should be carried out with a balloon catheter before proceeding in the newborn with useful but nontherapeutic intensive hemodynamic investigations.

The assessment of pulmonary artery pressures, pulmonary blood flow, and pulmonary vascular resistance is particularly important in older infants and children with ventricular septal defect, since advanced pulmonary vascular obstructive changes preclude safe corrective surgery at present. The pulmonary artery usually can be entered easily and directly during manipulation of the catheter in the right ventricle whenever a large VSD is present. When not entered by this route, and in TGA with IVS, the pulmonary artery can be entered from the left ventricle by resorting with gentle persistence to either a soft regular cardiac catheter coiled back upon itself within the left

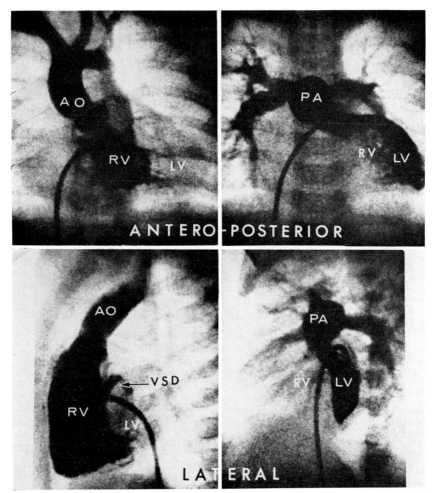

Figure 9. Selective right and left ventricular angiocardiograms in 11 week old infant with TGA and small ventricular septal defect. RV, right ventricle; LV, left ventricle; AO, aorta; PA, pulmonary artery; VSD, ventricular septal defect.

ventricle or to a flow-guided polyethylene tube, or directly by percutaneous suprasternal puncture.

It should be noted that the Fick principle is valid in calculating the systemic and pulmonary blood flow in TGA despite the parallel circuit configuration. However, limitations in analytical precision together with a very narrow pulmonary-arteriovenous oxygen saturation difference and the uncertainty of the volume of pulmonary collateral circulation preclude any high accuracy.

PALLIATIVE TREATMENT

The ingenious technique described by Rashkind and Miller [8] in 1966 has provided an effective and safe initial palliation in 90 per cent of our experience with 60 TGA infants. This atrial septostomy is performed by introducing a balloon-tipped catheter (preferably as large as feasible, 5.5 to 6.5 F) into the femoral vein and advancing the tip through the right atrium across the patent foramen ovale into the left atrium. The current balloons can be inflated with 2 to 5 ml. of dilute radiopaque material and should attain a diameter of at least 14 to 18 mm. to effect a satisfactory atrial septal defect (Fig. 10). The inflated balloon is forcefully and rapidly withdrawn from the left to the right atrium and thus tears the shunt-limiting septum primum flap covering the fossa ovalis (Fig. 11). Gratifying clinical improvement usually is noted immediately, with a fall in left atrial hypertension and a rise in systemic arterial oxygen saturation (Fig. 12). The procedure should be repeated several times in succession until a reasonably large and tense balloon (3-ml. volume, equivalent to about 15-mm. diameter) can be easily withdrawn across the interatrial opening. Certainty as to the placement of the balloon in the left atrium rather than in the right or left ventricle or pulmonary vein prior to inflation and withdrawal is essential to avoid serious cardiac trauma. A double lumen catheter with pressure monitoring is helpful, as is anatomic confirmation by viewing the catheter positioned posteriorly in the left atrium with the infant turned in the lateral view. Nonsurgical creation of an atrial septal defect has the obvious advantages of avoiding the risks of thoracotomy and general anesthesia in the critically ill infant and preserving the pericardium unscarred for later use in a definitive corrective operation.

A few clinics have reported satisfactory long-term palliation with this

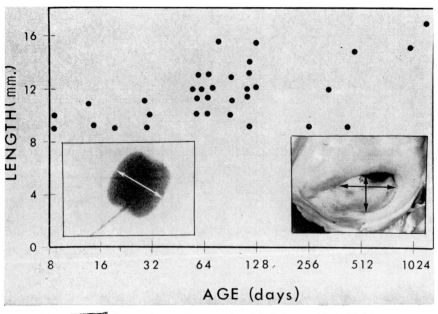

Figure 10. Fossa ovalis, maximum diameter (mm.) in infants with D-TGA. Septostomy catheter (6.5 F) with 4-ml. inflation of balloon, resulting in 17-mm. diameter.

224

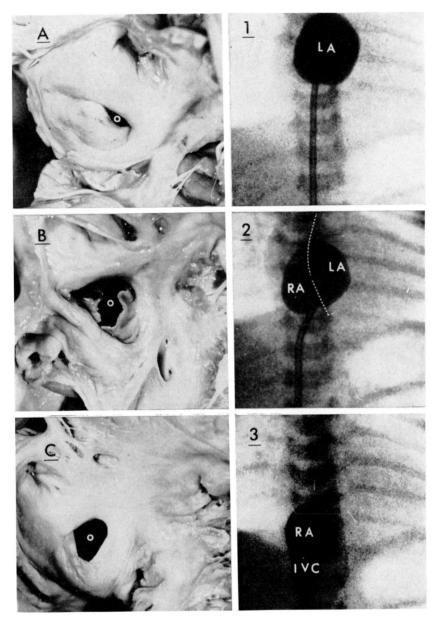

Figure 11. Nonsurgical creation or enlargement of atrial septal defect with balloon catheter. 1, 2, 3; individual cine frames illustrating atrial septostomy. 1, balloon inflated with 3 ml. radiopaque media in left atrium (LA). 2 and 3, balloon is withdrawn rapidly through patent foramen ovale into right atrium (RA) and inferior vena cava (IVC) with tearing of the shunt-limiting septum primum valve of the foramen ovale. A, B, C; pathology of foramen ovale openings, right atrial view. A, oval opening, patent foramen ovale (O) in 10-week-old infant with TGA and large VSD. The septum primum valve was unusually thick and fibrotic and resistant to balloon septostomy. B, infant with TGA and IVS, expired 6 hours after septostomy. Note long linear tear in septum primum valve. C, infant with TGA and IVS had a clinically successful septostomy at 7 days of age. A cerebral vascular accident and death occurred at 8 months of age. Note large nonsurgically created atrial septal defect.

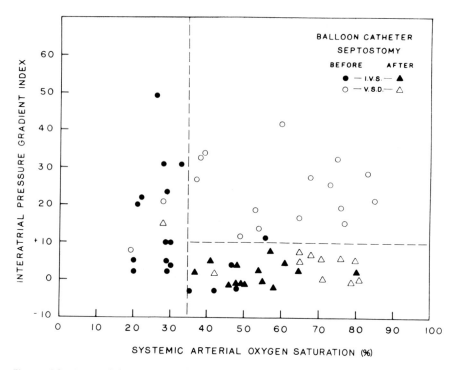

Figure 12. Interatrial pressure gradient index and systemic arterial oxygen saturation response to balloon atrial septostomy. Indices greater than 10 represent significant left atrial hypertension relative to right atrial pressures.

technique, permitting most of their patients to await corrective surgery at 18 or 24 months of age.[9] Other clinics, however, are continuing to resort to surgical creation of a larger atrial septal defect some time after the initial nonsurgical emergency atrial septostomy, because surgical septostomy provides higher, more nearly optimum systemic oxygen saturations (greater than 70 per cent oxygen saturation in TGA with IVS) and less symptomatic infants during the 2- to 3-year waiting interval.[10]

Our observations on 60 infants with TGA and balloon atrial septostomy confirm the dramatic, life-saving initial therapeutic value and the frequent long-term effective palliation, but in some infants, inadequate increases in systemic oxygen saturation have occurred despite vigorous and repeated application of the procedure, and surgical intervention was clearly indicated (Table 1). Atrial septostomy is indicated in TGA infants with VSD and relatively high systemic oxygen saturation, as well as in TGA infants with IVS, since the left atrial pressure falls equally in both groups (Fig. 12).

Surgical methods for producing atrial septal defects and other palliative venous return shunts are effective.[11, 12] The widely employed closed-heart procedure that excises the posterior aspect of the interatrial septum was described by Blalock and Hanlon in 1950. An alternative method utilizes systemic-venous inflow occlusion, right atriotomy, and direct excision of the

226

Table 1. Systemic blood oxygen saturation (per cent)

	TGA with IVS	TGA with VSD
Preseptostomy (mean ± SD (no. pts.))	31.1 ± 11.2(20)	56.2 ± 10.6(10)
Postseptostomy Immediate	56.6 ± 12.1(20)	70.4 ± 11.5(10)
Late: Highest Lowest	59.7 ± 9.6(27) 50.1 ± 9.7	74.5 ± 11.8(15) (14)

Note: Preseptostomy and immediate postseptostomy data were obtained during initial cardiac catheterization. Late postseptostomy data were obtained from femoral artery or heated heel capillary samples and represent highest and lowest values obtained from a series of samples obtained days, weeks, or months after balloon septostomy.

atrial septum. In some clinics, the operative and postoperative management techniques have improved to such an extent that infant survival with these atrial septectomy technics is about 90 per cent.

The patent ductus arteriosus (PDA) associated with TGA seldom is large and, in most instances, closes spontaneously. Surgical closure, often as an emergency procedure, as well as atrial septectomy or balloon septostomy, is indicated in the rare infant with a persistent large PDA, since it appears to contribute to marked congestive heart failure.

In infants with TGA and a persistent large VSD with pulmonary hypertension, surgical banding of the main pulmonary artery appears clearly indicated, probably before 6 to 9 months of age, to prevent irreversible advanced pulmonary vascular obstructive changes. Creation of an atrial septal defect, as discussed earlier, is also indicated in most infants with TGA and large VSD.

In patients with TGA, VSD, and PS with diminished pulmonary blood flow, palliative treatment requires establishing a systemic-to-pulmonary shunt to increase pulmonary blood flow. In infants, an ascending aorta to right pulmonary artery anastomosis usually is performed; but in older infants and children, superior vena cava to right pulmonary artery or subclavian to pulmonary artery shunts have been very effective.

The anatomical as well as physiological status of these infants must not be viewed as static.[13, 14] During a 4-year period of observation in 60 infants with atrial septostomy in our clinic, moderate and small-sized ventricular septal defects have closed (five infants) and quite significant left ventricular outflow tract (PS) stenosis has developed (five infants). In this interval of months or years that separates successful palliation from eventual corrective surgery, almost all patients demonstrate poor growth and cyanosis. Cerebral vascular accidents (four infants) with paralysis or death have been increasingly noted, and clinically silent thrombosis of the left pulmonary artery also has been detected (two infants). One would anticipate that optimum palliation with maximum systemic arterial oxygen saturation would minimize these serious complications. At present, it would appear judicious also to reassess the physiological and anatomical status of all patients before open-heart corrective surgery, irrespective of the initial early infancy findings.

DEFINITIVE SURGERY

The most widely practiced corrective surgical procedure, based on redirecting the systemic venous and pulmonary venous blood streams, was proposed in 1954 by Albert and successfully applied in 1964 by Mustard. During cardiopulmonary bypass, the atrial septum (or its remnants in a previously palliated patient) is excised and a baffle of pericardial tissue is fashioned and sutured to the atrial walls to redirect oxygenated pulmonary venous blood to the tricuspid valve, right ventricle, and aorta. Systemic venous return passes across the baffle and is directed to the mitral valve, left ventricle, and pulmonary artery (Fig. 13).

The most favorable surgical candidates at present are TGA patients with IVS (or very small VSD) approximately 2 years old or older, with normal or slightly elevated left ventricular and pulmonary artery pressures. These patients (group I) are indeed the most likely to die in the first days of life without prompt recognition and effective palliation. The results of corrective surgery are most gratifying for this group, with an estimated surgical mortality risk of about 15 per cent.

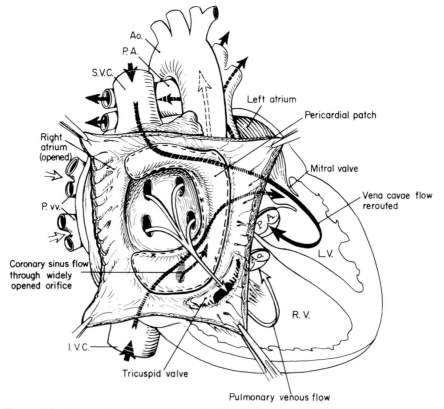

Figure 13. Correction of TGA by surgical procedure according to Mustard.[17]

The correction of TGA with large VSD is technically a more difficult and prolonged procedure, has had a more limited application, and has had less satisfactory results to date. Certainly patients with significant pulmonary vascular obstructive disease are unsuitable candidates. However, we should anticipate good results in children now accumulating with the pulmonary vascular bed protected by early palliative pulmonary artery banding. It is also anticipated that when cardiopulmonary bypass and the Mustard operation can be technically applied to the infant of about 6 months of age,[15] the surgeon will accomplish primary correction of TGA and the VSD before the development of irreversible pulmonary vascular obstruction.

The TGA patient with VSD and PS with diminished pulmonary blood flow presents yet another problem to the surgeon. The pulmonary stenosis may occur in various forms, at the pulmonary valve level or within the left ventricular muscular outflow tract, and it is difficult to approach because of the posterior orientation of the pulmonary outflow tract. At present, corrective surgical therapy should be postponed in most infants and younger children in favor of palliative systemic-to-pulmonary shunt procedures. New corrective procedures are being devised, and Rastelli et al.[16] have successfully used an intracardiac ventricular baffle and extracardiac aortic homograft to completely bypass severely stenosed left ventricular outflow tracts.

Thus, the results for palliative management and surgical correction of TGA have become quite gratifying. If one estimates an optimum 85 to 90 per cent survival rate after atrial septostomy and atrial septectomy, a 10 per cent incidence of serious intervening medical complications, and an optimum 85 to 90 per cent survival from corrective surgery, we can anticipate that about 70 of each 100 infants with TGA and IVS will approach a near normal childhood. It is a sharp contrast, indeed, to the totally hopeless prognosis for this group of infants a decade ago.

References

1. LIEBERMAN, J., CULLOM, L., AND BELLOC, N. B.: *Natural history of transposition of the great arteries. Anatomy and birth and death characteristics.* Circulation 40:237, 1969.

2. LAMBERT, E. C., CANENT, R. V., AND HOHN, A. R.: *Congenital cardiac anomalies in the newborn.* Pediatrics 37:343, 1966.

3. PAUL, M. H., VAN PRAAGH, R., AND VAN PRAAGH, S.: in Watson, H. (ed.): Transposition of the Great Arteries. *Pediatric Cardiology.* C. V. Mosby Co., St. Louis, 1968, pp. 567–610.

4. SHAHER, R. M.: *The hemodynamics of complete transposition of the great vessels.* Brit. Heart J. 26:343, 1964.

5. VILES, P. H., ONGLEY, P. A., AND TITUS, J. L.: *The spectrum of pulmonary vascular disease in transposition of the great arteries.* Circulation 40:31, 1969.

6. NOONAN, J. A., NADAS, A. S., RUDOLPH, A. M., AND HARRIS, G. B. C.: *Transposition of the great arteries. A correlation of clinical, physiologic, and autopsy data.* New Eng. J. Med. 263:592, 1960.

7. SHAHER, R. M., AND DEUCHAR, D. C.: *The electrocardiogram in complete transposition of the vessels.* Brit. Heart J. 28:265, 1966.

8. RASHKIND, W. J., AND MILLER, W. W.: *Creation of an atrial septal defect without thoracotomy: Palliative approach to complete transposition of the great arteries.* J.A.M.A. 196:991, 1966.

9. RASHKIND, W. J., AND MILLER, W. W.: *Transposition of the great arteries: Results of palliation by balloon atrioseptostomy in 31 infants.* Circulation 38:453, 1968.

10. PLAUTH, W. H., NADAS, A. S., BERNHARD, W. F., AND GROSS, R. E.: *Transposition of the great vessels.* Circulation 37:316, 1968.

11. WATSON, H.: *Palliative procedures for transposition of the great arteries.* Brit. Heart J. 31:407, 1969.

12. PAUL, M. H., MUSTER, A. J., COLE, R. B., AND BAFFES, T. G.: *Palliative management for transposition of the great arteries, 1957–1967.* Ann. Thorac. Surg. 6:321, 1968.

13. TYNAN, M., CARR, I., GRAHAM, G., AND BONHAM CARTER, R. E.: *Subvalvar pulmonary obstruction complicating the postoperative course of balloon atrial septostomy in transposition of the great arteries.* Circulation 39–40 (suppl. I):223, 1969.

14. PLAUTH, W. H., JR., FYLER, D. C., AND NADAS, A. S.: *Changing hemodynamics in transposition of the great arteries* (abstract). Amer. J. Cardiol. 23:132, 1969.

15. DOBELL, A. R. C., GIBBONS, J. E., AND BUSSE, E. F. G.: *Hemodynamic correction of transposition of the great vessels in infants.* J. Thorac. Cardiov. Surg. 57:108, 1969.

16. RASTELLI, G. C., WALLACE, R. B., AND ONGLEY, P. A.: *Complete repair of transposition of the great arteries with pulmonary stenosis: A review and report of a case corrected by using a new surgical technique.* Circulation 39:83, 1969.

17. MUSTARD, W. T.: *Successful two-stage correction of transposition of the great vessels.* Surgery 55:469, 1964.

Patent Ductus Arteriosus in Early Infancy

J. B. Kostis, M.D., and
A. N. Moghadam, M.D.

Ductus arteriosus is a vascular channel connecting the pulmonary artery to the descending aorta. During fetal life, it carries out the important function of delivering most of the blood entering the right ventricle to the aorta, thus bypassing the nonaerated lungs. After the onset of respiration and the subsequent increase in pulmonary blood flow occurring at birth, the ductus arteriosus loses its function and finally closes to become a ligament (ligamentum arteriosum). Patency of the ductus arteriosus persisting during extrauterine life creates important pathophysiological changes by connecting the high-pressure systemic circulation to the pulmonic circuit and constitutes one of the common congenital anomalies of the cardiovascular system.

INCIDENCE

Patent ductus arteriosus, occurring as a single lesion or accompanying other anomalies, occurs in 1 out of 2,500 to 5,000 births. It has been reported to occur in 5 to 20 per cent of cases with congenital heart disease. The incidence varies from one series to another, probably as a result of differences in the degree of application of certain diagnostic procedures, specialization of some centers on a particular group of lesions, and different age groups included in the statistics. Thus, in the neonatal period, patent ductus arteriosus is present in about 5 per cent of cases and ranks fifth or sixth in order of frequency among congenital anomalies of the heart. However, as a result of the death of infants with more serious cardiac malformations, at one year of age, patent ductus arteriosus is second in order of frequency (about 10 to 15 per cent), exceeded only by ventricular septal defect.[1-5] In a series of 1,000 cases with congenital heart disease catheterized at the Philadelphia General Hospital, patent ductus arteriosus was present in 9 per cent of the cases. Sixty per cent of the affected children were female and forty per cent, male. This sex predilection of patent ductus arteriosus with a female to male ratio of 2:1 to 3:1 has been noted by many investigators. However, it may not be true for cases resulting from maternal rubella, in which both sexes probably are affected with the same frequency.[1, 6-8]

FETAL ROLE AND POSTNATAL CLOSURE OF THE DUCTUS

Role in Fetus

During fetal life, the right ventricle receives the portion of blood entering the right atrium that does not pass to the left atrium across the foramen ovale. Because this right ventricular blood comes mainly from the head and upper extremities via the superior vena cava and, to a lesser extent, from the coronary sinus and inferior vena cava, it has a low oxygen saturation. From the right ventricle, the blood is ejected to the main pulmonary artery, where it can flow both to the pulmonary capillary bed via the right and left pulmonary arteries and to the systemic circulation via the ductus arteriosus and the descending aorta. The resistance to the flow of blood offered by the narrow arterioles of the collapsed lungs is much greater than the resistance of the systemic circuit, which includes the low-resistance placental circulation. For this reason, most of the blood entering the pulmonary artery flows through the ductus to the descending aorta, and only a minimal proportion reaches the lungs. Thus, the role of the ductus arteriosus in the fetus is to bypass the nonaerated lungs. By the same token, it contributes to the delivery of unsaturated blood to the placenta, which carries out the respiratory function in the fetus. More saturated blood entering the right atrium from the inferior vena cava goes to the left atrium through the foramen ovale and finally is delivered to the head and upper part of the body.[9, 10]

The Closure of Ductus Arteriosus

Since the beginning of the century, it has been recognized that the physiological closure of the ductus begins with the onset of respiration and the histological obliteration occurs later. Although constriction of the ductus is initiated by the first breath, complete functional closure takes place 15 to 20 hours later, and in rare cases, a few days after birth. A left-to-right shunt through the ductus usually is present during this period in healthy infants. A right-to-left or bidirectional shunt may be present only in the first few hours after birth. Because these shunts are of small magnitude, they usually are not associated with the clinical signs of patent ductus arteriosus in the normal newborn.[11-18]

Anatomic closure of the ductus is complete by the age of 2 weeks in 35 per cent of the cases, by 2 months in about 90 per cent, and at 1 year in 99 per cent. It rarely occurs later in life, though after the end of the first week, the opening is narrow, allowing the passage of only a 2 mm. wide probe.[19-22]

It is now generally accepted that the primary mechanism of early functional closure of the ductus is contraction of the muscular fibers of the media, which shortens, narrows, and distorts the lumen of the ductus. Changes in the position of the ductus in relation to the great vessels and in pressure relationships may play a minor role.

The main factor in triggering the constriction of the ductus appears to be the different response of the musculature of the pulmonary arterioles and the ductus to changes in arterial pO_2.[23-25] An increase in arterial pO_2 causes dilatation of the pulmonary arterioles and constriction of the ductus. With the initiation of breathing, the pulmonary vascular resistance falls while the lumen of the ductus narrows. This event results in an increase in blood flow to the lungs, which have assumed their respiratory function, and a decrease in the amount of blood shunted through the ductus. Since the lumen of the pulmonary arterioles increases gradually after birth, rather than suddenly, the pulmonary artery pressure remains higher than the systemic pressure during the first hours after birth, creating a right-to-left shunt. About 3 to 6 hours after birth, the pulmonary artery pressure becomes lower than the aortic pressure, and a left-to-right shunt is present. Finally, the ductus closes completely by contraction of its very muscular media. These changes depend on arterial pO_2 and initially are reversible. Closure of the ductus and abolition of the shunt during the first 8 hours of life has been obtained by breathing 100 per cent oxygen. On the contrary, hypoxia caused by breathing 13 per cent oxygen reopened the ductus and resulted in shunting again.[10, 23, 26]

The pronounced reactivity of the ductus to changes in pO_2 is present only very early in life. This occurrence may be related to the release of vasoactive kinins, which recently have been found to play an important role in the closure of the ductus. Bradykinin is capable of producing potent constriction of the ductus and remarkable dilatation of the pulmonary arterioles. These effects are oxygen-dependent in that they are minimum at pO_2 corresponding to fetal oxygen concentrations and near maximum at the pO_2 found in the newborn. Kinin is formed from a precursor, kininogen, by the action of an activated enzyme, kallicrein. Plasma kallicrein activation resulting in the formation of bradykinin is thought to result from the decrease of umbilical blood temperature at birth and exposure to granulocytes, which are present in increased numbers shortly after birth. Thus, in addition to the partial pressure of oxygen in the blood, vasoactive peptides may play a role in the pulmonary arteriolar dilatation and the constriction of the ductus occurring after birth.[23, 27, 28]

ETIOLOGY

Although no clear-cut etiological basis can be established for the majority of cases of patent ductus arteriosus, numerous authors have suggested an interplay of genetic and environmental factors as the cause.

Genetic Factors

The operation of genetic factors is suggested by the increased incidence of congenital heart disease in siblings and other relatives of patients with patent ductus arteriosus. Pedigrees suggesting autosomal recessive, autosomal dominant, and multifactorial inheritance were observed in a small number of families. In the great majority of cases, however, the data do not fit any simple mode of hereditary transmittance. For purposes of genetic counseling, one should consider that the siblings of a patient with patent ductus arteriosus have a probability of 1 to 2 per cent to be affected by some form of congenital malformation of the cardiovascular system.[1, 29–32]

Additional evidence of operation of genetic factors in the etiology of patent ductus arteriosus is the occurrence of the defect in patients with chromosomal aberrations. Patent ductus arteriosus is present in a considerable number of patients with trisomy 21, although it is less common than are endocardial cushion defects. In trisomy 18, patent ductus arteriosus is one of the most common associated cardiovascular malformations. However, in the majority of cases of patent ductus arteriosus, there are no chromosomal aberrations.[33, 34]

Environmental Factors

Rubella during the first trimester of pregnancy results in congenital anomalies such as cataracts, deafness, and cardiovascular malformations in a great proportion of the offspring. About 50 per cent of the affected children have congenital heart disease, and patent ductus arteriosus is the most common form (about 60 per cent of the cases). In our experience, the second cardiovascular abnormality in order of frequency is stenosis of the pulmonary artery branches. The actual percentage of cases of patent ductus arteriosus resulting from rubella probably is small (3 to 15 per cent, depending on the presence and severity of rubella epidemics). Because there are serious doubts about the effectiveness of maternal gamma globulin administration in preventing fetal malformations, therapeutic abortion and the recently developed rubella vaccine should be considered the main preventive measures.[35-37]

Residence at high altitudes has been implicated as another environmental factor causing patent ductus arteriosus. Higher incidence of the defect at high altitudes has been reported by several investigators. Whether this incidence is related to failure of the ductus to constrict after birth because of low oxygen tensions in these altitudes still is a matter of speculation.[38, 39]

Fetal distress, also, may participate in the causation of patent ductus arteriosus. Higher incidence of birth asphyxia and fetal distress has been found in patients with patent ductus arteriosus. In addition, the incidence of this lesion is higher in premature infants recovering from respiratory distress syndrome. In some of these infants, a large left-to-right shunt across the ductus could cause congestive heart failure. Inadequate development of the smooth muscle of the ductus and prolonged hypoxia have been proposed as causative factors in this group of patients.[29, 40-43]

EMBRYOLOGY AND ANATOMY

The ductus arteriosus develops from the distal portion of the sixth left aortic arch. The proximal portion of this arch contributes to the formation of the left pulmonary artery. During early infancy, the ductus appears as a continuation of the left pulmonary artery and may have a diameter equal to the main pulmonary artery or the aorta. This anatomic arrangement renders the recognition of the structures difficult and has resulted in occasional operative accidents when the left pulmonary artery was ligated and the ductus was left intact. Later in life, the anatomical relationships become clear.

There is great variation in the shape and size of the persistent ductus arteriosus. It usually is cylindrical, but it may have a conical shape with the base towards the aorta. It may have a small diameter (e.g., 1 mm.) or may be as wide as the aorta. The length of the ductus also varies from a few to 15 or 20 mm. When it is very short, it may create difficulties during the operation. The usual position of the patent ductus arteriosus is between the origin of the left pulmonary artery and the ventral aspect of the aorta, just distal to the origin of the left subclavian artery. Rare cases of bilateral or right-sided ductus arteriosus creating murmurs in unusual locations of the chest have been reported.

The histology of the ductus differs from that of the pulmonary artery and the aorta in that the media contains mainly muscular fibers and in that the intima is much thicker. These factors contribute to the postnatal closure of the normal ductus.[44, 45]

HEMODYNAMICS

Factors Affecting the Magnitude and Direction of the Shunt

Understanding of the hemodynamics of the various forms of patent ductus arteriosus is very important because they are the basis of clinical, X-ray, and electrocardiographic findings, and they determine the prognosis and treatment.

Because the ductus represents in essence an abnormal communication between the systemic and pulmonic circulations, it allows the creation of a shunt between them. The quantity and direction of the shunt are controlled by the relative magnitudes of the resistance * to flow offered by the systemic capillaries, the pulmonary capillaries, and the ductus itself. The resistance of the ductus depends on the length, internal cross-sectional area, and configuration of this vessel and affects only the magnitude but not the direction of the shunt. When the ductus is wide and short, it offers very low resistance and allows a large shunt across it. In such a situation, the pressures in the aorta and pulmonary artery are equal. When the ductus is narrow and long, it offers high resistance and, other factors being equal, determines a shunt of smaller magnitude. The direction and, to a great extent, the magnitude of the shunt are determined by the ratio of the pulmonary vascular resistance to the systemic vascular resistance. As there are only small variations in the systemic vascular resistance (usually slightly lower than normal in cases with patent ductus arteriosus), the magnitude of the pulmonary vascular resistance is of prime importance in determining the characteristics of the shunt.

Normal Hemodynamics

The normal and two examples of patients with patent ductus arteriosus are diagrammatically shown in Figure 1. The area of the chambers and great vessels has been drawn proportional to the relative volume of these structures. The thickness of the arrows is proportional to the blood flow. The magnitude of pressure is indicated by the density of the vertical lines, the thickness of the ventricular wall by the thickness of the sides of the squares that represent the ventricles. The peripheral and pulmonary resistances also have been drawn in proportion.

In the normal (Fig. 1A), the systemic and pulmonary circuits operate in series and the blood flow is equal in all chambers. Because the systemic resistance is higher than pulmonic, the left ventricle is forced to generate higher pressure to deliver the same flow against a higher resistance and thus becomes thicker than the right.

---

* For simplicity, only the viscous resistance to flow offered mainly by narrow conduits is taken into consideration. Effects resulting from the inertia of the blood and distensibility of the vessels contribute less to the total impedance of the circuits and are not mentioned in this discussion.[46]

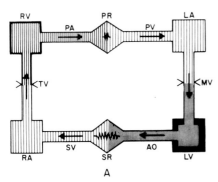

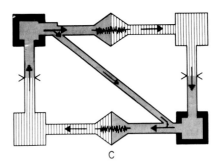

Figure 1. Diagrammatic representation of the normal circulation (A), a case of patent ductus arteriosus with left-to-right shunt (B), and a case of patent ductus arteriosus with right-to-left shunt (C). RV: right ventricle; LV: left ventricle; RA: right atrium; LA: left atrium; PDA: patent ductus arteriosus; PA: pulmonary arteries; PV: pulmonary veins; AO: aorta and systemic arteries; SV: systemic veins; MV: mitral valve; TV: tricuspid valve; PR: peripheral resistance; SR: systemic resistance. Volume, wall thickness, flow, and resistance have been drawn in proportion to representative values (see text for further explanation).

Left-to-Right Shunt

Figure 1B displays a patient with patent ductus arteriosus and pulmonary vascular resistance much lower than systemic. In such a situation, a great proportion of the left ventricular output is shunted across the patent ductus arteriosus to the low-resistance pulmonic circuit, while the rest flows normally to the systemic circulation and finally to the right atrium. The smaller the ratio of pulmonic to systemic resistance, the higher the proportion of left ventricular output that is shunted. Pulmonary to systemic blood flow ratios as high as 4:1 or 5:1 frequently are seen in clinical practice. Because the amount of blood that follows the normal pathways (i.e., to the systemic capillaries and then to the right atrium) is determined by the oxygen needs of the peripheral tissues via homeostatic mechanism, it cannot be reduced by any significant proportion. The left ventricle is obliged to eject the normal cardiac output plus the amount of blood that is shunted and, in order to accommodate this increased volume, dilates. If the magnitude of the shunt increases more, left ventricular failure occurs.

The stroke volume of the left ventricle increases to maintain the increased output of this chamber. The increased volume of blood that suddenly enters the aortic root produces a sharp elevation of the systolic pressure. Because of the rapid runoff through the low-resistance PDA-pulmonic circuit as well

237

as the peripheral runoff through a lowered systemic resistance, the pressure falls to low levels during diastole. The characteristic water-hammer pulse is thus created. The systemic resistance is decreased presumably because of reflex inhibition of arterial baroreceptors.

Because of the left-to-right shunt, the flow through the pulmonary arteries, pulmonary veins, left atrium, left ventricle, and aorta is increased, and this increase creates dilatation of these structures. Because these changes in volume are detectable by physical examination, electrocardiography, or radiography, they are very important in the evaluation of patients with patent ductus arteriosus. In addition, the increased pulmonary blood flow predisposes the lungs to infection.

Because the pulmonary vasculature retains its normal compliance, the increased flow across the pulmonic circuit is accommodated with only mild or moderate increase in the pulmonary artery and right ventricular pressures. The right ventricle remains normal. The flow across the patent ductus arteriosus from a high- to low-pressure circuit occurs during systole and diastole and creates a continuous murmur. The increased flow across the mitral valve may create a diastolic rumble because of relative mitral stenosis.[47]

Right-to-Left Shunt

At the opposite end of the spectrum of patients with patent ductus arteriosus are those with markedly increased pulmonic vascular resistance, i.e., with pulmonary resistance greater than systemic (Fig. 1C). In these patients, the shunt is from right to left, creating desaturation or even cyanosis of the lower part of the body. Because a proportion of the right ventricular output is shunted to the descending aorta, the pulmonary blood flow is decreased. The right ventricle hypertrophies, because it has to overcome the high pulmonary vascular resistance, but does not dilate, because it does not have to accommodate increased volume of blood. The main branches of the pulmonary artery are dilated because of the increased pressure. The left atrium and left ventricle do not dilate as they do not accommodate increased volume. Thus, the only abnormality on the chest X ray is the dilatation of the pulmonary artery and the decreased pulmonary blood flow, while the electrocardiogram shows right ventricular hypertrophy. The only auscultatory findings are the accentuation of the pulmonic second sound because of pulmonary hypertension and a systolic murmur created in the dilated main pulmonary artery.

Intermediate Forms

Between these two forms of patent ductus arteriosus are patients with transitional characteristics. When the pulmonary vascular resistance is elevated but slightly less than systemic, a left-to-right shunt of small magnitude may occur. These patients resemble the case described in Figure 1C in that they display right ventricular hypertrophy on the electrocardiogram, normal or slightly increased pulmonary blood flow, a heart of normal size on X ray, and only a systolic murmur and increased second heart sound on auscultation. However, cyanosis is absent. In other patients, the pulmonary vascular resistance is elevated but still significantly lower than systemic, so that a left-to-right shunt of considerable magnitude still is present while the pulmonary artery pressure is elevated.

Usual Forms of Patent Ductus Arteriosus in Infancy

In a number of cases, especially those with a ductus of relatively small diameter, a left-to-right shunt during the entire cardiac cycle and an almost normal pulmonary artery pressure are present (Fig. 1B). In another group of patients, especially with respiratory distress syndrome, markedly increased pulmonary vascular resistance, pulmonary hypertension, and bidirectional shunt exist (Fig. 1C). In other cases, especially those with large ductus, an intermediate form with pulmonary hypertension due to a combination of increased pulmonary blood flow and increased pulmonary vascular resistance is present. In these cases, it is very important to establish the degree of contribution of the above two factors in the creation of pulmonary hypertension because of the different prognosis, operative mortality, and morbidity associated with them. The factors that cause the marked elevation of the pulmonary vascular resistance seen in some patients have not been definitely elucidated. In many cases, the changes of the pulmonary arterioles responsible for this increased resistance appear to be caused by a previous large left-to-right shunt. In other cases, no such stage can be demonstrated, and the increased pulmonary resistance is thought to be of congenital origin.

CLINICAL MANIFESTATIONS

Symptoms

The infants with small patent ductus arteriosus are asymptomatic. Infants with large ductus and low pulmonary vascular resistance have a large left-to-right shunt and frequently show tachypnea, especially on feeding; tachycardia; excessive sweating; limitation of activity; and poor weight gain. Bouts of pneumonia are frequent. It is now widely accepted that left ventricular failure resulting from a large patent ductus arteriosus occurs in infancy. This fact should be always kept in mind when infants with respiratory difficulties are evaluated.[6, 8, 48–52]

General Physical Findings

Subnormal physical development, low body weight, and failure to thrive are seen commonly in infants with patent ductus arteriosus. In a significant percentage of the cases, this poor growth persists even after surgical correction of the lesion, indicating the operation of prenatal factors unrelated to the presence of shunt across the ductus. The age at the time of operation also may play a role, because heart failure and repeated respiratory infections may have an adverse effect during the period of rapid growth that is not easily overcome at an older age.

Cyanosis is absent in the uncomplicated patent ductus arteriosus with left-to-right shunt. When the pulmonary vascular resistance is high, mild transient cyanosis may appear during crying, respiratory infections, or failure.

Auscultation and Phonocardiography

The Continuous Murmur of Patent Ductus Arteriosus

The type of auscultatory and phonocardiographic findings directly depends on the hemodynamics of the individual case. The typical murmur of patent ductus arteriosus is a harsh, continuous machinery murmur best heard at the second left intercostal space near the sternum (Gibson murmur). Occasionally, it may be heard at the third left intercostal space. When loud enough, it radiates to the entire precordium and the suprasternal notch.

This murmur is present when a left-to-right shunt exists during systole and diastole, which requires an aortopulmonary pressure gradient during both parts of the cycle. It has been proved by intracardiac phonocardiography that the murmur is generated inside the pulmonary artery at the opening of the ductus, where turbulence is created by the abnormal flow (Fig. 2). The murmur begins a short time after the first heart sound. This time interval is taken by the isovolumetric contraction period during which the left ventricle develops adequate pressure to open the aortic valve, by the time needed for the transmission of the pressure wave from the aortic valve to the site of the ductus, and by a short interval during which adequate pressure gradient between the aorta and pulmonary artery is created. After the onset, the

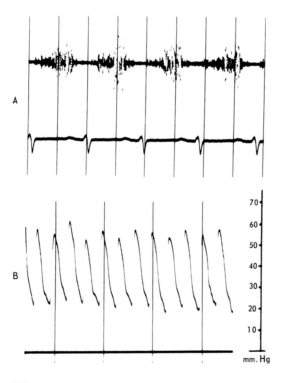

Figure 2. A, phonocardiogram at the left sternal border and simultaneous electrocardiogram on a 4-month-old patient with patent ductus arteriosus and left-to-right shunt. Note the continuous murmur of patent ductus arteriosus. B, Direct pressure tracing of the femoral artery on the same patient. Note the wide pulse pressure resulting mainly from lowering of the diastolic pressure.

murmur is crescendo because of the increasing pressure gradient between these two vessels, which creates an increasing flow across the ductus. The maximum intensity occurs near the second heart sound, again because of the time needed for transmission of the pulse wave from the heart to the area of the ductus. This late peak distinguishes the murmur of patent ductus arteriosus from other murmurs heard in the same area. During diastole, the murmur is decrescendo and finally disappears because of the decreasing aortopulmonary pressure gradient. The systolic component usually is louder than the diastolic. When the ductus is small, the murmur has a higher frequency and lasts throughout most of diastole. When the ductus is large, the murmur tends to have coarser quality and ends early in diastole as the pulmonary artery and aortic pressures equalize. The intensity of the murmur can be enhanced by increasing the pressure gradient across the ductus. The gradient can be increased either by increasing the aortic pressure (e.g., by methoxamine or other vasopressors) or by decreasing the pulmonary artery pressure (e.g., by inspiration). The continuous murmur of patent ductus arteriosus appears when the pulmonary vascular resistance is low enough to allow a left-to-right shunt during systole and diastole. In most infants, this happens at about 6 to 18 months of age, although it can occur even in neonates. In younger infants as well as older children with pulmonary arteriolar constriction, the pulmonary vascular resistance is relatively high, so that a significant aortopulmonary pressure gradient is present only during systole. In these cases, a significant shunt across the patent ductus arteriosus occurs only during systole, and only a systolic murmur is present. This systolic murmur usually has a crescendo configuration with a late systolic peak. However, it is in reality a continuous murmur, because a "spillover" during early diastole may be present in the phonocardiogram, although it cannot be detected by auscultation. In these cases, the phonocardiogram is a very helpful diagnostic tool. Similarly, in cases with a very large ductus and left-to-right shunt, the pressures in the aorta and the pulmonary artery rapidly become equal, so that the diastolic murmur becomes very short or is eliminated.

Immediately after birth, when the pressures of the pulmonary artery and aorta are about equal and the pulmonary and systemic resistances are of similar magnitude, no murmur usually is present because there is no significant flow across the defect.

Occasionally the continuous murmur may be present only intermittently or may vary from one examination to the other. This variation has been attributed to intermittent obliteration of the ductus either by kinking or by irregularities in the lumen. It should be kept in mind, because other causes of disappearance of the murmur, such as severe increase in the pulmonary vascular resistance and closure of the defect, either normal or thrombotic, have different prognostic and therapeutic implications.[50, 51, 53–58]

Other Murmurs

In patients with large left-to-right shunt, the increased flow across the mitral valve may create a mitral diastolic rumble best heard at the apex.

Although this murmur is very commonly heard in such instances, its absence does not exclude a large left-to-right shunt. This murmur may, on occasion, be very loud and may be heard in the absence of the characteristic continuous murmur in cases with a large ductus with pulmonary hypertension caused by a large left-to-right shunt.

In patients with markedly increased pulmonary vascular resistance and a small left-to-right or right-to-left shunt, no murmur is generated by the flow through the ductus. In these patients, only a nonspecific ejection murmur is generated in the dilated pulmonary artery. A decrescendo early diastolic murmur of pulmonic insufficiency also may be heard in such patients.[50, 59]

Heart Sounds

The first heart sound usually is normal or slightly accentuated. The pulmonic component of the second heart sound may be buried in the continuous murmur and usually is accentuated (Fig. 2). The intensity of this sound is related to the degree of pulmonary hypertension and is a very important auscultatory sign. However, quantitative inferences about the level of pulmonary artery pressure from the intensity of the pulmonic second sound have proven unreliable. The second heart sound usually is split. In the presence of severe pulmonary hypertension, the splitting may become close and fixed and the second sound very loud. In the presence of a large left-to-right shunt, the ejection period of the left ventricle may be prolonged and create a paradoxical splitting of the second heart sound. This phenomenon is best detected by phonocardiography. A third heart sound may be present also in cases with left-to-right shunt. Pulmonic or aortic systolic clicks are heard at the base in many cases of patent ductus arteriosus.[60]

Palpation

In about 50 per cent of the patients with a continuous murmur, a precordial thrill can be palpated. This thrill is systolic in most cases and continuous in a few. The thrill usually is present at the upper left sternal border, but in some cases, it may be felt all over the precordium. A hyperactive apical impulse may be palpated in patients with left-to-right shunt, while a parasternal heave resulting from right ventricular hypertrophy may be present in cases with pulmonary hypertension and right ventricular hypertrophy. The characteristic rapidly rising and then collapsing water-hammer pulse and the wide pulse pressure are present in the cases with significant left-to-right shunt (Fig. 2B). In some patients, visible capillary pulsations and the other peripheral signs usually associated with significant aortic regurgitation are present. As accurate determinations of the blood pressure are difficult in infancy, palpation of the femoral and axillary arteries may give an important diagnostic clue. The bounding pulse is present even in cases with congestive heart failure, but it is not pathognomonic of patent ductus arteriosus, because it may be present in other lesions with increased diastolic runoff. It is absent in the presence of pulmonary hypertension when the diastolic pressure of the pulmonary artery is elevated (Fig. 3).[6, 51, 52]

242

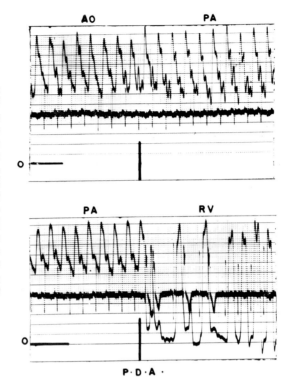

Figure 3. Continuous pressure recording during pullback of the catheter under fluoroscopic control from the aorta to the pulmonary artery through a patent ductus arteriosus on a patient with elevated pulmonary vascular resistance and bidirectional shunt. Note that the pressures in the pulmonary artery and aorta are equal and that the diastolic pressure is not low. A normal pulse pressure is present (compare with Figure 2B). AO: aorta; PA: pulmonary artery; RV: right ventricle.

ELECTROCARDIOGRAPHY AND VECTORCARDIOGRAPHY

The electrocardiogram of patent ductus arteriosus may be normal or display left, right, or biventricular hypertrophy, depending on the hemodynamics of the individual case.

In the cases with considerable left-to-right shunt, electrocardiographic abnormalities resulting from volume overload of the left ventricle and left atrium are present. Left ventricular volume overload is indicated by an increased amplitude of the R wave and Q wave and a tall upright T wave in the leads exploring the left ventricle. The mean QRS axis is usually normal in infancy. In these cases, the vectorcardiogram displays a magnified QRS loop oriented to the left, inferiorly, and posteriorly. The rotation of the loop is normal, i.e., counterclockwise in the frontal and horizontal planes and clockwise in the right sagittal. The QRS–T angle also is normal (Fig. 4). Left atrial enlargement is indicated by an increased duration and notching of the P wave in the limb leads and an increased area of negativity of the P wave in the right precordial leads.

Biventricular hypertrophy is present in most infants with large patent ductus arteriosus, left-to-right shunt, and elevation of the pulmonary artery pressure. Tall R or RS deflections are present in the right precordial leads, accompanied on occasion by positive T waves indicating right ventricular hypertrophy. In addition, tall R waves in the left precordial leads suggest

243

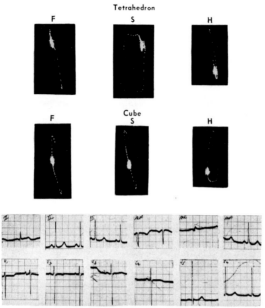

Figure 4. Vectorcardiogram and electrocardiogram of a 7-year-old patient with patent ductus arteriosus and left-to-right shunt, showing left ventricular hypertrophy ("volume overload").

V_1 to V_2 on Half Standardization

left ventricular hypertrophy (Fig. 5). In the vectorcardiogram, a significant proportion of the loop is anterior because of increased right ventricular forces. Isolated right ventricular hypertrophy of the systolic overload type is rare in uncomplicated patent ductus arteriosus. It is seen in patients with severe pulmonary hypertension resulting from increased pulmonary vascular resistance. In these cases, a QR pattern with tall R wave is present in the right precordial leads, while the left precordial leads show small RS complexes. Right axis deviation is present. The vectorcardiographic loop is anterior, inferior, and to the right. The rotation is clockwise in the horizontal plane.[6, 8, 50–52]

RADIOLOGICAL FINDINGS

The chest roentgenogram is helpful in the diagnosis and evaluation of the hemodynamic status of patients with patent ductus arteriosus. As expected from the discussion of Figure 1B, dilatation of the left atrium, left ventricle, aorta, pulmonary arteries, and pulmonary veins and increased pulmonary blood flow are present in patients with left-to-right shunt (Fig. 6). Cardiomegaly and engorged pulmonary vascularity in the anteroposterior view is seen in practically all infants with significant shunt. These findings, however, may be seen in cases with left-to-right shunt caused by other lesions (such as ventricular septal defect) and are not specific for patent ductus arteriosus. Radiographic diagnosis of specific chamber enlargement is difficult in infancy, especially in the presence of a markedly enlarged heart. Enlargement of the aortic shadow, which is not present in cases of ventricular septal defect and

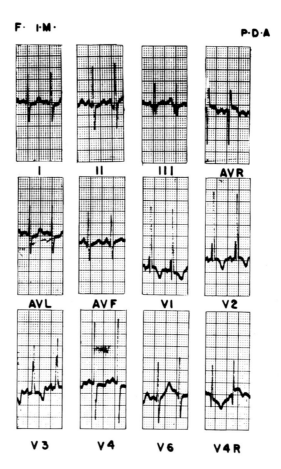

F· I·M·

P·D·A

Figure 5. Electrocardiogram of a 1-month-old infant with patent ductus arteriosus, left-to-right shunt, and pulmonary hypertension, showing right and probably left ventricular hypertrophy.

is a useful differential diagnostic sign in older patients, is infrequently seen in infants (Fig. 7). In a considerable number of patients, signs of left ventricular hypertrophy, such as leftward and downward bulging of the apex in the anteroposterior view and posterior enlargement in the left anterior oblique, are present and signify a large left-to-right shunt. Left atrial enlargement may also be recognized by an elevation of the left main stem bronchus and reduplication of the right heart border in the anteroposterior view and posterior displacement of the barium-filled esophagus in right anterior oblique view.

On fluoroscopy, increased pulsations of the left ventricle, aorta, and pulmonary artery are noted in patients with a considerable left-to-right shunt.

In patients with increased pulmonary resistance and reversed or minimal shunt, the radiological picture is quite different. The main pulmonary artery branches are dilated, in contrast to the decreased size of the peripheral vessels. As the right ventricle is obliged to generate high pressure but does not have to accommodate an increased volume of blood, it hypertrophies but, in the absence of heart failure, does not dilate. Consequently, in these

245

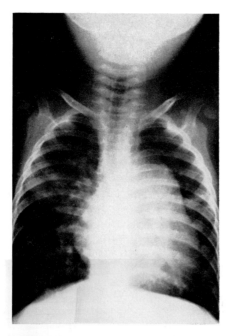

Figure 6. Chest roentgenogram on a 6-month-old patient with patent ductus arteriosus and left-to-right shunt. Note the increased heart size and the increased pulmonary blood flow.

cases, the involvement of the right ventricle is obvious in the electrocardiogram and only equivocable in the chest X ray.[51, 52]

CARDIAC CATHETERIZATION

Cardiac catheterization and related techniques are used for the confirmation of diagnosis, the detection of associated lesions, and the study of the

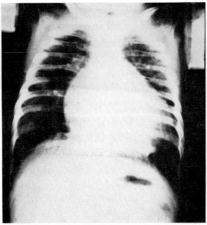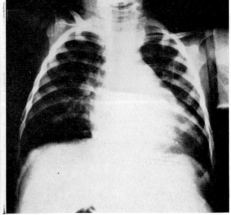

Figure 7. Chest roentgenograms of a patient with ventricular septal defect (*left*) and a patient with patent ductus arteriosus (*right*). In both patients, a left-to-right shunt was present, resulting in similar radiographic appearance, i.e., cardiac dilatation and increased pulmonary blood flow. It is difficult to recognize the aortic shadow, which could help in the differential diagnosis.

hemodynamic parameters, such as pulmonary vascular resistance and magnitude of shunt, of the particular patient. Catheterization should be done in infants with atypical features. These studies can be done safely and easily in a laboratory with experienced personnel.

Direct evidence of patency of the ductus is obtained by passage of the catheter from the pulmonary artery to the aorta (or from the aorta to the pulmonary artery) at the site where the ductus is expected to be. This characteristic course of the catheter is shown in Figure 8. An experienced operator should be able to enter the ductus in a great percentage of cases.

The pulmonary artery pressure, which is measured at the same time, is elevated but still lower than aortic pressure in most infants. In patients with a left-to-right shunt of adequate magnitude, a step-up in oxygen saturation in the pulmonary artery is detected during right heart catheterization. This sign, however, is not pathognomonic for patent ductus arteriosus, because an aortopulmonary window and a high ventricular septal defect may produce the same changes. In these cases, diagnosis can be made from other studies, such as angiography, intracardiac phonocardiography, or the course of the catheter.[50, 61]

In cases with only a systolic murmur on auscultation and conventional phonocardiography, the diagnosis may be made by intracardiac phonocardiography. In nine out of ten patients with a systolic murmur on conventional phonocardiography, a continuous murmur was revealed inside the pulmonary artery by intracardiac phonocardiography (Fig. 9). The location of this continuous murmur inside the pulmonary artery and the sharp disappearance in the right ventricle are diagnostic of aortopulmonary communication (Fig. 10).[62]

Visualization of the defect by angiocardiography provides definite diagnostic proof. This visualization can be done either by retrograde aortography or by selective cineangiography with injection into the left atrium or main pulmonary artery. Simultaneous opacification of the pulmonary artery and the aorta or reopacification of the pulmonary artery after injection into it

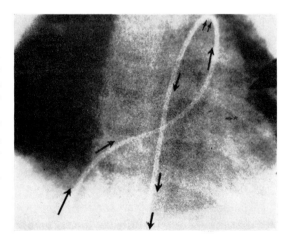

Figure 8. Course of the catheter in an infant with patent ductus arteriosus. The arrows indicate the course of the catheter from the inferior vena cava, to the right atrium, right ventricle, pulmonary artery, ductus arteriosus, thoracic descending aorta, and abdominal aorta. The double arrows indicate the site of the ductus.

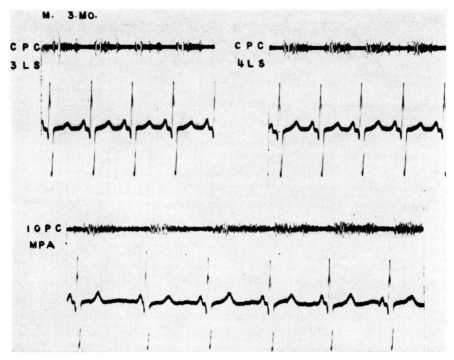

Figure 9. Chest phonocardiograms (CPC) at the third (3LS) and fourth (4LS) left intercostal space near the sternum and intracardiac phonocardiography (ICPC) inside the main pulmonary artery (MPA) of a 3-month-old infant with large patent ductus arteriosus. Note that the murmur is only systolic on the chest phonocardiograms, while it is continuous in the intracardiac phonocardiogram.

indicates the presence of left-to-right shunt at the level of injection or distally. With the high-quality equipment presently available, the actual shunt can be seen and accurately located in most cases.[63, 64]

Direct visualization of the ductus after injection in the aortic root or the left ventricle offers the advantage of differentiating the patent ductus arteriosus from other forms of aortopulmonary communication, such as aortopulmonary septal defect (Fig. 11). In the presence of right-to-left shunt, the preferable site of injection is the main pulmonary artery.[65–67]

DIAGNOSIS

Although the diagnosis of patent ductus arteriosus in infancy may present certain difficulties, it is by no means impossible. In the majority of cases, an accurate diagnosis of the lesion and the hemodynamic parameters may be made from the clinical examination, the chest X ray, and electrocardiogram. A characteristic continuous murmur with nearly normal X ray and electrocardiogram indicate that the ductus has a small diameter. When the continuous murmur is accompanied by evidence of left ventricular, left atrial, and aortic dilatation and increased pulmonary blood flow, a large

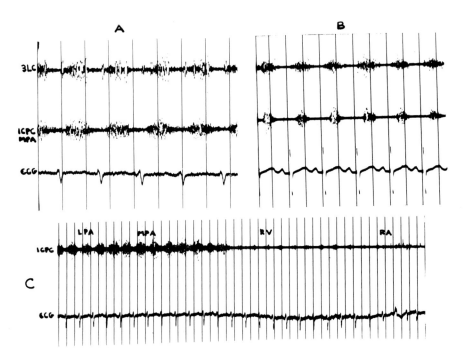

Figure 10. A, simultaneous recording of the chest phonocardiogram at the third left intercostal space (3LC), the intracardiac phonocardiogram in the main pulmonary artery (ICPC–MPA), and the electrocardiogram of a 4-month-old patient with patent ductus arteriosus and left-to-right shunt. Note the similarity of the continuous murmur in the two phonocardiograms. B, Similar tracing of a 3-month-old patient with large ductus and only a short diastolic component in both phonocardiograms. C, Intracardiac phonocardiogram in the case described in A, recorded continuously during pullback of the phonocatheter from the left pulmonary artery to the right atrium under fluoroscopic control. LPA: left pulmonary artery; MPA: main pulmonary artery; RV: right ventricle; RA: right atrium. Note the sharp disappearance of the murmur when the phonocatheter is withdrawn in the right ventricle.

left-to-right shunt is present. In infants with a large ductus and only a systolic murmur, the physical, electrocardiographic, and radiological findings are very similar to those of ventricular septal defect. In these cases, the differential diagnosis can be made from the bounding peripheral pulses and the phonocardiogram, which may demonstrate a short diastolic murmur not heard with the stethoscope. Definite diagnosis can be made by the use of cardiac catheterization, cineangiography, and intracardiac phonocardiography.

The presence of aortopulmonary fenestration and coronary arteriovenous fistulas may be suspected clinically and proven by aortography.

Arteriovenous fistula of the chest wall or in the left upper lobe also may produce a continuous murmur resembling the murmur of patent ductus arteriosus.

249

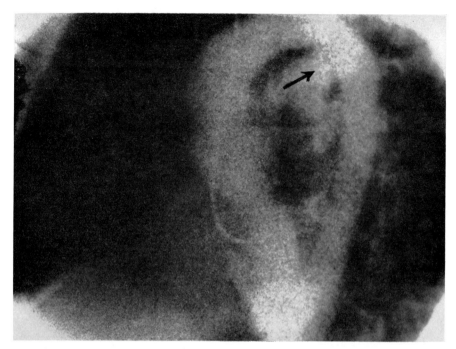

Figure 11. A frame of a cineangiogram taken after injection in the left ventricle of a patient with patent ductus arteriosus and left-to-right shunt. The catheter was guided from the right atrium to the left atrium through a patent foramen ovale and then into the left ventricle. Note the large patent ductus arteriosus (arrow) originating at the beginning of the descending aorta.

COURSE AND COMPLICATIONS

It has been recognized that patent ductus arteriosus is a more serious defect in early infancy than later in life. The life expectancy of patients with patent ductus arteriosus is definitely lower than normal. Death resulting from the defect usually occurs because of either heart failure or subacute bacterial endocarditis. Repeated bouts of congestive heart failure, often associated with pulmonary infections, are common in infants with large left-to-right shunt. We have observed heart failure caused by patent ductus arteriosus even in neonates (Fig. 12). Fifteen to twenty per cent of the patients with a large ductus develop congestive heart failure during the first 6 months of life. In many cases, the heart failure is resistant to medical treatment and may lead to death.

Subacute bacterial endocarditis is observed in infants also, but definitely less frequently than in older children. Another complication of patent ductus arteriosus in infancy is the development of an aneurysm of the ductus. The aneurysms may develop at the site of subacute bacterial endocarditis. They are important because they may rupture or exert pressure on surrounding structures.

Spontaneous closure of patent ductus arteriosus occurs in a small number of cases. This development, however, is relatively rare and should not be considered an argument against operative intervention.

Some infants (about 5 per cent of cases) with large patent ductus arteriosus and large left-to-right shunt develop a progressive increase in pulmonary vascular resistance. This increase ultimately results in permanent changes in the pulmonary arterioles, which cause elevation of the pulmonary vascular resistance to systemic levels and reversal of the shunt. Every effort should be made to identify such cases early, when operative intervention still is possible. The exact causes and mechanism of this complication are not well understood.

In summary, small numbers of patients with patent ductus arteriosus develop either spontaneous closure or progressive increase in pulmonary vascular resistance, while most probably develop congestive heart failure and subacute bacterial endocarditis.[50-52, 68-71]

TREATMENT

The mere presence of uncomplicated patent ductus arteriosus is an indication for its surgical treatment at the time of diagnosis or at a later date. Operative intervention carries very low mortality, but the life expectancy of patients with the uncorrected lesion is significantly reduced. Because the operative mortality is slightly higher in infancy than later in life, it is better to postpone the operation in asymptomatic infants until the age of 3 or 4 years. When cardiac failure, marked cardiac enlargement, repeated respiratory infections, or retardation of growth is present, the operation should be performed after establishment of the diagnosis at any age. Because of the possibility of recanalization, the original method of simple ligation has been largely replaced by multiple suture ligation or division.

In cases with left-to-right shunt and moderate elevation of the pulmonary artery pressure, improvement should be expected immediately after the operation (Fig. 12). The continuous murmur disappears, the heart size decreases, the pulmonary artery pressure becomes lower, and the electrocardiogram eventually returns to normal. Soft systolic murmurs may persist, probably because of persistent dilatation of the pulmonary artery. In some cases, the arterial pressure may increase and remain high for a few days after the operation. The mortality in such cases is about 1 per cent. The mortality of cases with severe pulmonary hypertension depends on the severity of the changes of the pulmonary arterioles. It should be kept in mind that when the pulmonary vascular resistance is less than systemic, a left-to-right shunt exists, and closure of the ductus is beneficial. When the pulmonary vascular resistance is higher than systemic, a right-to-left shunt is present, and closure of the ductus leads to increasing elevation of the pulmonary artery pressure and to death.[72-75] Estimation of the relative magnitude of the resistances can be made during cardiac catheterization. Temporary closure of the ductus, either during the operation or by a balloon catheter, may indicate the response of the pulmonary artery pressure to the correction of this defect.

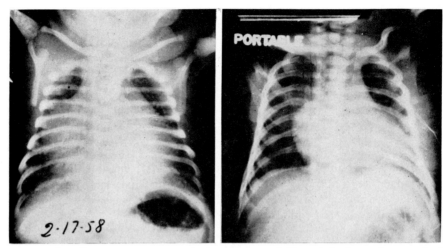

Figure 12. Chest roentgenogram before surgery (*left*) and 3 days after surgical closure (right) of a large patent ductus in a 3-week-old infant. Note the decrease in heart size.

In infants in heart failure with left-to-right shunt at two levels, such as ventricular septal defect and patent ductus arteriosus, a careful evaluation of the magnitude of shunts and the size of the defects is important. Closure of the ductus is recommended when the ductus is large and the ventricular septal defect small. On the other hand, when the ventricular septal defect is large and the ductus is small, one should consider closing the ductus and banding the pulmonary artery.

References
  1. ANDERSON, R. C.: *Causative factors underlying congenital heart malformations. I. Patent ductus arteriosus.* Pediatrics 14:143, 1954.
  2. ABBOTT, M. E.: *Atlas of congenital cardiac disease.* American Heart Association, New York, 1936.
  3. WOOD, P.: *Congenital heart disease.* Brit. Med. J. 1:1051, 1954.
  4. GARDINER, S. H., AND KEITH, T. R.: *Prevalence of heart disease in Toronto children.* Pediatrics 7:713, 1951.
  5. SCOTT, H. W., JR.: *Surgical treatment of patent ductus arteriosus in childhood.* Surg. Clin. N. Amer. 32:1299, 1952.
  6. ASH, R., AND FISCHER, D.: *Manifestations and results of treatment of patent ductus arteriosus in infancy and childhood.* Pediatrics 16:695, 1955.
  7. GROSS, R. E.: *The patent ductus arteriosus.* Amer. J. Med. 12:472, 1952.
  8. KROVETZ, L. S., AND WARDEN, H. E.: *Patent ductus arteriosus.* Dis. Chest 42:46, 1962.
  9. ADAMS, F. H.: *Fetal and neonatal cardiovascular and pulmonary function.* Ann. Rev. Physiol. 27:257, 1965.
 10. DAWES, G. S.: *Pulmonary circulation in the fetus and new-born.* Brit. Med. Bul. 22:61, 1966.
 11. GERARD, G.: *De l'oblitération du canal arteriel: Les théories et les faits.* Journal de l'Anatomie et de la Physiologie de l'Homme et des Animaux. 36:323, 1900.

12. BARKLAY, A. E., FRANKLIN, K. J., AND PRICHARD, M. M.: *The Fetal Circulation and Cardiovascular System and the Changes They Undergo at Birth*. Charles C Thomas, Springfield, Ill., 1945.

13. MOSS, A. J., EMMANOVILIDES, G., AND DUFFIE, E. R., JR.: *Closure of the ductus arteriosus in the newborn infant*. Pediatrics 32:25, 1963.

14. PREC, K. J., AND CASSALS, D. E.: *Dye dilution curves and cardiac output in newborn infants*. Circulation 11:789, 1955.

15. ADAMS, F. H., AND LIND, J.: *Physiologic studies on the cardiovascular status of normal newborn infants*. J. Pediat. 39:330, 1951.

16. ELDRIDGE, F. L., AND HULTGREN, H. N.: *The physiologic closure of the ductus arteriosus in the newborn infant*. J. Clin. Invest. 34:987, 1955.

17. ROWE, R. D., AND JAMES, L. S.: *The normal pulmonary arterial pressure during the first year of life*. J. Pediat. 51:1, 1957.

18. BURNARD, E. D.: *A murmur of the ductus arteriosus in the newborn baby*. Brit. Med. J. 1:806, 1958.

19. CHRISTIE, A.: *Normal closing time of the foramen ovale and the ductus arteriosus*. Amer. J. Dis. Child. 40:323, 1930.

20. MITCHELL, S. C.: *The ductus arteriosus in the neonatal period*. J. Pediat. 51:12, 1957.

21. DAWES, G. S.: *Changes in the circulation at birth*. Brit. Med. Bul. 17:148, 1961.

22. JAGER, B. V., AND WOLLERMAN, O. J., JR.: *An anatomical study of the closure of the ductus arteriosus*. Amer. J. Path. 18:595, 1942.

23. MOSS, A. J., EMMANOVILIDES, G. C., ADAMS, F. H., AND CHUANG, K.: *Response of the ductus arteriosus and pulmonary and systemic arterial pressure to changes in oxygen environment in newborn infants*. Pediatrics 33:937, 1964.

24. KENNEDY, J. A., AND CLARK, S. L.: *Observations on the ductus arteriosus of the guinea pig in relation to its method of closure*. Anat. Rec. 79:349, 1941.

25. BORN, G. V. R., DAWES, G. S., MOTT, J. C., AND RENNICK, B. R.: *The constriction of the ductus arteriosus caused by oxygen and by asphyxia in newborn lambs*. J. Physiol. 132:304, 1956.

26. EVANS, J. R., ROWE, R. D., DOWNIE, H. G., AND ROWSELL, H. C.: *Murmurs arising from ductus arteriosus in normal newborn swine*. Circ. Res. 12:85, 1963.

27. MELMON, K. L., CLINE, M. J., HUGHES, T., AND NIES, A. S.: *Kinins: Possible mediators of neonatal circulatory changes in man*. J. Clin. Invest. 47:1295, 1968.

28. CAMPBELL, A. G. M., DAWES, G. S., FISHMAN, A. P., HYMAN, A. I., AND PERKS, A. M.: *The release of a bradykinin-like pulmonary vasodilator substance in fetal and newborn lambs*. J. Physiol. 195:83, 1968.

29. POLANI, P. E., AND CAMPBELL, M.: *Factors in the causation of persistent ductus arteriosus*. Ann. Hum. Genet. 24:343, 1960.

30. EKSTROM, G.: *The surgical treatment of patent ductus arteriosus*. Acta Chir. Scand. suppl. 169, 1952.

31. KJAERGAARD, H.: *Patent ductus botali in three sisters*. Acta Med. Scand. 125:339, 1946.

32. LYNCH, H. T., GRISSOM, R. L., MAGNUSON, C. R., AND KRUSH, A.: *Patent ductus arteriosus. Study of two families*. J.A.M.A. 194:135, 1965.

33. ROWE, R. D., AND UCHIDA, I. A.: *Cardiac malformations in mongolism.* Amer. J. Med. 31:726, 1961.

34. WARKANY, J., PASSARGE, E., AND SMITH, L. B.: *Congenital malformations in autosomal trisomy syndromes.* Amer. J. Dis. Child. 112:502, 1966.

35. GREGG, N. M.: *Congenital cataract following german measles in the mother.* Trans. Ophthal. Soc. Aust. 3:35, 1941.

36. CAMPBELL, M.: *Place of maternal rubella in the etiology of congenital heart disease.* Brit. Med. J. 1:691, 1961.

37. JACKSON, B. T.: *The pathogenesis of congenital cardiovascular anomalies.* New Eng. J. Med. 279:80, 1968.

38. ALZAMORA-CASTRO, V., BATTILAVA, G., ABUGATAS, R., AND SIALER, S.: *Patent ductus arteriosus and high altitude.* Amer. J. Cardiol. 5:761, 1960.

39. PENALOZA, D., ARIAS-STELLA, J., SIME, F., RECAVARREN, S., AND MORTICORENA, E.: *The heart and pulmonary circulation in children at high altitudes.* Pediatrics 34:568, 1964.

40. RECORD, R. G., AND McKEOWN, T.: *Observations relating to the etiology of patent ductus arteriosus.* Brit. Heart J. 15:376, 1953.

41. DANILOWICZ, D., RUDOLPH, A. M., AND HOFFMAN, J. I. E.: *Delayed closure of the ductus arteriosus in premature infants.* Pediatrics 37:74, 1966.

42. JEGIER, W., KARN, G., AND STERN, L.: *Operative treatment of patent ductus arteriosus complicating respiratory distress syndrome of the premature.* Canad. Med. Assoc. J. 98:105, 1968.

43. SIASSI, B., EMMANOVILIDES, G. C., CLEVELAND, R. J., AND HIROSE, F.: *Patent ductus arteriosus complicating prolonged assisted ventilation in respiratory distress syndrome.* J. Pediat. 74:11, 1969.

44. HARLEY, H. R. S.: *The development and anomalies of the aortic arch and its branches.* Brit. J. Surg. 46:36, 1959.

45. KELSEY, J. R., JR., GILMORE, C. E., AND EDWARDS, J. E.: *Bilateral ductus arteriosus representing persistence of each sixth aortic arch.* Arch. Path. 55:154, 1953.

46. MORRIS, J. A., BEKEY, G. A., ASSALI, N. S., AND BECK, R.: *Dynamics of blood flow in the ductus arteriosus.* Amer. J. Physiol. 208:471, 1965.

47. JARMAKANI, M. M., EDWARDS, S. B., SPACH, M. S., CANEHT, R. V., CAPP, M. P., HAGAN, M. J., BARR, R. C. AND JAIN, V.: *Left ventricular pressure-volume characteristics in congenital heart disease.* Circulation 37:879, 1968.

48. ADAMS, P., JR., ADAMS, F. H., VARCO, R. L., DAMMANN, J. F., JR., AND MULLER, W. H.: *Diagnosis and treatment of patent ductus arteriosus in infancy.* Pediatrics 12:664, 1953.

49. LYON, R. A., AND KAPLAN, S.: *Patent ductus arteriosus in infancy.* Pediatrics 13:357, 1954.

50. RUDOLPH, A. M., MAYER, F. E., NADAS, A. S., AND GROSS, R. E.: *Patent ductus arteriosus: A clinical and hemodynamic study of 23 patients in the first year of life.* Pediatrics 22:892, 1958.

51. ZIEGLER, R. F.: *The importance of patent ductus arteriosus in infants.* Amer. Heart J. 43:553, 1952.

52. KROVETZ, L. J., LESTER, R. G., AND WARDEN, H. E.: *The diagnosis of patent ductus arteriosus in infancy.* Dis. Chest 42:241, 1962.

53. GIBSON, G. A.: *Persistence of the arterial duct and its diagnosis.* Edinburgh Med. J. 8:1, 1900.

54. HARING, O., LUISADA, A. O., AND GASUL, B. M.: *Phonocardiography in patent ductus arteriosus.* Circulation 10:501, 1954.

55. CREVASSE, L. E., AND LOGUE, R. B.: *Atypical patent ductus arteriosus. The use of a vasopressor agent as a diagnostic aid.* Circulation 19:332, 1959.

56. KEITH, T. R., AND SAGARMINAGA, J.: *Spontaneously disappearing murmur of patent ductus arteriosus.* Circulation 24:1235, 1961.

57. SHAPIRO, W., SAID, S. I., AND NOVA, P. L.: *Intermittent disappearance of the murmur of patent ductus arteriosus.* Circulation 22:226, 1960.

58. HYRSKE, I., LANDTMAN, B., LOUHIMO, I., AND TOUTERI, L.: *Intermittent disappearance of the continuous murmur of patent ductus arteriosus.* Acta Paediat. Scand. 54:593, 1965.

59. RAVIN, A., AND DARLEY, W.: *Apical diastolic murmurs in patent ductus arteriosus.* Ann. Intern. Med. 33:903, 1950.

60. HUBBARD, T. F., AND NEIS, D. D.: *The sounds at the base of the heart in cases of patent ductus arteriosus.* Amer. Heart J. 59:807, 1960.

61. GRAYSEL, J., AND JAMESON, A. G.: *Optimum criteria for the diagnosis of patent ductus arteriosus from measurements of blood oxygen saturation.* Amer. Heart J. 67:23, 1964.

62. MOGHADAM, A. N., KHALIL, E. F., AND MATTIOLI, L. F.: *Intracardiac phonocardiography in the diagnosis of large patent ductus arteriosus in early infancy.* J. Pediat. 67:214, 1965.

63. DOTTER, G. T., AND STEINBERG, I.: *Angiocardiography in congenital heart disease.* Amer. J. Med. 12:219, 1952.

64. LIND, J., ROCHA, M., AND WEGELRUS, C.: *The value of fast angiocardiography in the early diagnosis of patent ducts arteriosus.* Amer. J. Roentgen. 77:235, 1957.

65. BAVERSFELD, S. R., ADKINS, P. C., AND KENT, E. M.: *Patent ductus arteriosus in infancy.* J. Thorac. Cardiov. Surg. 33:123, 1957.

66. CARTWRIGHT, R. S., AND BAVERSFELD, S. R.: *Thoracic aortography in infants and children.* Ann. Surg. 15:266, 1959.

67. SINGLETON, E. B., McNAMARA, D. G., AND COOLEY, D. A.: *Retrograde aortography in the diagnosis of congenital heart disease in infants.* J. Pediat. 47:720, 1955.

68. CAMPBELL, M.: *Natural history of persistent ductus arteriosus.* Brit. Heart J. 30:4, 1968.

69. PATE, J. W., AND AINGER, L. E.: *Aggressive approach to malignant patent arteriosus.* Surgery 53:811, 1963.

70. GROSS, R. E., AND LONGINO, L. A.: *The patent ductus arteriosus: Observations from 412 surgically treated cases.* Circulation 3:125, 1957.

71. SELLORS, T. H.: *Surgery of the persistent ductus arteriosus.* Lancet 1:615, 1945.

72. GERBODE, F., O'BRIEN, M. F., KERTH, W. J., AND ROBINSON, S. S.: *Surgical aspects of heart disease in infants under the age of two years.* Amer. J. Surg. 108:224, 1964.

73. HARDY, J. D., WEBB, W. R., TIMMIS, H., WATSON, D. G., AND BLAKE, T. M.: *Patent ductus arteriosus: Operative treatment of 100 consecutive patients with isolated lesions without mortality.* Ann. Surg. 164:877, 1966.

74. KIMBALL, K. G., AND McILROY, M. B.: *Pulmonary hypertension in patients with congenital heart disease.* Amer. J. Med. 41:883, 1966.

75. TRUSLER, G. A., ARAYANGKOON, P., AND MUSTARD, W. T.: *Operative closure of isolated patent ductus arteriosus in the first year of life.* Canad. Med. Assoc. J. 99:879, 1968.

Congenital Heart Disease in Adults

Albert N. Brest, M.D.

The diagnosis of congenital heart disease comes quickly to mind in the infant with a heart murmur and signs of cardiac distress. In contrast, the diagnosis is frequently overlooked in the adult patient. In young adults, the cardiac malformation is frequently misdiagnosed as a rheumatic lesion, while in older patients, presenting signs are often attributed to arteriosclerotic heart disease. The reason for this diagnostic credibility gap is related mainly to the lack of familiarity with the natural history of the various congenital cardiac malformations.

LENGTH OF SURVIVAL OF PATIENTS WITH MAJOR CARDIAC MALFORMATIONS

Investigations into the natural history of congenital cardiac disease indicate that most patients born with cardiac malformations die within the first year of life. However, certain persons with major cardiac anomalies may live for long periods. The studies of Fontana and Edwards,[1] Leech,[2] and Clawson[3] demonstrate that survivals beyond the age of 50 years are by no means rare.

Of the 357 cases studied by Fontana and Edwards,[1] only about one third of the patients lived beyond their tenth birthday, and less than one quarter lived to be adults; however, it is noteworthy that more than 10 per cent of those persons born alive lived for 50 years or more. Leech[2] reported a series of 75 patients with major cardiac malformations; of the latter group, 12 per cent lived to be adults, and 3 patients (4 per cent) lived more than 50 years. Clawson studied 141 patients with major malformations. He found that less than 20 per cent lived beyond 10 years, and less than 15 per cent lived to be adults. Three patients in the latter study lived to be more than 50 years old.

The advent of modern cardiac surgery has improved markedly the prognosis for patients with congenital heart disease. Most of the major cardiac malformations are amenable to surgical repair. As a result, there now exists a substantial population of patients with corrected congenital cardiac anomalies whose life span has been significantly prolonged beyond that which could be anticipated from the natural history of the disorder.

FREQUENCY OF OCCURRENCE OF VARIOUS ANATOMIC TYPES OF MALFORMATIONS

Although the exact frequency of occurrence of each type of cardiac malformation cannot be stated categorically, it is quite clear that certain types of malformations tend to occur much more commonly than others. Among 10 pathological studies in the literature,[1-10] six types of single malformations tended to predominate, i.e., ventricular septal defect, atrial septal defect, patent ductus arteriosus, tetralogy of Fallot, coarctation of the aorta, and complete transposition of the great vessels. The combined incidence of these six conditions accounts for about 50 per cent of all cardiac anomalies.

Certain disparities are evident when clinical and pathological studies of congenital cardiac malformations are compared. For example, both in pathological studies and in clinical studies of infants and children,[11] complete transposition of the great vessels is one of the most frequently encountered congenital lesions. In contrast, this anomaly is observed infrequently in clinical studies dealing with older children or adults.[12] The obvious reason for the discrepancy is that most patients with this disorder succumb during infancy or early childhood. On the other hand, pulmonary stenosis with intact ventricular septum is relatively uncommon (about 2 per cent) in pathological studies, whereas in clinical studies [13] it has generally been encountered much more often (about 8 per cent). Again, the apparent discrepancy can be explained by the fairly long survival usually observed among patients with this latter condition.

LENGTH OF SURVIVAL WITH VARIOUS TYPES OF CONGENITAL CARDIAC ANOMALIES

The discussion that follows deals with the six common cardiac malformations. Attention is focused on clinical aspects that apply particularly to adult patients.

Atrial Septal Defect

Atrial septal defect is compatible with a long life span. About 50 per cent of patients who have this malformation live more than 40 years, and survivals longer than 70 years are not uncommon.[14–17] In fact, in many instances death is unrelated to the atrial septal defect, even when the defect is relatively large. When death is related to the anomaly, it is usually caused by cardiac failure.[1] Although bacterial endocarditis and cerebral abscess may complicate this malformation, these complications are relatively uncommon.

In patients with atrial septal defect, symptoms are often insignificant until congestive heart failure develops.[18] In other patients, symptoms may be initiated by the development of arrhythmias and, in fact, irregularities in rhythm often predispose to or presage heart failure.

Following is the case history of an adult patient with atrial septal defect who was asymptomatic until age 48 when he developed recurrent atrial arrhythmias, the latter leading to discovery of the disorder and subsequent surgical correction.

S. B., a 48-year-old male, was discovered to have a heart murmur at age 10. However, he was asymptomatic until 1 month earlier when he suffered a bout of rapid heart action. Electrocardiograms indicated the presence of paroxysmal atrial tachycardia, which was controlled by rapid digitalization. Subsequently he experienced two additional episodes of atrial arrhythmia.

Physical examination was unremarkable except for the cardiac findings: Heart rate and rhythm were normal; grade 1 systolic murmur was heard at the pulmonary area; fixed splitting of the second sound was noted; PMI was not felt.

Chest X rays revealed moderate cardiomegaly with enlargement of the pulmonary artery and its main branches. The electrocardiogram disclosed complete right bundle branch block.

Cardiac catheterization revealed evidences of an atrial septal defect, with normal pulmonary artery pressure and normal cardiac output.

Because of recurrent bouts of atrial tachycardia, the patient was subsequently submitted to successful open-heart surgical repair of the atrial septal defect.

Ventricular Septal Defect

Ventricular septal defect frequently leads to death at an early age, often during the first year of life.[3, 5, 19, 20] However, occasional patients reach adult life, and survivals as long as 79 years have been reported.[21, 22] When death is the result of the cardiac malformation, it is usually caused by cardiac failure or bacterial endocarditis.[1] Cardiac failure is the more frequent cause of death among those who die young, while the likelihood that bacterial endocarditis will develop becomes greater as length of survival increases.

There appears to be a definite relationship between the size of the defect and the length of survival of patients who have ventricular septal defect. This is in contrast with atrial septal defect where there is no definite association between the size of the defect and the length of survival. Hemodynamic differences undoubtedly account for this disparity.

Following is the clinical resumé of a 51 year old patient with ventricular septal defect who was completely asymptomatic until 10 years earlier.

H. C., a 51-year-old male, had a known heart murmur since birth. However, he was asymptomatic until age 41 years, when cyanosis was noted and he began to experience progressive exertional dyspnea, intermittent episodes of hemoptysis, and occasional ankle edema. Other complaints included infrequent exertional angina and several short bouts of paroxysmal tachycardia.

Physical examination was unremarkable except for cyanosis of the lips and nail beds, digital clubbing of the fingers and toes, and the following cardiac findings: Heart rate and rhythm were normal; grade IV pansystolic murmur best heard at the fourth left interspace was transmitted to the apex and base of the heart.

Chest X rays revealed moderate cardiac enlargement with prominence of the main pulmonary artery segment, left ventricle, and right ventricle; in addition, there was slight engorgement of the vasculature in the lungs. The electrocardiogram disclosed biventricular hypertrophy. Hemoglobin was 17.4 gm. per 100 ml., hematocrit 61 per cent.

Hemodynamic studies disclosed the presence of a ventricular septal defect with a bidirectional shunt. The pulmonary arterial pressure was equal to that of the systemic (brachial artery) pressure, and arterial oxygen saturation was significantly decreased.

In view of the advanced hemodynamic changes that resulted from the ventricular septal defect, the operative risk was considered to be inordinately high, and it was decided to manage the patient conservatively.

Patent Ductus Arteriosus

About 50 per cent of patients with patent ductus arteriosus live to reach adult life. There are, in fact, many recorded instances of patients with proved patent ductus arteriosus who lived more than 60 years.[23-26] White and associates recently reported a patient who lived to the age of 90 years.[27]

It is now generally recognized that isolated patent ductus arteriosus may cause death during infancy. The infant who dies as a result of this disorder usually has a ductus that is rather large in comparison to the size of the aorta.[1] In these cases, the usual cause of death is cardiac failure, and this often is associated with a marked degree of pulmonary edema. In contrast, in the adult patient with patent ductus arteriosus in whom heart failure

260

develops, manifestations of right heart failure usually predominate. Whereas bacterial endocarditis rarely develops in infants with patent ductus arteriosus, this complication is one of the leading causes of death in those patients who survive infancy.

The following patient, like the two preceding ones, remained asymptomatic for more than 40 years. The subsequent 10-year history of symptoms was followed by discovery of the underlying congenital lesion, as a result of a complete diagnostic survey.

C. T., a 55-year-old female, was asymptomatic until 10 years earlier, when she began to note easy fatigue and progressive exertional dyspnea. She denied any significant chest pain, orthopnea, ankle edema, cough, or hemoptysis.

Physical examination was unremarkable except for blood pressure of 160/70 mm. Hg and a continuous murmur best heard at the second left intercostal space.

Chest X rays revealed prominence of the left ventricle, pulmonary outflow tract, and aorta. Electrocardiogram disclosed left ventricular hypertrophy.

Cardiac catheterization and catheter ascending aortography disclosed the presence of patent ductus arteriosus with left-to-right shunt and mild pulmonary hypertension (34/20 mm. Hg).

The patient underwent successful surgical ligation of the ductus. During the ensuing months, substantial clinical improvement was noted.

Tetralogy of Fallot

Most patients who have this malformation die during childhood. However, long survivals of patients with tetralogy of Fallot are not rare. Bain [28] reported a patient with this anomaly who died at the age of 69 years as a result of metastatic disease secondary to carcinoma of the prostate gland. White and Sprague [29] reported a case in which a famous American composer who had tetralogy of Fallot died at the age of 59 years.

Patients with this disorder may die suddenly during periods of intense cyanosis. Death may result also from cardiac failure, pneumonia, bacterial endocarditis, or cerebral complications, including abscess or infarction. Among the 357 cases of congenital heart disease studied by Fontana and Edwards,[1] cerebral abscess occurred twice as often in patients with tetralogy of Fallot as it did in patients with any other type of cardiac malformation.

The following patient with tetralogy of Fallot lived well into adult life without any cardiac manifestations except for a single bout of bacterial endocarditis. The latter was treated successfully, and she remained asymptomatic for another 10 years before the onset of symptoms related to the defect per se. Subsequent diagnostic workup established the correct diagnosis. Although a surgical candidate, the patient declined any operative intervention.

H. H., a 38-year-old female, had a known heart murmur since childhood. Except for some easy fatigue, she was essentially asymptomatic until 3 months earlier, when she began to note shortness of breath, intermittent orthopnea, and occasional syncopal episodes. She denied any cyanosis, chest pain, peripheral edema, or palpitation. Past medical history was unremarkable except for a bout of bacterial endocarditis at age 28.

The physical examination was unremarkable except for the cardiac findings: Heart rate and rhythm were normal; grade 5 systolic murmur starting at S1 and ending beyond A2 was heard throughout the precordium, best at the pulmonary area and third left sternal border; right ventricular heave was palpable.

Chest X rays revealed moderate cardiac enlargement. The electrocardiogram disclosed right ventricular hypertrophy. Cardiac catheterization revealed infundibular pulmonic stenosis and ventricular septal defect with right-to-left shunt.

Coarctation of the Aorta

As with patent ductus arteriosus, about 50 per cent of patients in whom coarctation of the aorta exists as a single malformation live to reach adult life.[1] Among patients with coarctation of the aorta who survive beyond infancy, the major causes of death are cardiac failure, rupture of the aorta, bacterial endocarditis or endarteritis, and cerebral hemorrhage.[30]

Cardiac failure and rupture of the aorta are, in a sense, mechanical complications of coarctation of the aorta. Heart failure results chiefly from the accompanying hypertension, while rupture of the aorta usually occurs proximal to the site of coarctation. The relatively high incidence of intracranial hemorrhage is also related, at least in part, to the hypertension. However, another factor contributing to the high incidence of intracranial hemorrhage is the increased prevalence of aneurysms of the circle of Willis. There is also a distinct tendency for congenital bicuspid aortic valve to be associated with coarctation of the aorta. As a result, bacterial endocarditis usually involves the aortic valve, and especially the congenitally bicuspid valves. In contrast, bacterial endarteritis (aortitis) is somewhat less common than endocarditis.

Although it might be understandable that a cardiac murmur (due to a congenital heart lesion) might be overlooked or, more to the point, misdiagnosed as an innocent murmur, it seems much less plausible to overlook, or at least fail to explain, the occurrence of hypertension in a child or young adult. The following is an example of a patient who had a known heart murmur and hypertension since childhood, and both signs were overlooked until the patient was more than 40 years of age. Undoubtedly, the patient pays a penalty when the congenital cardiac lesion remains undiagnosed for long periods, and surgery has to be undertaken at an advanced age. In the case of coarctation of the aorta, it has been established that the extent by which surgical correction lowers the blood pressure is proportional to the magnitude of the hypertension before the operation; and the greater the hypertension preoperatively, the greater the residual hypertension postoperatively.[31] After about 15 years of age, the blood pressure may reach levels from which a complete return to normal is unlikely.

O. S., a 44-year-old female, had a known heart murmur and hypertension since age 9. Easy fatigue was noted for many years, but she was otherwise asymptomatic until 1 year earlier, when she experienced frequent episodes of lightheadedness.

On physical examination, the blood pressure was 170/80 in the upper extremities but not obtainable in the lower extremities. Arterial pulses were palpable, but markedly diminished in both lower extremities. The heart rate and rhythm were normal; grade III midsystolic ejection murmur best heard at the base of the heart was transmitted to the carotid vessels and also well heard over the interscapular region. The findings were otherwise not remarkable.

Chest X rays revealed mild cardiac enlargement, prominence of the aortic knob, and rib notching. Electrocardiogram disclosed left ventricular hypertrophy.

Catheter thoracic aortography revealed coarctation of the aorta just beyond the origin of

262

the left subclavian artery. The study also disclosed the presence of an anatomically abnormal aortic valve, with the posterior cusp larger than normal and the right and left coronary cusps very small. There was, in addition, a suggestion of valvular "doming" during systole.

Complete Transposition of the Great Vessels

Patients with this malformation usually die early in infancy. About one half of the patients who have this anomaly die before the end of the third month of life, and relatively few patients live beyond the age of 1 year. Cardiac failure is the cause of death in most instances.

Long survivals of patients with this malformation are the exception, but have been reported by several investigators. Messeloff and Weaver [32] reported a patient with this defect who died at the age of 38 years. Other long survivals have been reported by Nichol and Segal [33] (26 years), Vogelsang [34] (19 years), Pung and associates [35] (18 years), Alexander and White [36] (17 years), and Keith [37] (16 years).

Patients with complete transposition of the great vessels cannot survive after birth unless some form of communication exists between the systemic and pulmonary circulations. Various studies indicate that the life expectancy of these patients is dependent upon the type of communication. Most patients with long survival have an associated ventricular septal defect. The outlook for survival is less favorable if a patent ductus arteriosus or an atrial septal defect is the only means of communication.

SUMMARY

Occasional instances of long survival have been reported with virtually all of the congenital cardiac anomalies. However, the three malformations that tend to predominate among patients who live 20 years or more are: (1) atrial septal defect, (2) patent ductus arteriosus, and (3) coarctation of the aorta. The ability of many patients to lead long, active lives is impressive.

Age per se should not be considered an important differential diagnostic point to be used in the exclusion of congenital heart disease. On the contrary, special diagnostic consideration should be given in the older patient with unexplained heart disease, so as not to overlook a potentially correctable (or at least remediable) cardiac disorder.

References

1. FONTANA, R. S., AND EDWARDS, J. E.: *Congenital Cardiac Disease: A Review of 357 Cases Studied Pathologically.* W. B. Saunders Co., Philadelphia, 1962.
2. LEECH, C. B.: *Congenital heart disease: Clinical analysis of seventy-five cases from the Johns Hopkins Hospital.* J. Pediat. 7:802, 1935.
3. CLAWSON, B. J.: *Types of congenital heart diseases in 15,597 autopsies.* Lancet 64:134, 1944.
4. ABBOTT, M. E.: *Atlas of Congenital Cardiac Disease.* The American Heart Association, New York, 1936.

5. GIBSON, S., AND CLIFTON, W. M.: *Congenital heart disease: A clinical and postmortem study of one hundred and five cases.* Amer. J. Dis. Child. 55:761, 1938.

6. SOMMERS, S. C., AND JOHNSON, J. M.: *Congenital tricuspid atresia.* Amer. Heart J. 41:130, 1951.

7. MCALEESE, J. J.: *A survey of congenital heart disease in a children's hospital: With special reference to surgical treatment.* Amer. J. Surg. 83:755, 1952.

8. WHITE, P. D.: *The natural history of congenital cardiovascular defects,* in *Congenital Heart Disease: Report of the Fourteenth M and R Pediatric Research Conference.* M & R Laboratories, Columbus, Ohio, 1955, pp. 61–70.

9. OBER, W. B., AND MOORE, T. E., JR.: *Congenital cardiac malformations in neonatal period: Autopsy study.* New Eng. J. Med. 253:271, 1955.

10. KEITH, J. D.: *Congenital heart disease,* in Parsons, L.: *Modern Trends in Pediatrics.* Paul B. Hoeber, Inc., New York, 1941, pp. 75–122.

11. STUCKEY, D.: *The pattern of congenital heart disease in infancy and children.* Aust. Med. J. 2:433, 1954.

12. BLUMENTHAL, S.: *The incidence of congenital cardiac malformations.* Trans. Amer. Coll. Cardiol. 3:209, 1953.

13. ABRAHAMS, D. G., AND WOOD, P.: *Pulmonary stenosis with normal aortic root.* Brit. Heart J. 13:519, 1951.

14. STANNUS, D. G., LANSMAN, W., AND REED, F. A.: *Atrial septal defect in a seventy year old patient.* J. Florida Med. Assoc. 41:947, 1955.

15. TINNEY, W. J., JR.: *Interatrial septal defect.* Arch. Intern. Med. 66:807, 1940.

16. TARNOWER, H., AND WOODRUFF, I. O.: *Widely patent foramen ovale: Case report with discussion of diagnosis.* Amer. Heart J. 12:358, 1936.

17. ELLIS, F. R., GREAVES, M., AND HECHT, H. H.: *Congenital heart disease in old age: Interauricular septal defect with mitral and tricuspid valvulitis.* Amer. Heart J. 40:154, 1950.

18. MARK, H., AND YOUNG, D.: *Congenital heart disease in the adult.* Amer. J. Cardiol. 15:293, 1965.

19. MARQUIS, R. M.: *Ventricular septal defect in early childhood.* Brit. Heart J. 12:265, 1950.

20. ENGLE, M. A.: *Ventricular septal defect in infancy.* Pediatrics 14:16, 1954.

21. SELZER, A.: *Defect of the ventricular septum: Summary of twelve cases and review of the literature.* Arch. Intern. Med. 84:798, 1949.

22. SELZER, A., AND LAQUEUR, G. L.: *The Eisenmenger complex and its relation to the uncomplicated defect of the ventricular septum: Review of thirty-five autopsied cases of Eisenmenger's complex, including two new cases.* A.M.A. Arch. Intern. Med. 87:218, 1951.

23. LINDERT, M. C. F., AND CORRELL, H. L.: *Rupture of pulmonary aneurysm accompanying patent ductus arteriosus: Occurrence in 67 year old woman.* J.A.M.A. 143:888, 1950.

24. FISHMAN, L., AND SILVERTHORNE, C.: *Persistent patent ductus arteriosus in the aged: Including the report of the oldest case on record with diagnosis confirmed post mortem.* Amer. Heart J. 41:762, 1951.

25. HOLMAN, E., GERBODE, F., AND PURDY, A.: *The patent ductus: A review*

of seventy-five cases with surgical treatment including an aneurysm of the ductus and one of the pulmonary artery. J. Thorac. Surg. 25:111, 1953.

26. STORSTEIN, O., HUMMERFELT, S., MULLER, O., AND RASMUSSEN, H.: *Patent ductus arteriosus in a woman aged 72 years.* Brit. Heart J. 14:276, 1952.

27. WHITE, P. D., MAZURKIE, S. J., AND BOSCHETTI, A. E.: *Patency of the ductus at 90.* New Eng. J. Med. 280:146, 1969.

28. BAIN, G. O.: *Tetralogy of Fallot: Survival to seventieth year: Report of a case.* A.M.A. Arch. Path. 58:176, 1954.

29. WHITE, P. D., AND SPRAGUE, H. B.: *The tetralogy of Fallot: Report of a case in a noted musician who lived to his sixtieth year.* J.A.M.A. 92:787, 1929.

30. ABBOTT, M. E.: *Coarctation of the aorta of the adult type. II. A statistical study and historical retrospect of 200 recorded cases with autopsy, of stenosis or obliteration of the descending arch.* Amer. Heart J. 33:146, 1947.

31. SELLORS, T. H., AND HOBSLEY, M.: *Coarctation of the aorta: Effect of operation on blood pressure.* Lancet 1:1387, 1963.

32. MESSELOFF, C. R., AND WEAVER, J. C.: *A case of transposition of the large vessels in an adult who lived to the age of 38 years.* Amer. Heart J. 42:467, 1951.

33. NICHOL, A. D., AND SEGAL, A. J.: *Complete transposition of the main arterial stems: Report of a case.* J.A.M.A. 147:545, 1951.

34. VOGELSANG, A.: *Transposition of the great arteries with patent foramen ovale.* Canad. Med. Ass. J. 69:625, 1953.

35. PUNG, S., GOTTSTEIN, W. K., AND HIRSCH, E. F.: *Complete transposition of great vessels in a male aged eighteen years.* Amer. J. Med. 18:155, 1955.

36. ALEXANDER, F., AND WHITE, P. D.: *Four important congenital cardiac conditions causing cyanosis to be differentiated from the tetralogy of Fallot: Tricuspid atresia, Eisenmenger's complex, transposition of the great vessels, and a single ventricle.* Ann. Intern. Med. 27:64, 1947.

37. KEITH, A.: *Six specimens of abnormal heart.* J. Anat. Physiol. 46:211, 1912.

Medical Management of the Patient with Congenital Heart Disease

Mary Allen Engle, M.D.

The goals of medical management are to enable the individual born with a cardiac anomaly to perform at the peak of his physical capacity and to encourage him to be a happy and effective member of his peer group. These goals are as applicable to the nursery schooler as to the businessman and housewife.

This medical management is a lifetime affair. It begins as soon as the cardiac condition is recognized (usually when a murmur is first detected) and, unless the condition is completely corrected and the heart is then entirely normal, it continues until death. The management is of several forms: diagnostic, expectant, preventive, and therapeutic.

Optimal management of that individual depends on a knowledge of the type and severity of his specific lesion(s), superimposed on what is known of the natural history of that defect as growth, development, and ageing take place.[1-3] In general, the newborn infant is at greatest risk of being affected by his malformation or of dying from it.[4] Though the incidence of congenital heart disease is 8 per 1,000 live births,[5, 6] the prevalence in school-aged children is only about 4 per 1,000.[7, 8] This mortality rate of 50 per cent occurs in the first year of life and chiefly in the first 3 months of life. The childhood years are relatively benign, with few complications and with freedom from symptoms except for those who are cyanotic. It is during late adolescence and early adult life that in some patients symptoms and disability become evident again. With few exceptions, most of the common malformations follow this pattern. Exceptions are the condition of atrial septal defect, which causes no difficulty in the first year of life and, indeed, is rarely recognized that early. An exception too, but in the opposite direction, is a malformation common in infancy but rarely encountered later unless surgery has intervened to make it possible: complete transposition of the great arteries.

TOOLS OF DIAGNOSIS

Frequently Used

Fortunately, the correlations that have been made between findings at the bedside and those from pathophysiological studies plus contrast visualization of the cardiovascular system have rendered increasingly accurate the information the physician can obtain from simple and readily available tools: a careful *physical examination* abetted initially and serially as indicated by *electrocardiogram* and *cardiac series of chest roentgenograms*.[9] This last consists of four views (frontal, right-anterior-oblique, left-anterior-oblique, and lateral) with barium swallow in each view. In this way, all four cardiac chambers and both great arteries can be evaluated. These three tools, together with a blood count, can be utilized at frequent intervals throughout the long-term followup of the patient so that the physician can, with confidence in his knowledge of his patient's status, recommend the appropriate management. This may take the form of hospitalization for specialized cardiac diagnostic studies or for surgery or for treatment of complications. Such an event looms large when it is advised for special indication, but this is an infrequent recommendation in the life-long management of the individual born with a cardiovascular defect.

Infrequently Used

The indications for *cardiac catheterization with contrast visualization* are for full evaluation in the following circumstances:

Infancy

Catheterization is performed on strong indications and often as an emergency procedure.

TREATMENT FOR CARDIAC FAILURE. Whether medical management will be continued or surgical intervention is required, it is important to document the lesions and their effects when the infant's heart fails. Sometimes several malformations coexist, and some of them may be masked by the presence of the others. Sometimes even the major lesion cannot be distinguished from other similar ones without these studies. This is particularly true when there is pulmonary hypertension together with a large left-to-right shunt at the ventricular level or beyond. The differential diagnosis among a ventricular septal defect and truncus arteriosus, aortic septal defect, and patent ductus arteriosus is a common one in the noncyanotic baby admitted for cardiac failure.

A DEEPLY CYANOTIC NEWBORN. Cyanotic congenital heart disease is the most common cause of persistent cyanosis in the newborn but occasionally cannot be differentiated by bedside techniques from pulmonary or peripheral circulatory causes for desaturation in the sick cyanotic newborn. Cardiac catheterization may be needed to settle the question and to determine proper management of the baby.

More often, the physician is sure that the infant has cyanotic congenital heart disease and has made a preliminary sorting out between that group with diminished pulmonary blood flow and that without by examining the chest roentgenograms for the status of the pulmonary vasculature. Excessively clear lung fields imply severe pulmonary stenosis or atresia. This infant is likely a candidate for early, even emergency cardiac surgery. If the lung fields of the newborn are congested, this usually indicates pulmonary venous obstruction, as from left ventricular failure or anomalous drainage of pulmonary veins. If in addition, the base of the heart is abnormally narrow in the frontal view and twice as wide in an oblique view, one makes the diagnosis of complete transposition of the great arteries. After six or more weeks of age, the baby with congested lung fields usually has overcirculation from a large left-to-right shunt, most likely at the ventricular or aorticopulmonary area. Under any of these situations, the physician desires anatomic delineation; often this is in anticipation of surgery.

Childhood, Adolescence, Adulthood

    a. Preoperative assessment in anticipation of surgery
    b. Postoperative evaluation of results of surgery

c. Clarification of an obscure or complex condition
d. Followup of a specific problem, such as pulmonary hypertension
e. Documentation of the malformation in the adolescent or adult for such purposes as athletic competition, insurability, or job placement
f. Long-term evaluation of the effects of the defect

When these studies are performed by a skilled and experienced team, the information gained is considerable and the risks are minimal.[10] Morbidity and mortality from the study are highest in the youngest patients.[11, 12] This is not surprising, for one would not study a sick newborn unless the information sought was critical for his immediate medical or surgical management.

EXPECTANT MANAGEMENT

This term most closely describes what the physician does on his regular checkups of his patient's condition and progress. Expectant management is age related.

Infancy

Since the pediatrician knows that many babies with congenital heart disease do satisfactorily, yet that the greatest risk of death for them is in the first few months of life, he expects the best but is on the alert for the worst. He arranges to see the baby often enough to detect any warning signs of failure to thrive or of cardiac failure so that he may take appropriate action. If he finds that the baby's progress is good, he passes this reassuring news on to the parents. The usual well-baby care and immunizations are given as for any other baby.

Once the period of greatest likelihood of cardiac difficulty is safely passed, examinations can be at longer intervals for the second 6 months, perhaps twice a year for the second year, and usually annually thereafter until adolescence. On each visit, the physician notes any changes in heart size, heart sounds and murmurs, and he pays close attention to the rate of weight gain and growth. A change from the previous growth curve may be the first signal of worsening or of improvement. During the first year an electrocardiogram every 3 or 4 months is helpful in judging whether the baby's tracing follows the expected pattern of regression of right ventricular dominance or whether hypertrophy of any cardiac chamber is present. From the second year on, records once a year usually suffice. Radiological studies are obtained less often still, for one wants to avoid undue radiation in an individual destined for long-term followup over many years. Considerable irradiation is involved when cardiac catheterization, angiocardiography, and surgery are performed; so it seems wise to hold the number of X-ray films down to the minimum consistent with good care.

Childhood

Even if the baby has not done well in the first year of life and perhaps has required treatment for cardiac failure, almost always there is improvement after the first year. By the second year, parents and physicians alike are

270

impressed by the energy and activity of the toddler. The childhood years are generally free of symptoms, unless the child is cyanotic; so the doctor must look beyond the lack of symptoms and examine closely for signs of cardiac enlargement or overactivity and for radiological or electrocardiographic evidence of a cardiac or pulmonary burden.

Though the childhood years are a benign time from a cardiac standpoint, it is during this period that we recommend surgery electively for certain conditions: before starting to school for the child with a patent ductus arteriosus or large ventricular septal defect, before the adolescent growth spurt for coarctation of the aorta, and at any convenient time from 5 years on for closure of an atrial septal defect or relief of moderately severe valvular pulmonic stenosis. Surgery for more serious degrees of pulmonic stenosis and for severe aortic stenosis is performed whenever the condition is recognized. Open repair of cyanotic conditions such as tetralogy of Fallot is not scheduled until around the age of 6 years. Such surgical procedures are well tolerated by the child who has been prepared for them psychologically and who is handled with understanding and kindness in the postoperative period.

Beginning when the child is 4 or 5 years old, we inform the parents about penicillin prophylaxis for dental extractions or tonsillectomy and adenoidectomy, and we remind them on each visit.

Full activity is permitted except for those with cardiac enlargement, moderately severe aortic stenosis, or complete heart block. Then we restrict competitive team sports or activities that require long sustained, strenuous effort.

Adolescence

Typically the time of rebellion, these few years pose a problem for physicians, chiefly when teen-aged boys with mild to moderate aortic stenosis want to go out for the basketball or track team or, perhaps still worse, a body-contact sport like football. The unwed teen-aged mother with congenital heart disease poses another problem. It has been suggested that some actually seek to become pregnant as proof to themselves that they are as "normal" and healthy as their friends. In our cardiac clinic, we have a separate afternoon session each week for adolescents with congenital heart disease so they "don't have to come with the little kids." We schedule fewer patients than usual for the doctors so that there is ample time for communication. Eligibility for the draft and suitability for college or a job or marriage are frequent topics of conversation. Patients are counselled in the type of job appropriate for their physical condition. These youngsters usually attend clinic alone. We interpret to them their cardiac status and offer encouragement and reassurance when things are going well. Unless they have special problems, we extend the interval between visits to 2 or 3 years. They too are reminded about dental care and penicillin prophylaxis for oral procedures.

Adulthood

As pediatric cardiologists, we try to have the individual in the best shape possible before he enters the adult world with its many responsibilities.

Elective and indicated cardiac surgery is performed in childhood or adolescence to avoid the psychological and medical handicaps of that undertaking after he has the responsibilities of a job and family.

Marriage and a family are important considerations for the young man and woman with congenital heart disease. Their parents have usually asked long ago about these possibilities for their child. We have observed that even cyanosis and considerable cardiac disability have been no barrier to falling in love and having a happy marriage. The young woman who has had remedial or palliative cardiac surgery or whose cardiac condition is so mild that surgery is not indicated has an excellent chance of an uneventful pregnancy and a healthy baby. The cyanotic woman has a better than average chance to miscarry or to have a baby with low birth weight.[13] Prospective parents sometimes ask if their baby will have congenital heart disease. No one can tell this in advance, but if there is no family history of congenital heart disease, their risk of a malformed child is somewhat greater than average, but nonetheless, their chances of having healthy offspring are excellent. If there is a family history of cardiac malformation, the risk is increased further.[14] If the malformation is of a common type in one or more relatives, the chances of a malformation in the baby are increased about fourfold.[15]

Bacterial endocarditis occurs more often in adults than in children, probably because there are more years of adulthood than childhood; the patient is at risk for a longer time.[16, 17] Prophylaxis against this infection should continue to be stressed.

PREVENTIVE MANAGEMENT

Psychological Considerations

The label "cardiac cripple" need rarely be applied in modern times, because physicians can be deservedly optimistic in their expectant handling of the individual with congenital heart disease. Knowledge is much more secure now than in earlier days concerning the excellent life expectancy of those with mildly to moderately severe congenital heart disease. For practically all those who need help, it is available, either medically or surgically. The informed physician does not overlay the many with the blanket of worry that should be reserved for only a few. Psychologically as well as physically, much has been gained in these last 20 years in the management of the person with congenital heart disease. Emotional cardiac cripples can be prevented by the manner in which the physician handles the patient.

Bacterial Endocarditis

Bacterial endocarditis can almost always be prevented at times of predictable risk, such as following dental extractions, by use of penicillin in therapeutic doses immediately before and for 3 days after the procedure. Equal attention should be given at the time of vaginal delivery or genitourinary surgery.[18] Endocarditis does still occur unpredictably, and there

272

is little one can do in preventive medicine, except to encourage good dental hygiene at all times.[19] The physician can, however, do the next best thing: recognize early any suggestion of bacterial endocarditis so that he can begin appropriate treatment. Patients can be asked to report promptly any febrile illness. The physician should refrain from prescribing penicillin for the patient with congenital heart disease unless he knows he is treating a specific condition, such as streptococcal sore throat or pneumococcal pneumonia. Treatment with penicillin for an unexplained fever will only temporarily suppress bacterial endocarditis and prolong the period when cardiac damage and other complications can occur with ongoing, inadequately treated endocarditis.

Cerebral Abscess or Thrombosis

The cyanotic individual is susceptible to two cerebral complications: brain abscess and cerebral thrombosis.[20–23] The former is rare before school age; the latter is apt to occur in the anemic, hypoxic infant and in the teen-ager or young adult who is polycythemic. Both complications are related to a pathway for venoarterial shunting. If this communication were abolished, such a condition could be prevented. However, this is not possible for some cyanotic individuals. Attention to good dental hygiene should minimize the risk of brain abscess, and attention to the blood count (the patient should be neither anemic nor excessively polycythemic) should minimize the risk of cerebral thrombosis. Treatment with iron is indicated for the cyanotic baby with hypochromic anemia. Plasmapheresis may help keep the polycythemia of the older individual at a safe level.

Pulmonary Vascular Obstruction

A great fear exists among many doctors who take care of infants, children, and adults with a left-to-right shunt that pulmonary vascular obstruction may develop. Actually, this fear is unfounded except for the relatively small number of infants and children who have a large ventricular septal defect or patent ductus big enough for systolic pressures to approximate across the communication. With atrial septal defects, pulmonary vascular disease is not apparent until a number of years have passed; some young adults around the age of 30 years or beyond become symptomatic from it.[24] Surgery in childhood, while the pulmonary hypertension is hyperkinetic, should prevent the possibility of pulmonary vascular obstructive disease in adult life.

Premature Cardiac Disability and Death

The whole plan of medical management of the person with congenital heart disease is to prevent premature cardiac disability and death and to enable him during his life span to lead as full and active a life as is possible with the developments of medical sciences. The expectant and preventive approaches to management described above, together with indicated therapy to be discussed below, should accomplish this goal for most patients.

THERAPEUTIC MEASURES

At important but infrequent times in the life of the individual with congenital heart disease, there arise certain situations calling for specific treatment. These include cardiac failure, bacterial endocarditis, arrhythmias and conduction disturbances, cyanotic "spells," and cerebrovascular complications.

Selection for surgery is a combined medical-surgical decision, as is the pre- and postoperative care of the patient. Most postoperative complications require medical management: the postpericardiotomy syndrome; the post-perfusion syndrome of fever, hepatosplenomegaly and lymphocytosis; arrhythmias; heart block; intravascular hemolytic anemia; post-surgical endocarditis; and pulmonary dysfunction. The postoperative syndrome of fever and mesenteric vasculitis experienced by some children following resection of coarctation of the aorta may need a combined medical and surgical approach; so may the rarely encountered "anterior compartment syndrome." This occurs immediately after cardiopulmonary bypass and is characterized by intense swelling and pain with later neuromuscular wasting of the lower leg. We shall discuss some of these in more detail.

Cardiac Failure

For the entire life span, the greatest risk of occurrence of cardiac decompensation in the individual with congenital heart disease is in the first few months of life.[25] The next greatest time of risk is in the post-surgical period, and the third time is in mid and late adult life.[26]

In babies, the symptoms and signs of cardiac failure are more subtle than at older ages.[27] Usually tachypnea in the newborn and fatigue on feeding are the two main manifestations. Though their dyspnea is due to left-sided failure, rales in the lungs are rare. Hepatomegaly with rounded edge is the sign of right-sided failure, while edema of the extremities is rare. There may be slight generalized edema, best detected by an ususually "good" weight gain on the physician's scale, but also noticed as puffiness of the eyelids.

Treatment of cardiac failure at any age depends on digitalization, calculated in the infant and child according to weight and adjusted according to his response.[27-29] Diuretics and restriction of sodium are helpful. In the infant these measures usually are not needed beyond the acute phase of treatment. Electrolyte imbalance can occur from chronic use, and the results can be disastrous, especially for a baby. Additional measures that are used in the acute period for those with left-sided failure are oxygen and an orthopneic position. For the dyspneic infant, a baby seat that can be adjusted to a comfortable angle is used.

Once the cardiac failure is under control, one determines the cause for

274

the failure and then corrects or improves that if possible. In the baby, cardiac catheterization is utilized to rule in or out the suspected diagnosis and to define the problem. If the decompensation results from patent ductus arteriosus, ligation of the ductus is performed. If the diagnosis is ventricular septal defect, then medical management is continued, usually for the first year of life. The indication for surgery in babies with that condition is the failure of medical management. Such failure is indicated by return of cardiac decompensation (despite adequate medication), persistent poor weight gain, or repeated pneumonia. If pulmonic or aortic stenosis is the cause of the failure, open-heart surgery is indicated, despite its relatively greater difficulties in small subjects.

In children, cardiac failure is rare, and then it is usually a postoperative event. For example, in a patient with tetralogy of Fallot, the heart may fail after a palliative procedure in which too large an aorticopulmonary anastomosis has been made, or after open heart surgery through an extensive right ventriculotomy if there are a residual ventricular septal defect and pulmonic regurgitation. In situations such as these, medical measures and the healing effects of time usually suffice to improve the patient. Occasionally more surgery must be undertaken if the failure cannot be controlled.

In the adult with congenital heart disease, cardiac failure is apt to be the end stage of a long-standing cardiac overload, accentuated by the ageing process, coronary arterial involvement, arrhythmias, or infection. Prognosis usually is not good, although medical management may improve the patient for a number of years. Surgery has less to offer here than in younger age groups, and its risk is higher, but successful operations have lessened the symptoms and improved the life expectancy for a number of people middle aged or older.[30, 31]

For all these age groups, digitalis is continued until the cause for the failure has been corrected or improved and the size of the heart has decreased toward normal.

Bacterial Endocarditis

Unexplained, persistent, or recurrent fever in a person of any age with congenital heart disease is suspect as the sign of endocarditis until proved otherwise.[32, 33] Fever with some malaise and tender splenomegaly are often the only evidence of the illness. Petechiae, anemia, Osler's nodes, hematuria, and embolic phenomena or cardiac failure are late signs and are not often encountered. Proof of diagnosis is by blood cultures, usually four, obtained over a 24- to 48-hour period.

Once the organism has been recovered and its sensitivities to antibiotics tested, one can adjust the medication and the duration of therapy accordingly. If the cultures are still negative after 48 hours and no other cause for the fever has been identified, one should begin treatment with large doses of intravenous penicillin (20,000,000 units for an adult) and intramuscular streptomycin as though the organism were resistant to antibiotics. The streptomycin can be stopped after 2 weeks and the penicillin after 4 weeks. If the organism recovered is the usual pencillin-sensitive Streptococcus viridans, the streptomycin may be discontinued sooner.

Post-surgical endocarditis in the patient treated prophylactically [34] with massive doses of antibiotics is apt to be due to a different organism, such as the Staphylococcus or an unusual gram-negative bacillus.[35] Most of these organisms are highly resistant to common antibiotics, but new drugs are becoming available to be used according to the sensitivities of the organism in question. Though the term "bacterial" endocarditis is the one commonly employed, fungi too may cause the infection, particularly in the postoperative period.

It is hoped that infective endocarditis will be prevented, but that if it occurs, it will be recognized early enough for treatment to be effective before complications occur, such as embolic phenomena, valvular insufficiency, or myocardial failure.

Arrhythmias

Some patients with congenital heart disease are susceptible to spontaneous attacks of paroxysmal tachycardia, both supraventricular and ventricular. For reasons that are not altogether clear, adults with atrial septal defect, for example, may develop atrial tachycardia, flutter, or fibrillation. Under anesthesia and in the early postoperative period, this tendency to arrhythmias may be enhanced.[36–38] This seems to be true for adults more than for children. Paroxysmal tachycardia is not well tolerated after surgery nor by the individual who has symptoms even when in normal rhythm. Prompt treatment is indicated to terminate the attack by medications (digitalization for supraventricular tachycardia, intravenous lidocaine for ventricular tachycardia) or by D.C. conversion if the condition is critical. Attention is then directed to prevention of recurrences, e.g., by continuing digitalis in maintenance doses or by correcting the cause of the arrhythmia, if such can be found. In the early postoperative patient, the arrhythmia may be associated with impaired ventilation.[39] If the latter can be corrected, the former also will improve. Children with certain malformations are especially prone to postoperative arrhythmias, in particular those undergoing the Mustard procedure for complete transposition of the great arteries. They need prolonged maintenance digitalis.[40]

Conduction Disturbances

Intraventricular conduction disturbances are common and of no consequence so far as management is concerned. Incomplete right bundle branch block is almost always found in patients with atrial septal defect and in those who have successfully undergone pulmonary valvotomy for valvular pulmonic stenosis. Complete right bundle branch block is present after repair of most ventricular septal defects.

Atrioventricular conduction disturbances are far less common but of much greater concern. They may be present with some malformations from birth and are an added handicap to that baby's survival. Heart block may be acquired spontaneously, especially in patients with "corrected" or L transposition and ventricular inversion, or postoperatively, when a ventricular septal defect or atrioventricular canal is repaired. Although spontaneously acquired complete heart block may be well tolerated for years, acutely induced surgical heart block may be disastrous in the immediate postoperative period and even in the first few years after surgery.[41]

Medical management of complete heart block, e.g., with isoproterenol sublingually, is generally unsatisfactory. If the patient needs help, as he surely does just after cardiac surgery or if he has shown symptoms of fatigue, cardiac failure, or Stokes-Adams attacks, then an artificial pacemaker should be implanted transvenously or surgically. Artificial pacemakers may be life saving, but they add other problems in the management of the person with congenital heart disease. The power pack may fail, wires break, or fibrosis occur about the myocardial electrodes. Children seem to tolerate pacemakers less well than adults, probably because their activities and games put greater stress on the wires and connections. In the situation of surgically induced heart block, prevention is better than treatment. Great effort should be made in the operating room to avoid this complication.

Cyanotic Spells

Infants with severe pulmonary stenosis and a right-to-left shunt at the ventricular level (as with tetralogy of Fallot) or at the atrial level (as with tricuspid atresia) may suffer attacks of deep cyanosis, dyspnea, and anxiety. These spells occur spontaneously, or on slight provocation, and frequently in the early morning. Parents often consider that they represent colic or temper tantrums. In reality, they represent sudden additional restriction of pulmonary blood flow because of infundibular spasm, with direction of practically the entire cardiac output into the systemic circulation. The drop in systemic oxyhemoglobin saturation may be profound, so that loss of consciousness or convulsions occur.

Management of the immediate episode consists of holding the baby in a knee-chest position. If a physician or nurse is present during a severe or prolonged attack, an injection of morphine sulfate, 0.2 mg. per kg., affords prompt relief. Oxygen administration is not of much help during an attack because the pulmonary blood flow is so reduced then.

Iron-deficiency anemia may increase the tendency to spells; so treatment with iron or transfusions may help the infant through this difficult period. If the hypoxic infant who is anemic is treated with iron, it is important to follow the hemoglobin and hematocrit closely so that no overshoot occurs and results in excessive polycythemia. Use of propranolol,[42] intravenously in an acute attack and orally for weeks or months, has improved the symptoms of cyanotic spells in certain babies and children, for whom there is reason to defer surgery.

These forms of medical management do help, but early surgical intervention is usually indicated when an infant or child has cyanotic spells: a systemic-to-pulmonary arterial anastomosis unless the child is around 6 years of age and has anatomy suitable for open repair.

Cerebrovascular Complications

The two chief cerebrovascular complications of patients with congenital heart disease are brain abscess and cerebral thrombosis or embolization. Both occur chiefly in individuals with a route for right-to-left shunting. It is important to distinguish the two, because their management is quite different. Certain features are helpful in this regard. Brain abscess is rarely seen before the age of 2 years, whereas thromboembolism occurs most often in the first 2 years and again in early adulthood. The onset of symptoms of brain abscess is insidious, while that of thromboembolism is sudden. The cerebrospinal fluid in abscess shows an increase in pressure and protein, and if there has been rupture, in white cells. With thromboembolism, however, the pressure and protein generally are normal and, depending on communication with the subarachnoid space, red cells may be found. The electroencephalogram shows a localized abnormality with brain abscess but a more diffuse one in the other condition.

Brain Abscess

Persistent, localized headache is the presenting symptom. Somnolence, convulsions, localizing neurological signs, and death may occur in frighteningly rapid sequence. A high index of suspicion, careful neurological examination, lumbar tap, electroencephalogram, and echoencephalogram permit diagnosis. Management begins with neurosurgical consultation. Massive doses of intravenous antibiotics and surgical drainage are needed. If organisms are recovered, antibiotic therapy can be adjusted appropriately. With early recognition and both medical and surgical management, survival rate is about 75 per cent.

Cerebral Thrombosis or Embolism

Those at greatest risk of this complication are the anemic, hypoxic infant and the excessively polycythemic young adult. Careful attention in cyanotic patients to maintaining the hemoglobin and hematocrit in the range between these two extremes should prevent some of these accidents. Administration of iron is indicated for the anemic, hypoxic baby until his hemoglobin reaches about 16 to 17 gm. and the hematocrit 48 to 52. For the excessively polycythemic older individual who is not a candidate for palliative or corrective surgery, repeated plasmaphereses should be employed at intervals sufficient to keep the blood count in a safe range.

If a sudden cerebrovascular accident has occurred, treatment is supportive, with attention paid to fluid and electrolyte balance. Rehabilitation with physical therapy begins as soon as the situation is stable and the patient can tolerate it.

278

Postoperative Complications [43]

Postpericardiotomy Syndrome

This febrile illness with pericardial and sometimes pleural reaction occurs in about one quarter of the patients undergoing surgery that involves wide incision of the pericardium.[44, 45] In this setting, diagnosis is based on identifying the signs of pericarditis by physical examination, ECG, and X ray and on excluding other causes of postoperative fever, such as endocarditis. The most effective management is rest in bed and restriction of activities until the condition spontaneously subsides. The danger of this complication is that pericardial fluid may accumulate and cause life-threatening cardiac tamponade. Pericardiocentesis is then indicated, sometimes as an emergency procedure. If the effusion reaccumulates so that repeated taps are necessary, we consider this the indication for steroid therapy to suppress the manifestations of the reaction. The patient's response determines how quickly it can be withdrawn. Treatment is continued for a week in most instances. Recurrences, usually mild, with precordial pain and fever, may continue into the first or second year after operation.

Postperfusion Syndrome

This postoperative complication is self limited and is noted about 6 weeks after surgery in which the heart-lung machine is used. It is characterized by fever, hepatosplenomegaly, and lymphocytosis.[46, 47] It is self limited and requires no management other than the exclusion of bacterial endocarditis.

Hemolytic Anemia

Intravascular hemolysis sufficient to produce severe anemia with hemosiderinuria and hypochromia was first reported after surgery for atrioventricular canal in which the mitral cleft was sutured and a Teflon patch was used to close the ostium primum defect.[48] The hemolytic anemia has since been encountered in other postoperative situations, such as insertion of a prosthetic aortic valve, and it has been identified in mild form in some unoperated patients with aortic stenosis or regurgitation.[49] For patients with mild to moderate anemia, iron therapy to correct the hypochromia may be the only management needed to improve the situation. After a period of months or years, the hemolytic anemia may gradually lessen and even disappear. For patients with severe anemia and marked symptoms unrelieved by transfusion and iron supplementation, reoperation may have to be undertaken.

Pulmonary Dysfunction

Optimal respiratory management in the operating theater and in the recovery room is essential for success of the operation.[50, 51] For infants and for children and adults undergoing complicated open-heart surgery, it is important to monitor arterial and venous pH and blood gases at frequent intervals before they leave the operating room and while they require intensive care. Only in this way can the adequacy of pulmonary function and the effects of metabolic adjustments be evaluated in the sick individual.

We prefer to have most infants and children so lightly anesthetized at the end of the procedure that they are practically awake and are extubated by the time they arrive in the recovery room. Endotracheal tubes can obstruct the airway because of their small size in relation to the trachea, and they can become completely obstructed by incompletely suctioned secretions. Respirator therapy should be reserved for those who demonstrate by blood gas determinations an inability to ventilate and oxygenate adequately. Under these circumstances, a tracheostomy is done and the respirator adjusted according to the patient's size and response. Very frequent and promptly reported determinations of arterial pH, pO_2, and pCO_2 are essential for the physician to manage the patient whose respirations have been taken over by a machine.

The "pump lung" problem of hemorrhagic atelectasis, manifested by some children after open-heart repair of tetralogy of Fallot, for instance, may prove lethal in the first days after surgery or may gradually improve, partially or completely.[52] We have recently studied two children with open repair of the tetralogy who underwent tracheostomies and respirator therapy for more than a week after surgery and who have, on postoperative catheterization, pulmonary hypertension that was not present before surgery. Meticulous attention to postoperative respiratory function is essential to avoid the problems of respirators and the risk of death or of temporary or permanent pulmonary dysfunction.

Postcoarctectomy Syndrome

The syndrome occurs chiefly in young children and is characterized by fever, abdominal pain, and in its severe form by hypertension even higher than that measured preoperatively, by ileus, and by infarction of the intestines.[53] Surgery is needed, if infarction occurs, to resect the nonviable segments. Fistulae have been reported to develop in later weeks or months. The pathologic process is an intense vasculitis. Management is expectant and supportive unless signs appear that suggest gangrene of the bowel, in which case resection is performed. This complication is a rare occurrence in our experience, possibly because we defer elective surgery for coarctation to the age of 10 to 14 years.

The "Anterior Compartment" Syndrome

We have observed four children who had open-heart surgery with cardiopulmonary bypass and perfusion into a femoral artery and who in the first hours postoperatively showed rapidly progressing and intensely painful swelling of the calf of the perfused leg. Arterial pulses were lost in the popliteal space and foot. The edema became stony hard, and the patient could not tolerate active or passive movement of that painful foot and leg. We think that whatever produced this reaction caused both the arterial and venous channels to become compromised in association with the intense brawny edema and that damage to nerves and muscles occurred at the same time.

280

Fasciotomy to release the tension was performed in two children. Exploration of the vessels of the groin did not help the one child in whom it was performed. Anticoagulation with heparin and then dicoumarol was used in two, who improved more promptly than the other two. All sustained injury to nerve and muscle, with foot drop and wasting of the muscles of the calf. Physiotherapy was instituted as soon as the pain subsided enough for passive and active movement, and it was continued for several weeks to a few months. One child recovered completely, another almost so, and the remaining two still have considerable muscular wasting and some problem with foot drop. We think that the best management for this unusual complication consists of fasciotomy and anticoagulation, followed by physiotherapy.[54]

Selection of Patients for Cardiac Surgery

This important decision in the life of the patient with congenital heart disease is arrived at by physician and surgeon together, and that team approach to care continues throughout the period of hospitalization for surgery. Though we have just discussed prevention and management of postoperative complications, we should put these in the total perspective of what cardiac surgery, both palliative and corrective, can do for the patient. The complications are few, and the marvelous and gratifying results are many.

Here are a cardiologist's indications for surgery in the most common malformations of the heart and great vessels.

Ventricular Septal Defect

INFANCY. Intensive medical management usually succeeds, but if it should not after a fair trial, then banding of the pulmonary artery to produce a 75 per cent constriction should be done. Narrowing the lumen to one fourth of its diameter causes a drop in pressure distal to the band by about 50 per cent and reduces pulmonary overcirculation.

CHILDHOOD. A large left-to-right shunt and a demonstrable left ventricular enlargement as evidence of overload are the criteria for open repair. The pulmonary arterial pressure is rarely normal under these circumstances, unless pulmonary stenosis coexists. Usually there is pulmonary hypertension equal to 50 to 100 per cent of the systemic systolic pressure.

ADOLESCENCE AND ADULTHOOD. Most large ventricular septal defects have already been corrected by the time the individual reaches this age. The indications are the same as for children.

Patent Ductus Arteriosus

INFANCY. Cardiac failure is the indication for ligation of the ductus.

CHILDHOOD. Surgical obliteration of a patent ductus is so safe and so effective that we believe that all children with this diagnosis should be operated upon. If the condition has been recognized in infancy and the child is thriving, the operation can be planned for the age of 3 or 4 years, before he starts school. If the rate of growth begins to lag, if cardiac enlargement increases, or if repeated respiratory infections occur, operation can be performed earlier than age 3.

ADOLESCENCE AND ADULTHOOD. As we enter the thirty-second year after a ductus was successfully ligated, it is unlikely that there will be many adults who have not been operated upon already. If such there be, operation is indicated to prevent bacterial endocarditis or any late effects of a cardiac or pulmonary burden. The contraindication to surgery is pulmonary vascular obstructive disease.

Atrial Septal Defect

INFANCY. An uncomplicated atrial septal defect causes no problems and, indeed, is rarely recognized.

CHILDHOOD. Closure of an atrial septal defect by open heart surgery has as low a mortality rate and is as effective as surgery for a patent ductus. The chief differences are the risk of postpericardiotomy syndrome and the slight risk inherent in the mechanics of cardiopulmonary bypass. We recommend closure of the atrial septal defect during childhood years unless the shunt is very small. Surgery is advised in childhood to prevent the complications some adults have because of arrhythmias, cardiac failure, or pulmonary hypertension.

ADOLESCENCE. Surgery is recommended as for children.

ADULTHOOD. Operation is advised for those young adults who do not have pulmonary vascular obstructive disease. Adults who have reached middle age or beyond and are still asymptomatic have passed the time when the complications would have occurred that surgery is undertaken to prevent. Operation in this group is more debatable than in the younger or more symptomatic patients.

Pulmonic Stenosis

INFANCY. Severe pulmonic stenosis, with or without cardiac failure, is the indication for surgery of valvular and subvalvular stenosis.

CHILDHOOD. Severe and moderate pulmonic stenosis should be operated on with the timing of the procedure being quite elective in the latter case.

ADOLESCENCE AND ADULTHOOD. Severe stenosis should be surgically relieved. Some middle-aged and older adults become symptomatic with moderate stenosis and can be benefited by surgery.

Aortic Stenosis

At any age, patients with severe stenosis should be operated upon. Operation is contraindicated for mild and moderate degrees of congenital aortic stenosis.

Coarctation of Aorta

INFANCY. Cardiac failure with lack of response to intensive medical management is the indication for repair of coarctation in a baby. Often there are

282

coexisting defects of even greater significance than the coarctation when this happens.

CHILDHOOD. Surgery is electively advised around the age of 10 to 14 years for all with a significant coarctation. Indications for earlier surgery are marked hypertension, increasing left ventricular enlargement, or electrocardiographic signs of left ventricular strain.

ADOLESCENCE AND ADULTHOOD. Premature degenerative changes in the aorta and aneurysms of the aorta or intercostal arteries increase the risk of surgery, but operation should still be considered if significant hypertension in the arm is present.

Tetralogy of Fallot

INFANCY. Attacks of paroxysmal dyspnea (cyanotic spells) are the indication for creation of an artificial ductus. Our preference is for anastomosis of the ascending aorta and right pulmonary artery.

CHILDHOOD. Before the age of 6 or 7 years, increasing symptoms or excessive polycythemia are the indications for a shunt procedure. After that age, open repair should be undertaken if the anatomy is suitable and the surgical team has had good experience with this difficult anomaly.

ADOLESCENCE AND ADULTHOOD. The same considerations for open repair apply as in childhood. If the anatomy is unsuitable for that and the patient is symptomatic, a shunt procedure should be undertaken.

Complete Transposition of the Great Arteries

INFANCY. A communication at the atrial level should be created in all when the diagnosis is made. This can be done by balloon septostomy or by the Blalock-Hanlon surgical technique. If a large ventricular septal defect is present, the pulmonary artery should be banded.

CHILDHOOD. Redirection of the venous return within the atria by the Mustard technique should be performed by a highly skilled surgical team. Coexisting ventricular septal defect and pulmonic stenosis can be corrected at the same time if physiologically significant.

SUMMARY AND CONCLUSIONS

Medical management of the patient with congenital heart disease has matured and flourished in the last three decades. Such management, combined with surgery at the proper time if indicated, has made life for these individuals not just possible but as normal as possible. Their destiny is not to be invalids but to be active and effective men and women.

References

1. DuShane, J., and Weidman, W. H. (eds.): *Five congenital cardiac defects. A study of the profile and natural history of aortic stenosis, atrial septal defect—primum type, atrial septal defect—secundum type, pulmonic stenosis, ventricular septal defect.* Circulation 31–32 (suppl. 3):1, 1965.

2. ENGLE, M. A., ITO, I., AND EHLERS, K. H.: *Ventricular septal defect. Progress of the past decade.* Advan. Pediat. 13:65, 1964.

3. ENGLE, M. A., ITO, T., AND GOLDBERG, H. P.: *Fate of the patient with pulmonic stenosis.* Circulation 9:632, 1964.

4. LAMBERT, E. C., CANENT, R. V., AND HOHN, A. R.: *Congenital cardiac anomalies in the newborn.* Pediatrics 37:343, 1966.

5. CARLGREN, L. E.: *The incidence of congenital heart disease in Gothenburg.* Proc. Assoc. Europ. Cardiol. 5:2, 1969.

6. RICHARDS, M. R., MERRITT, K. K., SAMUELS, M. H., AND LANGMANN, A. G.: *Congenital malformations of the cardiovascular system in a series of 6,053 infants.* Pediatrics 15:12, 1955.

7. MORTON, W. E., AND HUHN, L. A.: *Epidemiology of congenital heart disease: Observations in 17,366 Denver school children.* J.A.M.A. 195: 1107, 1966.

8. QUINN, R. W., AND CAMPBELL, E. S.: *Heart disease in children: Survey of school children in Nashville, Tennessee.* Yale J. Biol. Med. 34:370, 1961–2.

9. ENGLE, M. A.: *Roentgenology in congenital heart disease.* In Luisada, A. (ed.), *Cardiology,* McGraw-Hill Blakiston, New York, 1959, pp. 133–151.

10. BRAUNWALD, E., AND SWAN, H. J. C.: *Cooperative study on cardiac catheterization.* Circulation 37–38 (suppl. 3):1, 1968.

11. RUDOLPH, A.: *Complications occurring in infants and children. Cooperative study on cardiac catheterization in the newborn.* Circulation 37–38 (suppl. 3):59, 1968.

12. VARGHESE, P. J., CELERMAJER, J., IZUKAWA, T., HALLER, J. A., AND ROWE, R. B.: *Cardiac catheterization in the newborn: Experience with 100 cases.* Pediatrics 44:24, 1969.

13. NEILL, C. A., AND SWANSON, S.: *Outcome of pregnancy in congenital heart disease.* Circulation 24:1003, 1961.

14. EHLERS, K. H., AND ENGLE, M. A.: *Familial congenital heart disease: 1. Genetic and environmental factors.* Circulation 34:503, 1966.

15. NORA, J. J.: *Multifactorial inheritance hypothesis for the etiology of congenital heart diseases.* Circulation 38:604, 1968.

16. BLUMENTHAL, S., GRIFFITHS, S. P., AND MORGAN, B. C.: *Bacterial endocarditis in children with heart disease. A review based on the literature and experience with 58 cases.* Pediatrics 26:993, 1960.

17. PANKEY, G. A.: *Acute bacterial endocarditis at the University of Minnesota Hospitals, 1939–1959.* Amer. Heart J. 64:583, 1962.

18. COMMITTEE ON PREVENTION OF RHEUMATIC FEVER AND BACTERIAL ENDOCARDITIS OF THE COUNCIL ON RHEUMATIC FEVER AND CONGENITAL HEART DISEASE OF THE AMER. HEART ASSOC.: *Statement on prevention of bacterial endocarditis,* 1965.

19. CHAMBERLAIN, F. L.: *Management of medical-dental problems in patients with cardiovascular disease.* Mod. Conc. Cardiov. Dis. 30:697, 1961.

20. TYLER, H. R., AND D. B. CLARK: *Loss of consciousness and convulsions with congenital heart disease.* A.M.A. Arch. Neurol. and Psychiat. 79: 506, 1958.

21. MARTELLE, R. R., AND LINDE, L. M.: *Cerebrovascular accidents with tetralogy of Fallot.* Amer. J. Dis. Child 101:206, 1961.

22. McDonald, R., and Harris, F.: *Cerebral complications of cyanotic congenital heart disease.* S. African Med. J. 37:296, 1963.

23. Raimondi, A. J., Matsumoto, S., and Miller, R. A.: *Brain abscess in children with congenital heart disease.* J. Neurosurg. 23:588, 1965.

24. Campbell, M., Neill, C., and Suzman, S.: *The prognosis of atrial septal defect.* Brit. Med. J. 1:1375, 1957.

25. Keith, J. D.: *Congestive heart failure.* Pediatrics 18:491, 1956.

26. Mark, H., and Young, D.: *Congenital heart disease in the adult.* Amer. J. Cardiol. 15:293, 1965.

27. Engle, M. A.: *Cardiac failure in infancy: Recognition and management.* Mod. Conc. Cardiov. Dis. 32:825, 1963.

28. Engle, M. A.: *Treatment of the failing heart,* in Cassels, D. E. (ed.), *Symposium on Cardiovascular Therapy.* Pediat. Clin. N. Amer. 11:247, 1964.

29. Engle, M. A.: *Heart Failure,* in Gellis, S. and Kagan, F. (eds.), W. B. Saunders Co., Philadelphia, 1968, ed. 3, pp. 184–190.

30. Bloodwell, R. D., Hallman, G. L., Beall, A. C., and Cooley, D. A.: *Correction of congenital cardiovascular defects in patients over fifty years of age.* Amer. J. Surg. 114:751, 1967.

31. Austen, W. G., and Scannell, J. G.: *Surgical correction of congenital intracardiac defects in adult patients.* Heart Bull. 17:51, 1968.

32. Kerr, A.: *Bacterial endocarditis revisited.* Mod. Conc. Cardiov. Dis. 33:831, 1964.

33. Gersony, W. M., and Nadas, A. S.: *Treatment of endocarditis in congenital heart disease.* Pediatrics 35:704, 1965.

34. Nelson, R. M., Jenson, C. B., Peterson, C. A., and Sanders, B. C.: *Effective use of prophylactic antibiotics in open heart surgery.* Arch. Surg. 90:731, 1965.

35. Linde, L. M., and Heins, H. L.: *Bacterial endocarditis following surgery for congenital heart disease.* New Eng. J. Med. 263:65, 1960.

36. Dripps, R. D., Strong, M. J., and Price, H. L.: *The heart and general anesthesia.* Mod. Conc. Cardiov. Dis. 32:805, 1963.

37. Erlanger, H.: *Cardiac arrhythmias in relationship to anesthesia: Past and present concepts.* Amer. J. Med. Sci. 243:651, 1962.

38. Gomez, G., Gonzales, F., Adams, P., and Anderson, R. C.: *Electrocardiographic findings after open heart surgery in children.* Amer. Heart J. 64:730, 1962.

39. Ayres, S. M., and Grace, W. J.: *Inappropriate ventilation and hypoxemia as causes of cardiac arrhythmias.* Amer. J. Med. 46:495, 1969.

40. Aberdeen, E., and Carr, I.: *Transposition of the great arteries,* in Wooler, G. H., and Aberdeen, E. (eds.), *Modern Trends in Cardiac Surgery.* Appleton-Century-Crofts, New York, 1968, pp. 182–199.

41. Lauer, R. M., Ongley, P. A., DuShane, J. W., and Kirklin, J. W.: *Heart block after repair of ventricular septal defect in children.* Circulation 22:526, 1960.

42. Eriksson, B. O., Thoren, C., and Zetterqvist, P.: *Long-term treatment with propranolol in selected cases of Fallot's tetralogy.* Brit. Heart J. 31:37, 1969.

43. Engle, M. A.: *Postoperative syndromes,* in Moss, A. J., and Adams, F. H. (eds.), *Heart Disease in Infants, Children and Adolescents.* The Williams & Wilkins Company, Baltimore, 1968, pp. 1087–1101.

44. ITO, T., ENGLE, M. A., AND GOLDBERG, H. P.: *Postpericardiotomy syndrome following surgery of nonrheumatic heart disease.* Circulation 17:549, 1958.

45. ENGLE, M. A., and ITO, T.: *The postpericardiotomy syndrome.* Amer. J. Cardiol. 7:73, 1961.

46. ANDERSON, R., AND LARSON, O.: *Fever, splenomegaly, and atypical lymphocytosis after open-heart surgery.* Lancet 2:947, 1963.

47. HOLSWADE, G. R., ENGLE, M. A., REDO, S. F., GOLDSMITH, E. I., AND BARONDES, J. A.: *Development of viral disease and a viral disease-like syndrome after extracorporeal circulation.* Circulation 27:812, 1963.

48. SAYED, H. N., DACIE, J. V., HANDLEY, D. A., LEWIS, S. M., AND CLELAND, W. P.: *Haemolytic anaemia of mechanical origin after open heart surgery.* Thorax 16:356, 1961.

49. BRODEUR, M. T. H., SUTHERLAND, D. W., KOLER, R. D., STARR, A., KIMSEY, J. A., AND GRISWOLD, H. E.: *Red blood cell survival in patients with aortic valvular disease and ball-valve prostheses.* Circulation 32:570, 1965.

50. TAYLOR, L. M., THEYE, R. A., DEVLOO, R. A., AND KIRKLIN, J. W.: *Patterns of acid-base changes during surgical convalescence.* Surg. Gynec. Obstet. 114:97, 1962.

51. DAMMANN, J. F., JR., THUNG, N., CHRISTLIEB, I. I., LITTLEFIELD, J. B., AND MULLER, W. H., JR.: *The management of the severely ill patient after open-heart surgery.* J. Thorac. Cardiov. Surg. 45:80, 1963.

52. BAER, D. D., AND OSBORN, J. J.: *The postperfusion pulmonary congestion syndrome.* Amer. J. Clin. Path. 34:442, 1960.

53. LOBER, P. H., AND LILLEHEI, C. W.: *Necrotizing panarteritis following repair of coarction of aorta: Report of two cases.* Surgery 35:950, 1954.

54. HERMAN, B. E., WALLACE, H. W., GADBOYS, H. L., AND LITWAK, R. S.: *Anterior crural syndrome as a complication of cardiopulmonary bypass.* J. Thorac. Cardiov. Surg. 52:755, 1966.

Surgical Management of Congenital Heart Disease: Viewpoint of the Surgeon

Dwight C. McGoon, M.D.

The heart is a mechanical organ, and its sole function is to propel blood under sufficient pressure to allow perfusion of the systemic and pulmonary circulations. Most of the congenital deformities of the heart, therefore, are structural and are manifested by alterations in cardiac dynamics. Surgery is a mechanically oriented mode of treatment and is that branch of medical therapeutics dealing primarily with structure. It is not unexpected, therefore, that the most important modality for the treatment of congenital heart disease is surgical, and conversely, that congenital heart deformities are eminently suitable for surgical therapy. Other modes of therapy, though of great importance, were inevitably destined to a supportive role rather than to a primary therapeutic one.

Notwithstanding this natural affinity between congenital heart disease and surgical treatment, the heart was the last organ of the body to be approached confidently by surgeons. The development of cardiac surgery by necessity awaited ancillary technical developments. These included anesthetic and ventilatory techniques that allowed safe thoracic surgery, the successful employment of heparin and multiple transfusions; but the primary developments were those of heart-lung machines and the safe institution of extracorporeal circulation.

Now that a decade and a half of experience with open-heart surgery have elapsed, surgical correction of most congenital cardiac deformities can be accomplished with considerable confidence and success by highly skilled teams. The endeavor, however, is complex and requires an accurate performance by a large number of participants and successful execution of many individual steps and manipulations. Thus, success in cardiac surgery depends on the efficient, skillful, and harmonious performance of the many members of the surgical team, who, in the sum of their efforts, accomplish the therapeutic goal. Particular emphasis must be given to the necessity for technical perfection in the cardiac repair, accomplished with the utmost gentleness and respect, since a perfect surgical repair is the one most essential requirement for the attainment of an ideal result.

A review of the more common forms of congenital heart disease and their suitability for surgical repair is given in Table 1 and confirms that the majority can be corrected by operative intervention. Conditions that remain inoperable are primarily hypoplasia or atresia of one or the other atrioventricular valves, resulting in serious underdevelopment of the respective ventricle. Thus, absence of hypoplasia or disease of the myocardium itself defies corrective surgical intervention thus far. The common ventricle, which is not an unusual lesion, is the one deformity that still has evaded correction by the cardiac surgeon, and though it, too, is characterized by an extensive deficiency of myocardium (the entire interventricular septum), the theoretical likelihood of its correctability poses a particular challenge to the cardiac surgeon today.

The decisions relating to whether or not a congenital cardiac deformity should be treated surgically, and if so, at what time and by what specific technique, can be approached both in general and in particular. The general

288

Table 1. Congenital diseases of the heart and great vessels

Disease	Present status of surgical therapy *
Defects in partitioning of pulmonic and systemic circulations	
Atrial septal defect (secundum)	A
Partial anomalous pulmonary venous connection	A
Endocardial cushion defects	A
Common atrium	A
Ventricular septal defect	A
Common ventricle	DP
Aortopulmonary window	A
Truncus arteriosus	A
Total anomalous pulmonary venous connection	A
Congenital valve deformities	
Tricuspid atresia and stenosis	EP
Mitral atresia	E
Ebstein's malformation	B
Pulmonic stenosis	A
Trilogy	A
Tetralogy	A
Mitral stenosis and insufficiency	B
Aortic stenosis	A
Aortic insufficiency	B
Nonvalvular obstructions	
Peripheral pulmonary artery stenosis	A
Cor triatriatum	A
Supravalvular aortic stenosis	A
Subaortic stenosis (diffuse)	B
Subaortic stenosis (localized)	A
Coarctation of aorta	A
Transposition of great vessels	
Levotransposition	E
Dextrotransposition	A
Double-outlet right ventricle	A
Coronary artery disease	
Origin from pulmonary artery	A
Arteriovenous fistulas	A
Diseases of myocardium	E
Complete heart block	B

* A = Corrective operation clearly established as treatment of choice whenever lesion is present and significant (contraindications in specific instances may exist). B = Corrective operation clearly established as advisable, provided certain additional indications are present (usually progressive disability). C = Surgical corrective methods available, but it has not been clearly established that operation is in toto beneficial. (None included among these congenital cardiac defects.) D = Surgical corrective methods that have been tried, but with no real success as yet. E = No surgical approach now possible. P (after D or E) = Palliative approach possible.

indications for an operation designed to correct a given deformity may be related to the disability that the deformity causes the patient, or may be related to the pathophysiology of the lesion, even in an asymptomatic patient. In either situation, consideration is given to the balance between the natural history of the disease and the degree of safety and success that the respective operative procedure was achieved. Thus, correction of many acquired cardiac lesions is delayed until significant and progressive disability is manifested by the patient, largely because the operations designed to correct acquired lesions, such as valvular deformity, are not as highly curative as many of the procedures for congenital deformities. Thus, operation is advised for the child with a large, simple, atrial septal defect, even when asymptomatic, on the grounds that the operative procedure is highly safe and essentially completely curative and that most patients with this condition will experience progressive disability in later years. Similar considerations are appropriate for coarctation, patent ductus arteriosus, and even supravalvular aortic stenosis. However, the factor of potential spontaneous regression or healing of the lesion in other conditions, such as small or asymptomatic ventricular septal defect when it is manifested in infancy and early childhood, may require postponement of operation. Particularly difficult is the decision regarding timing of operation for aortic stenosis, because complete cure of the valvular deformity is infrequently accomplished, and full knowledge of the natural history of the condition itself is not available. In lesions of this type, careful analysis of the various factors must be brought to bear on the specific characteristics of the individual case if one is to achieve a wise decision regarding the indications and timing of operation.

It is prudent, therefore, that parents, patients, cardiologists, and surgeons approach the surgical treatment of congenital heart disease with the prospect of accomplishing correction or palliation, but seldom complete cure. For example, the tetralogy of Fallot can be corrected with confidence, but seldom cured—a systolic murmur, a deformed pulmonary valve, and irregular right ventricular outflow tract usually persist. Similarly, a ventricular septal defect can be readily closed, but some element of residual pulmonary vascular obstructive disease often indicates the presence of the previous lesion, and in general, complete resolution of this vascular alteration after operation does not occur. The various operations for congenital heart disease thus range from cure through correction to palliation.

With regard to the proper timing of surgical intervention, generalities and specifics must again be considered. All else being equal, the ideal age for operative correction of congenital heart defects is when the patient is between 5 and 10 years of age. The heart and great vessels are well developed and of the size convenient to manipulate, in addition to being elastic and pliable, whereas in an older patient, such conditions as myocardial hypertrophy, marked development of collateral circulation, or secondary vascular changes may increase technical difficulties. In a child less than 6 months old, open-heart surgery seems to be less well tolerated, particularly with respect to the pulmonary and vascular systems. After the age of 6 months has been reached, cardiac surgery is better tolerated and can be undertaken with confidence in instances where further postponement either is not possible or is inadvisable.

The correct timing for operation may be dictated by the specific congenital deformity. For example, complete transposition of the great vessels results in the death of a large proportion of infants in the first few weeks of life, and only a small percentage survive the first year. Thus, there is no alternative to an early and aggressive surgical approach involving the palliative procedure of either banding the pulmonary artery or creating an atrial septal defect, or both, in anticipation of corrective surgery at a later date. The timing of operation for the tetralogy of Fallot is entirely dependent on the severity of the pulmonary stenosis. If this is so severe that pulmonary flow is restricted to the point of producing severe cyanotic "spells," surgical intervention is required even before the child is 4 or 5 years old, in which circumstance a palliative shunt procedure to improve pulmonary perfusion is preferred. If operation is not required before this age, the corrective procedure is indicated. These, then, are two examples of conditions in which staging of the repair, with a preliminary palliative procedure and a later definitive intervention, are practiced. In general, however, staging of operations is undesirable and historically has in most instances been superseded by a one-stage definitive procedure.

For some conditions, there is not unanimity of opinion among various authorities as to whether the two-stage or the single-stage procedure is indicated: for example, the infant with ventricular septal defect who fails to respond to medical measures for congestive heart failure could be treated either by a pulmonary arterial banding procedure, followed at an older age by closure of the ventricular septum and "debanding" of the pulmonary artery, or by a definitive intracardiac repair at the initial operation. Almost surely, the latter approach will ultimately prove the better, dependent only on further technical improvements to allow greater tolerance of intracardiac repair.

Gradual progress continues in the elucidation of contraindications to operation for conditions that are anatomically operable. Of chief concern is the presence of pulmonary vascular obstructive disease and its importance in the selection of patients for operation. Increased pulmonary vascular resistance exists so commonly in patients with congenital heart deformities, particularly in the presence of increased pulmonary blood flow, that an understanding of the basic features of this condition is essential. When the resistance to flow through the lungs (pulmonary resistance) approaches the resistance to flow through the body (systemic resistance), it is true both in theory and in practice that closure of the defect of partitioning between the left and right sides of the heart and corresponding great arteries would not significantly reduce the pulmonary arterial pressure or flow. If the pulmonary resistance exceeds systemic resistance, closure of the defect would cause the pulmonary pressure to exceed systemic pressure. Thus, when pulmonary resistance becomes elevated to or above systemic levels, surgery for closure of the defect and partitioning is contraindicated. Experience has shown that when pulmonary resistance is greater than about 0.7 times systemic resistance, the benefit and advisability of surgical closure of the defect are highly doubtful. With this fact in mind, emphasis cannot be given to the presence or absence of pulmonary hypertension with respect to operability (though it does have relevance to the operative risk), but rather the degree of elevation of pulmonary vascular resistance should be recognized as the crucial factor relative to operability. In many more patients who are not candidates for operation for congenital heart disease, it is pulmonary vascular obstructive disease, rather than the anatomic nature of the cardiac malformation, which is the contraindication.

NEWER CORRECTIVE OPERATIONS

There is neither a requirement nor space here to review the status of surgical treatment for the various forms of congenital heart disease. Rather, recent advances in technique and concept in three types of congenital cardiac disease are described.

An Operation for the Correction of Truncus Arteriosus

Truncus arteriosus constitutes less than 1 per cent of all congenital cardiac defects. The anomaly is characterized anatomically by the presence of a single artery that takes origin from the base of both ventricles by way of a single semilunar valve. A high ventricular septal defect is characteristic. The pulmonary artery or arteries take origin from the truncus arteriosus in a variable manner: [1] In type I truncus arteriosus, a single main pulmonary trunk connects the right and left pulmonary arteries to the truncus. In type II, the right and left pulmonary arteries originate directly from a common orifice in the left dorsal aspect of the truncus. In type III, the right and left pulmonary arteries originate separately from the lateral aspects of the truncus. In type IV, the pulmonary circulation derives from large vessels originating from the descending portion of the aorta. The anomaly thus causes mixing of the systemic and pulmonary circulations, with the result that bidirectional shunting of blood occurs, and hence there is always some degree of systemic arterial desaturation. Pulmonary blood flow is increased unless severe stenosis of the pulmonary arteries or severe pulmonary vascular obstructive disease is present.

In theory, persistent truncus arteriosus should be correctable. Attempts at repair were not successful until it had been demonstrated by Rastelli and associates [2] in the laboratory animal that the outflow tract of the right ventricle and main pulmonary artery could be replaced with a homograft of ascending aorta and aortic valve. This favorable experience motivated the attempt, in September 1967, to correct the truncus deformity in a patient by using the homograft of ascending aorta with integral aortic valve.[3] That operation proved successful, and at the present time, 19 such operations have been accomplished at the Mayo Clinic.

The operation consists of three major steps: after extracorporeal circulation is established, the pulmonary arteries are disconnected from the truncus, and the resulting opening in the truncus is repaired (Fig. 1). Through a circular right ventriculotomy, the ventricular septal defect is closed by attaching a patch of Teflon cloth to the septal rim of the defect caudally and to the deep margin of the ventriculotomy adjacent to the annulus of the truncal valve superiorly (Fig. 2). The homograft, consisting of aortic valve and ascending aorta, is anastomosed to the pulmonary artery distally and to the margins of the ventriculotomy proximally. This latter step is facili-

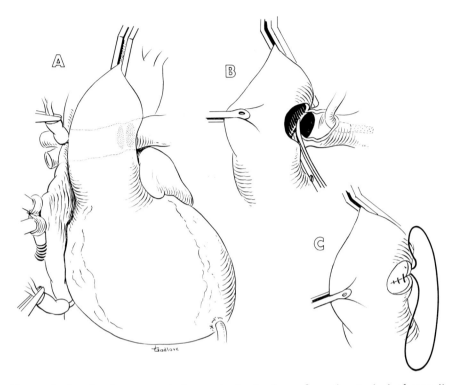

Figure 1. Repair of truncus arteriosus. A, Anatomic configuration typical of type II truncus. B, Detachment of pulmonary arteries from truncus. C, Repair of defect in wall of truncus (now aorta). (From McGoon, D. C.: *Technics of Open-Heart Surgery for Congenital Heart Disease.*[4])

tated by leaving the anterior mitral leaflet of the donor heart as part of the homograft to act as a gusset to reach to the caudal rim of the ventriculotomy.

The advisability of placing a valve in the newly fashioned right ventricular outflow tract is based on the theoretical consideration that in the presence of increased pulmonary vascular resistance, absence of such a valve would impose a highly significant additional burden on the right ventricle.

The 19 operations of this kind that have been performed at the Mayo Clinic have included operations for each of the four types of truncus arteriosus. Five hospital deaths have occurred in the entire series, only one of which occurred in the last 10 operations. In addition, there has been one late death (which occurred 3 months after operation) due to tachycardia, which developed during an influenza-like illness. All of the 13 surviving patients are clinically well. The principal concern regarding the late condition of the surviving patients is the appearance of calcification in the media of the homograft, which has become detectable within a few months after operation. There has been no calcification in the cusps of the homograft valve in either the clinical or the experimental series.

In selecting patients with this anomaly for operation, the criterion relative

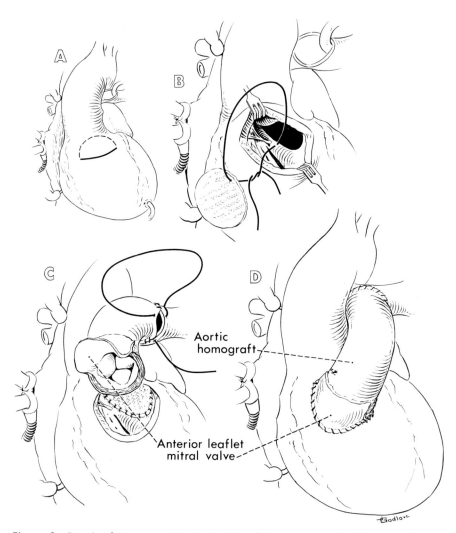

Figure 2. Repair of truncus arteriosus. A, Site of transverse ventriculotomy, with portion of anterior wall of right ventricle excised to create an outflow tract. B, High ventricular septal defect caudal to truncus valve and extending dorsally to level of papillary muscle of conus. C, Defect closed so that truncus valve (now aortic valve) is entirely to left of patch. D, Proximal anastomosis completed, with use of anterior mitral leaflet of homograft as an extension or gusset to allow homograft valve to assume a more transverse position. (From McGoon, D. C.: *Technics of Open-Heart Surgery for Congenital Heart Disease.*[1])

to the hemodynamic state is anticipated to be the same as for any patient having a defective separation of systemic and pulmonary circulations: pulmonary vascular resistance should be less than about 0.75 times the systemic vascular resistance. The only previously available surgical procedure for this condition, namely, banding of the pulmonary arteries, was palliative. It would seem at this time that the banding procedure should be reserved

294

for those patients who are less than 6 months old, who are in intractable failure with pulmonary consolidation or collapse, and who are, therefore, not candidates for open-heart surgery.

Transposition of the Great Arteries

Complete transposition of the great arteries became amenable to correction with the introduction of various techniques for transposing the venous return,[5, 6] operations that are regularly in use at all cardiac surgical centers. However, the application of these techniques to the repair of complete transposition of the great arteries when associated with severe pulmonary stenosis has carried a high and nearly prohibitive surgical mortality rate. Indeed, no series of attempted repairs of the transposition when associated with severe subpulmonic stenosis are recorded in the literature. In the experience of my colleagues and myself, the Mustard operation for the repair of complete transposition associated with valvular pulmonary stenosis usually resulted in a successful outcome, but when subvalvular pulmonary stenosis was present, the hospital mortality rate increased steeply to 61 per cent.[7] Residual pulmonary stenosis appeared to be the major cause of failure in most patients. Because of the technical inability to restore an adequate outflow tract to the left ventricle in these patients, a different operative approach was conceived by Rastelli,[8] again utilizing an aortic homograft with integral valve to fashion an entirely new outflow tract leading to the pulmonary artery.

This operation was first performed clinically in July 1968 by Wallace at the Mayo Clinic.[7] It consists of three principal steps (Fig. 3). First, through a right ventriculotomy, the ventricular septal defect is closed with a patch in such a way that the left ventricle drains behind the patch into both the aorta and pulmonary artery. Second, the pulmonary artery is divided just beyond its origin, and the proximal stump is closed by suturing. Third, the right ventriculotomy is enlarged, and a homograft of ascending aorta that incorporates the aortic valve of the donor heart is inserted to connect the right ventricle with the distal pulmonary artery. This operation, therefore, is more completely corrective than are the operations that accomplish venous transposition, in that the right ventricle now ejects into the pulmonary artery and the left ventricle into the aorta, which of course is the normal sequence.

At the present time, three such operations have been performed without hospital mortality and with clinically successful results in each. These patients are considered to be unusually ideal candidates for correction, because their pulmonary circulation has not been subjected to increased flow and there is freedom from significant pulmonary vascular obstructive disease.

Complete Atrioventricular Canal

Repair of the complete form of persistent common atrioventricular canal has proved a formidable task for the cardiovascular surgeon. The surgical

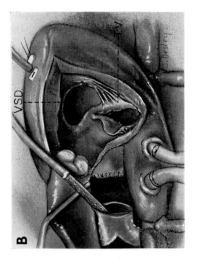

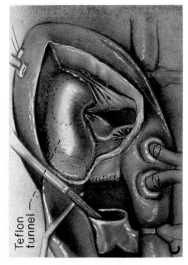

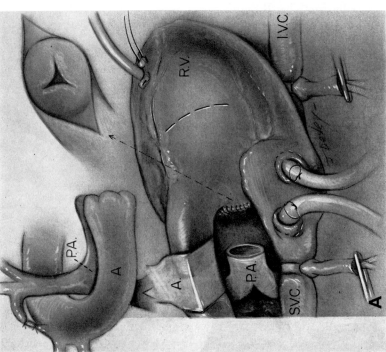

Figure 3. Drawings illustrating steps in surgical repair. A, Left Blalock anastomosis is ligated (upper left). Pulmonary valve, inspected through pulmonary arteriotomy, shows moderate fusion of cusps (upper right). Main pulmonary artery is divided, and proximal end is oversewn. Broken line indicates ventriculotomy. A=aorta; PA=pulmonary artery; RV=right ventricle; IVC=inferior vena cava; SVC=superior vena cava. B, Drawing illustrates inside of right ventricle and relationship of ventricular septal defect (VSD), aortic valve, and tricuspid valve (TV). C, Teflon tunnel is constructed to connect left ventricle and aorta. D, Homograft of aorta, including aortic valve and anterior leaflet of mitral valve, is sutured to distal end of main pulmonary artery. Portion of anterior wall of right ventricle is excised around ventriculotomy. E, Proximal anastomosis is carried out, with the use of homograft's mitral anterior leaflet to complete apical aspect of anastomosis. (From Rastelli, G. C., Wallace, R. B., and Ongley, P. A.: Complete repair of transposition of the great arteries with pulmonary stenosis: A review and report of a case corrected by using a new surgical technique.[7]

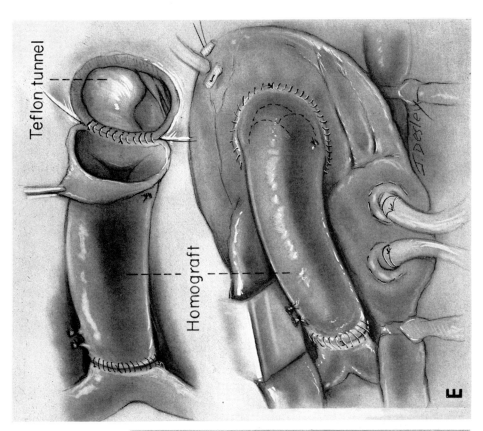

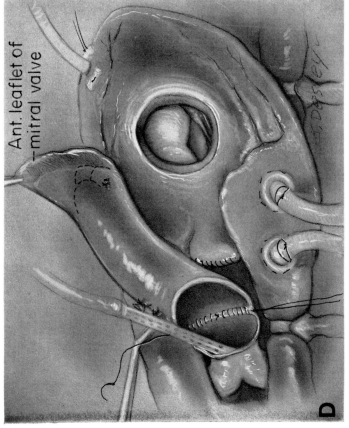

mortality rate for all reported cases was 62 to 75 per cent, with the exception of Gerbode and Sabar's [9] exemplary experience of one surgical death in 13 operations. The risk of this repair prior to 1964 in the hands of my colleagues and myself had been at the discouragingly high level of 60 per cent, with the deaths believed to be primarily the result of continuing incompetence of the atrioventricular valves after operation. An improved technique of repair was instituted in 1964; it has resulted, in the subsequent 5 years, in a striking reduction in the operative mortality rate of 15 per cent.

Concomitantly, elucidation of the anatomic characteristics of complete atrioventricular canal by Rastelli, Kirklin, and Titus [10] and recognition of the three anatomic types gave support to the validity of the improved surgical technique. These three types of complete atrioventricular canal can be recognized on the basis of the anatomy of the anterior common atrioventricular leaflet and the extent and site of interventricular communication (Fig. 4). In type A, the anterior common atrioventricular leaflet is divided into two portions, one mitral and one tricuspid, both attached medially to the muscular septum. In this type, the membranous septum has formed, and the inter-

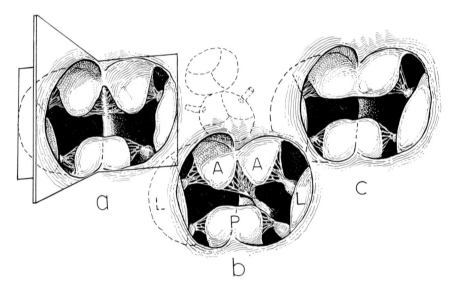

Figure 4. Three varieties of complete atrioventricular canal. A, In type A, anterior common leaflet is divided into a "mitral" and a "tricuspid" portion which are medially attached to crest of ventricular septum via separate chordae tendinae. B, In type B, anterior common leaflet is divided but attaches medially not to the ventricular septum but to an anomalous papillary muscle located in right ventricle. C, In type C, anterior common leaflet is not divided and is not attached to ventricular septum but bridges over it. In B, A indicates anterior and P posterior common leaflets, and L lateral or mural leaflets. (From Rastelli, G. C., Ongley, P. A., and McGoon, D. C.: Surgical repair of complete atrioventricular canal with anterior common leaflet undivided and unattached to ventricular septum.[11])

298

ventricular communication does not extend to the vicinity of the aortic cusps. In type B, the anterior common atrioventricular leaflet is divided into two portions unattached to the septum, but both are attached medially to an anomalous papillary muscle in the right ventricle, adjacent to the septum. In type C, the anterior common atrioventricular leaflet is undivided and is not attached to the septum but freely floats above it. In types B and C, the interventricular communication extends beneath the common anterior leaflet to the proximity of the aortic cusps.

Type A is the most common when there are no associated lesions such as pulmonary stenosis, but type C is the most common when associated conditions exist.

The first type (type A) of complete canal deformity is repaired [12] by first reconstructing the mitral valve and approximating its two components at their base with a few interrupted stitches (Fig. 5). A single autogenous pericardial or Teflon patch is then placed to repair the persistent atrioventricular canal. The medial edge of the reconstructed mitral leaflet is attached to the patch with interrupted sutures before closure of the atrial portion of the defect is completed. In patients in whom the posterior common leaflet is attached to the interior septum by a continuous membrane or by fused chordae, it may be preferable to suture the patch directly to the atrial surface of the leaflet tissue. This technique avoids suturing in the area of the bundle of His.

For correction of the type C deformity,[11] the mitral components of the anterior and posterior common leaflets are first approximated with interrupted sutures (Fig. 6). Next, the anterior common leaflet is incised at its midpoint from the free margin to the annulus of the atrioventricular valve. The posterior common leaflet is similarly incised. A Teflon patch is then fashioned to the size of the septal defect and sutured to the right side of the crest of the ventricular septum. These sutures all are placed before the patch is lowered into position. Next, both incised edges of the anterior common leaflet are attached with a single row of interrupted mattress sutures to their respective sides of the Teflon patch at the level estimated to be in the same plane as the annulus of the common atrioventricular valve. This is usually about 6 to 10 mm. above the lower margin of the patch. The components of the split, posterior, common leaflet are similarly attached to the patch. Finally, the atrial component of the defect is closed by suturing the patch to the rim of the atrial septal defect.

We have not encountered the type B deformity in our surgical practice since 1964.

After repair by these methods, there often is a slight to moderate residual mitral insufficiency, as is true for repair of the partial atrioventricular canal, but the rarity of persistent severe mitral insufficiency in our experience suggests that prosthetic replacement of the atrioventricular valves in complete atrioventricular canal is rarely indicated.

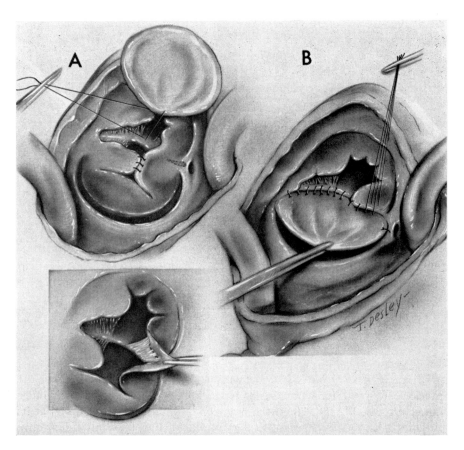

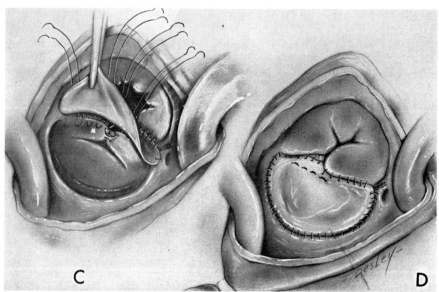

Figure 5. A, Mitral portions of anterior and posterior common leaflets are approximated; a single patch is used and sutures are started midway in muscular septum to right of crest. B, Patch first is sutured between chordal attachment of anterior mitral and tricuspid leaflets. In area of posterior common leaflet, in absence of interventricular communication below this leaflet (*inset*), sutures are placed (while heart is beating) onto leaflet tissue without incorporating underlying muscular septum, thus avoiding stitches in area of bundle of His. C, After lower edge of patch is sutured in place, upper portion is folded back into right atrium. Medial edge of reconstructed anterior mitral leaflet is then attached with interrupted mattress sutures to patch at height it reaches without tension on underlying chordae tendineae. D, Closure of atrial portion of defect is completed with continuous sutures. (From Rastelli, G. C., Ongley, P. A., Kirklin, J. W., and McGoon, D. C.: Surgical repair of the complete form of persistent common atrioventricular canal.[12])

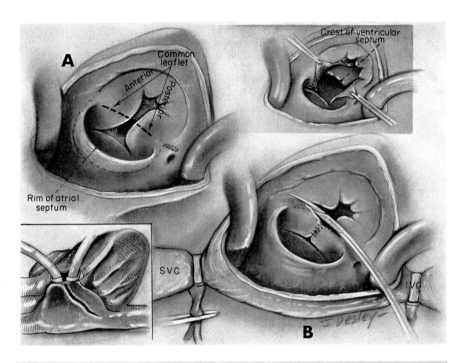

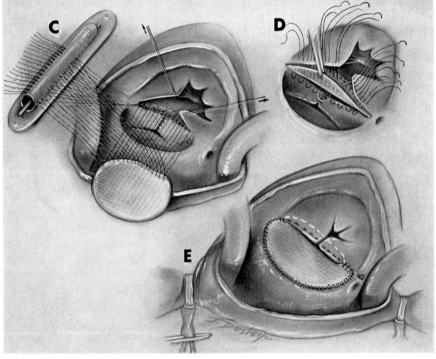

Figure 6. Surgical repair of type of complete atrioventricular canal defined in Figure 4C. A, Heavy broken line indicates line of division of common atrioventricular leaflets. B, Anterior leaflet of mitral valve is reconstructed by approximating "mitral" components of anterior and posterior common leaflets, which are split along midline. C, Sutures are placed in ventricular septum before lowering of patch. "Tricuspid" components of anterior and posterior common leaflets are retracted. D, Sutures attaching patch to ventricular septum have been tied and medial edges of reconstructed anterior mitral leaflet and tricuspid counterparts are attached to patch by means of mattress sutures. E, Repair is completed by suturing remaining circumference of patch to rim of atrial septum. Interrupted sutures placed superficially are used in area of bundle of His. (From Rastelli, G. C., Ongley, P. A., and McGoon, D. C.: Surgical repair of complete atrioventricular canal with anterior common leaflet undivided and unattached to ventricular septum.[11])

303

CONCLUDING REMARKS

To summarize, the viewpoint of the cardiovascular surgeon with respect to the surgical treatment of congenital heart disease is one of optimism and enthusiasm. Congenital malformations of the heart are inherently suited to operative correction, and this fact offers the chief hope of attaining a full life, which these children are so often otherwise incapable of attaining. Though there remains much to be achieved, the surgery of congenital heart disease holds the prospect of enduring value and gratifying reward.

References

1. COLLETT, R. W., AND EDWARDS, J. E.: *Persistent truncus arteriosus: A classification according to anatomic types.* Surg. Clin. N. Amer. 29:1245, 1949.

2. RASTELLI, G. C., TITUS, J. L., AND McGOON, D. C.: *Homograft of ascending aorta and aortic valve as a right ventricular outflow: An experimental approach to the repair of truncus arteriosus.* Arch. Surg. (Chicago) 95:698, 1967.

3. McGOON, D. C., RASTELLI, G. C., AND ONGLEY, P. A.: *An operation for the correction of truncus arteriosus.* J.A.M.A. 205:69, 1968.

4. McGOON, D. C.: *Technics of open-heart surgery for congenital heart disease.* Curr. Probl. Surg., April 1968, 3–42.

5. SENNING, Å.: *Surgical correction of transposition of the great vessels.* Surgery 45:966, 1959.

6. MUSTARD, W. T., KEITH, J. D., TRUSLER, G. A., FOWLER, R., AND KIDD, L.: *The surgical management of transposition of the great vessels.* J. Thorac. Cardiov. Surg. 48:953, 1964.

7. RASTELLI, G. C., WALLACE, R. B., AND ONGLEY, P. A.: *Complete repair of transposition of the great arteries with pulmonary stenosis: A review and report of a case corrected by using a new surgical technique.* Circulation 39:83, 1969.

8. RASTELLI, G. C.: *A new approach to "anatomic" repair of transposition of the great arteries.* Mayo Clin. Proc. 44:1, 1969.

9. GERBODE, F., AND SABAR, E. F.: *Endocardial cushion defects: Diagnosis and surgical repair.* J. Cardiov. Surg. 5:223, 1964.

10. RASTELLI, G. C., KIRKLIN, J. W., AND TITUS, J. L.: *Anatomic observations on complete form of persistent common atrioventricular canal with special reference to atrioventricular valves.* Mayo Clin. Proc. 41:296, 1966.

11. RASTELLI, G. C., ONGLEY, P. A., AND McGOON, D. C.: *Surgical repair of complete atrioventricular canal with anterior common leaflet undivided and unattached to ventricular septum.* Mayo Clin. Proc. 44:335, 1969.

12. RASTELLI, G. C., ONGLEY, P. A., KIRKLIN, J. W., AND McGOON, D. C.: *Surgical repair of the complete form of persistent common atrioventricular canal.* J. Thorac. Cardiov. Surg. 55:299, 1968.

Surgical Management of Congenital Heart Disease: Viewpoint of the Pediatric Cardiologist

Henry Kane, M.D.

An increasing interest in congenital heart disease was stimulated by the successful correction of a patent ductus in 1938 by Dr. Robert Gross.[1] New diagnostic techniques, such as cardiac catheterization, angiocardiography, dye-dilution studies, and intracardiac phonocardiography, have made it possible to obtain extremely accurate physiological and anatomical diagnoses of most malformations. Advances in surgical techniques, especially the use of hypothermia [2] and extracorporeal pump oxygenators,[3] have made it possible to correct most abnormalities. The major problem now is not what can be done (although this is too often still a problem) but when is the most appropriate time to intervene and perform a surgical procedure, i.e., when will surgical intervention provide the most benefit and the least risk? This question must be considered in the light of knowledge concerning the nature and severity of the malformation and the expected course of the specific abnormality.

The malformations of the heart can be divided into groups by their functional derangements and by the type of therapy that will be necessary [4] as follows.

Simple Communications Between Systemic and Pulmonary Circulations. These are corrected by surgical procedures that interrupt or close the communication. Examples of this group include patent ductus arteriosus, ventricular septal defects, atrial septal defects, and more uncommon malformations, such as pulmonary-aortic windows and coronary arteriovenous fistulas.

Obstruction to Flow. Surgery for this group requires removal of the obstruction and, at times, careful reconstruction or replacement of a valve. This group includes pulmonary stenosis, aortic stenosis, mitral stenosis, tricuspid stenosis, and coarctation of the aorta.

Insufficient Valves. These require reconstruction or replacement of a valve. Included are aortic and mitral insufficiency, pulmonary and tricuspid insufficiency, and Ebstein's malformation.

Combinations of Obstructions to Flow and Intracardiac Communications. Corrective procedures for this group require interruption of the communication and removal of the obstruction. When correction is impossible or unduly risky, a bypass procedure may be expedient or necessary. Examples are tetralogy of Fallot, pulmonary atresia with and without a ventricular septal defect, and tricuspid atresia.

Combinations of Intracardiac Communications and Insufficient Valves. Correction of this group of malformations requires interruption of the communication and repair of the valve. This category includes ostium primum defect and ventricular septal defect with aortic insufficiency.

Complex Abnormalities. This group requires correspondingly complex operative procedures to correct or improve these defects. Included in this group are transposition of the great vessels, total anomalous pulmonary venous return, truncus arteriosus, and atrioventricularis communis defects.

Proper management demands a diagnosis sufficiently detailed to provide an adequate estimate of prognosis. Knowledge of both the anatomical nature of the abnormality and the pathophysiological status of the patient may be required. The specific needs depend on the clinical situation. Physical examination, clinical history, electrocardiographic and roentenographic studies may be satisfactory when the findings reveal a diagnosis with a high degree of probability; but when there is a significant doubt concerning the diagnosis or when the physiological status must be known, cardiac catheterization and angiocardiography are indicated. In stable patients, these studies are electively performed at 3 to 5 years of age. Diagnostic studies are indicated immediately if there is (1) a life-threatening situation, such as the presence of congestive failure; (2) a deteriorating condition, such as increasing symptoms, enlarging heart size, or progressive ECG abnormalities; or (3) cyanosis, congestive failure, anoxic spells, or severe respiratory distress. The risk of performing diagnostic or therapeutic procedures must be weighed against the risk of waiting with a particular disorder. In the newborn period, these problems dictate the need for accurate evaluation, although the risks of the diagnostic procedures are increased.[5, 6] The presence of a heart murmur in an otherwise normal infant permits clinical evaluation and postponement of special studies until the patient is older.

Each patient must be carefully evaluated, with consideration of the specific or probable diagnosis and the severity of the condition. Surgery is advisable when the surgical procedure is less dangerous than is continued medical management and delay would increase the operative risk.

Examples of some of the common malformations and other interesting problems will be discussed.

SIMPLE COMMUNICATIONS

Patent Ductus Arteriosus

Patent ductus arteriosus, the second most common malformation, is seen in about 12 per cent of children with congenital heart disease.[7] The ductus arteriosus is a communication between the descending aorta and the main pulmonary artery (Fig. 1). This vessel usually closes off during the first few weeks after birth. A patent ductus arteriosus permits a shunt from the aorta to the pulmonary artery. The size of the shunt depends on the size of the vessel and the pulmonary vascular resistance. The lesion results in increased pulmonary blood flow, increased venous return to the left atrium, increased

Figure 1. A, patent ductus arteriosus. B, ductus arteriosus, divided and sutured.

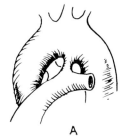 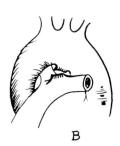

A   B

left ventricular work, and dilatation of the ascending aorta. Large communications subject the pulmonary vascular bed to systemic pressures. Elevated pressures and large flows induce intimal changes in the pulmonary vessels.[8] These obstructive lesions cause exertional dyspnea, easy fatigability, retardation of weight gain and growth, frequent respiratory infections, and congestive failure.

The clinical findings include a continuous machinery-like murmur, bounding peripheral pulses, X-ray evidence of increased pulmonary blood flow, and electrocardiographic or X-ray evidence of left or biventricular hypertrophy. With these findings, the clinical diagnosis can be made with a high degree of accuracy. Cardiac catheterization will demonstrate a step-up of oxygen saturation at the level of the main or left pulmonary artery. The pulmonary arterial pressures can be measured and the pulmonary vascular resistance calculated. Selective angiography demonstrates the patent ductus arteriosus.

Surgical correction is indicated when a patent ductus with a left-to-right shunt is demonstrated. Surgical correction is recommended between 3 and 5 years of age for asymptomatic patients. Surgery is recommended at any age, including infancy, if the patent ductus is the cause of congestive failure, retardation of growth, or symptoms. Surgical ligation and division and suture are equally effective. The operative risks are low, and the results are excellent.[4]

Ventricular Septal Defect

The ventricular septal defect is the most common defect seen in childhood. It occurs in about 25 per cent of children with congenital heart disease.[7] The direction and magnitude of flow are dependent on the size of the defect and the relative pulmonary and systemic vascular resistances. Usually, there is a left-to-right shunt. This shunt causes increased pulmonary blood flow, increased pulmonary venous return, dilatation of the left ventricle, and increased left ventricular work. In infants with large defects, the pulmonary vascular bed is subjected to systemic pressures; as a result the thick-walled pulmonary vessels persist, and the pulmonary vascular resistance remains high.[8] When the pulmonary vascular resistance becomes greater than the systemic vascular resistance, a right-to-left shunt develops.

Large left-to-right shunts cause dyspnea, easy fatigability, frequent respiratory infections, retardation of growth and weight gain, and congestive failure. Patients with large shunts often have problems during the first year of life. If they survive the first year, these patients usually remain satisfactory until the late teens. Studies of patients with ventricular septal defects have revealed that about 25 per cent of patients may undergo spontaneous closure of the defect.[9, 10, 11] This number includes some patients whose large defects caused failure during infancy. In addition, narrowing or relative decrease in the size of the defect may occur with growth.[12]

The shunt usually causes a holosystolic murmur associated with a thrill.

The murmur is loudest along the lower left sternal border and radiates over the entire precordium and back. The second sound is accentuated and normally split. An apical diastolic murmur may be audible because of large flow across the mitral valve. Chest X rays demonstrate increased pulmonary vascular markings and cardiac enlargement, with moderate or large shunts. Electrocardiograms show biventricular or left ventricular hypertrophy. If the pulmonary vascular resistance is greatly elevated, right ventricular hypertrophy is noted. The diagnosis of ventricular septal defect often can be made clinically on the basis of the aforementioned findings. Confirmation of the diagnosis is made by cardiac catheterization and angiography.

Surgical correction of ventricular septal defect is indicated if the defect permits a left-to-right shunt great enough to cause cardiac enlargement and evidence of increased pulmonary blood flow or pulmonary hypertension.[13-15] Surgery is not indicated in patients who have small defects, with the ratio of the pulmonary to systemic flow less than 1.3:1. For infants who develop intractable congestive failure or evidence of increasing pulmonary vascular resistance, a pulmonary artery banding procedure is advisable. This procedure diminishes the pulmonary blood flow and protects the pulmonary vascular bed from hypertension.[16] For older children, the presence of increased pulmonary artery pressure makes the closure of ventricular septal defect more hazardous, and banding can be considered a temporary palliative procedure, since the regression of the pulmonary vascular changes has been demonstrated following it.[17] Subsequent surgical correction by means of open-heart surgery is indicated. The optimum time for surgical correction is considered to be from 4 to 6 years of age. The presence of marked pulmonary vascular changes and a right-to-left shunt is a contraindication for corrective surgery.

Atrial Septal Defect

Atrial septal defect is the third most common abnormality seen during childhood, occurring in 10.6 per cent of children with congenital heart disease.[7] This defect permits a shunt that usually flows from the left atrium to the right. The size of the shunt varies with the size of the defect and the resistance to flow into the respective ventricles. There may be no shunt at birth, but with increasing age, an increasingly large shunt develops. Rarely, the left-to-right shunt may cause problems during infancy.[18, 19] Thirty per cent of all atrial septal defects are estimated to close spontaneously.[20, 21]

A left-to-right shunt at the atrial level produces dilatation of the right atrium, increased right ventricular work, and increased pulmonary blood flow. A pulmonary ejection murmur, which is widely transmitted, usually is audible. An accentuated second sound at the pulmonary valve area with wide fixed splitting is noted. With a large shunt, a mid-diastolic murmur may be present low along the left sternal border because of increased flow across the tricuspid valve.

X-ray studies reveal evidence of increased pulmonary blood flow and enlargement of the right atrium and right ventricle. Evidence of right axis deviation, incomplete right bundle branch block, and right ventricular hypertrophy (diastolic overload type) is noted in the electrocardiogram. The diagnosis can be made with high accuracy on the basis of the clinical findings. Cardiac catheterization and angiocardiography confirm the diagnosis.

Surgical correction of an atrial septal defect is indicated if the defect is large enough to produce a shunt that causes cardiac enlargement. In this situation, the pulmonary blood flow usually is twice the systemic flow or greater. The ideal age for surgical correction is 4 to 6 years. The defect is repaired by suturing under direct vision, employing a pump oxygenator or hypothermia. The surgery usually is curative, and the risks are low.[22, 23]

OBSTRUCTION TO FLOW

Pulmonary Stenosis

Pulmonary stenosis is seen in about 10 per cent of patients with congenital heart disease.[7] Pulmonary stenosis usually is valvular in nature, with a dome-shaped diaphragm caused by fusion of the pulmonary valve leaflets (Fig. 2). Infundibular stenosis combined with valvular stenosis often is seen with severe pulmonary stenosis. Isolated infundibular stenosis is rare. Significant obstruction of the pulmonary valve or right ventricular outflow tract causes decreased right ventricular emptying. When the right ventricle can no longer empty adequately because of the obstruction, congestive failure occurs.

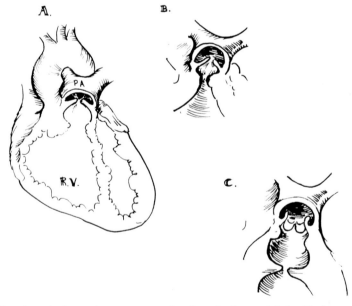

Figure 2. A, valvular pulmonary stenosis. B, valvular and infundibular pulmonary stenosis. C, infundibular pulmonary stenosis.

Pulmonary stenosis causes a harsh systolic murmur with an associated thrill, heard loudest at the pulmonary valve area and transmitted over the entire precordium. The duration of the murmur and the peak of intensity are related to the severity of the stenosis. The second sound is widely split and the pulmonary component diminished. The delay in pulmonary valve closure is related directly to the severity of the stenosis. Severe pulmonary stenosis may be associated with an elevation in right atrial pressure; and it is accompanied by a prominent jugular A wave and an audible fourth heart sound.

X-ray changes, i.e., post-stenotic dilatation of the pulmonary artery and cardiac enlargement, especially right atrial enlargement, are dependent on the severity of the stenosis. The electrocardiogram also varies with the degree of stenosis. An R wave greater than 20 mm. in V_1 suggests that the right ventricular systolic pressure is greater than systemic and forewarns of impending congestive failure.

Patients with stenotic lesions tend to grow worse when the demands for cardiac output are increased, especially during periods of active growth and motor activity;[23] but a sizeable group of patients have remained stable and even improved with growth. Indications for surgery include cyanosis, hypoxic spells, or evidence of right ventricular failure. These findings require surgery immediately, at any size or age. If there is electrocardiographic evidence of right ventricular hypertrophy and strain, impending failure is suggested, and corrective surgery should be planned in the immediate future. If catheterization data reveal a systolic pressure gradient of 60 mm. Hg or more, surgical correction is indicated as an elective procedure.

Surgical repair of pulmonary stenosis requires removal of the obstruction, and this task may be approached in various ways. For the critically ill patient, transventricular approach is desirable;[24] the use of hyperbaric oxygen offers an improved chance for these patients.[25] An approach to the pulmonary obstruction via the pulmonary artery using hypothermia or a pump oxygenator usually is preferred;[26] but an infundibular stenosis requires a transventricular approach.[26] Surgery is relatively safe when performed as an elective procedure, but the mortality rate increases substantially when the patient is in congestive failure.

Aortic Stenosis

Aortic stenosis is seen in about 5.5 per cent of children with congenital heart disease.[7] Obstruction of the outflow tract of the left ventricle may result from abnormalities of the aortic valve, supravalvular stenosis, or subvalvular stenosis. Subvalvular stenoses of several types have been described, including subvalvular fibrous bands and hypertrophic muscular subaortic stenosis. Aortic stenosis causes increased left ventricular work, and this work results in hypertrophy of the left ventricle. Aortic stenosis tends to grow more significant with increasing age. Problems occur at times of active growth and increasing physical activity. The left ventricular pressures increase with increasing stenosis, and late in the course of the disorder, dilatation of the left ventricle and congestive failure occur.

Aortic stenosis may be associated with exertional dyspnea and easy fatigability. Anginal pain may be produced by myocardial ischemia, and syncope may be caused by Stokes-Adams attacks resulting from arrhythmias.

Blood flow across the stenosis causes a harsh ejection systolic murmur, loudest at the second interspace at the right sternal border. The murmur is transmitted up the great vessels of the neck and usually is audible over the bony prominences of the chest, back, and head. A systolic thrill is palpable over the base and in the suprasternal notch. The second sound may be paradoxically split because of the prolongation of the left ventricular ejection time. The presence of an atrial sound (fourth heart sound) is suggestive of severe aortic stenosis. This sound also is associated with delayed upstroke of the arterial pulse.

X rays may demonstrate prominence of the ascending aorta. The heart size usually is normal. Concentric hypertrophy is difficult to demonstrate by chest films, but dilatation occurs with cardiac decompensation. The electrocardiogram reveals left ventricular hypertrophy. A normal electrocardiogram does not exclude the presence of severe aortic stenosis. ST-segment depression suggests left ventricular strain. Cardiac catheterization seldom is necessary to make the diagnosis of aortic stenosis, but left-sided studies distinguish the type of stenosis and demonstrate its severity.

Patients with mild to moderate aortic stenosis usually are asymptomatic. The presence of congestive failure, syncope, or anginal attacks suggests very severe aortic stenosis. Congestive failure is most commonly seen in infants with severe stenosis. Sudden death is always threatened in severe aortic stenosis.

Surgery is indicated in all patients who have symptoms of aortic stenosis and in patients who have laboratory evidence of severe aortic stenosis: cardiac catheterization data revealing a systolic pressure gradient of 50 mm. Hg or more, a functional aortic valve area less than 0.7 cm.^{2}/m.^{2} of body surface area, or electrocardiographic evidence of left ventricular strain.[27] The risk of surgery is increased after patients have developed congestive failure or angina. Surgery is not indicated for mild aortic stenosis.

Although the optimum age for surgery, because of the need for a pump oxygenator or hypothermia, is 4 to 6 years, the presence of severe obstruction dictates the need for surgery at any size or age. Valvulotomy under direct vision is the procedure of choice. Occasionally, replacement of the valve with a prosthesis or homograft is necessary. When signs of severe aortic stenosis are present, the risks of surgery are less than is the risk of continued medical management.

Coarctation of the Aorta

Coarctation of the aorta is seen in about 5 per cent of all patients with congenital heart disease.[7] This malformation is characterized by a con-

312

striction in the lumen of the aorta, usually for a short distance, distal to the origin of the left subclavian artery (Fig. 3). The obstruction causes the arterial pressure below the constriction to be diminished and damped, and usually there is significant hypertension in the part of the body supplied by the aorta proximal to the left subclavian. The ductus may enter proximal or distal to or directly into the narrowed area. Usually, there are collaterals between the proximal and distal aorta that supply most of the blood to the abdomen and the lower half of the body. The major collaterals, branches of the subclavian and axillary arteries, join branches of the intercostal and epigastric arteries from below. Variations or malformations of the aorta may change the picture and produce hypotension in the right or left arm as well as in the lower extremities. Frequently associated lesions are ventricular septal defect, aortic stenosis resulting from bicuspid aortic valve, and endocardial fibroelastosis.

Coarctation may cause congestive failure in infancy, but children who pass infancy relatively symptom-free remain undetected unless hypertension or murmurs resulting from associated defects are noted. The diagnosis of coarctation can be made by demonstrating a 20 mm. Hg drop in systolic pressure from the arms to the legs. The X-ray findings may reveal evidence of cardiac enlargement and left ventricular hypertrophy, if the obstruction is severe. Rib notching caused by prominent intercostal collaterals may be evident. The presence of pre- and post-stenotic dilatation of the aorta may be evidenced by pressure upon the barium-filled esophagus. The electrocardiogram in adults and older children usually demonstrates left ventricular hypertrophy. In infants who have evidence of cardiac failure, right ventricular hypertrophy usually is present.

Most patients with aortic coarctation do well throughout childhood, but a significant percentage develop evidence of congestive failure during

Figure 3. Coarctation of aorta.

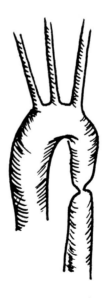

infancy. These usually have a preductal type of coarctation and associated defects. Medical management often is satisfactory in those patients with cardiac failure and is advisable during infancy. Surgical correction usually consists of excision of the stenosis and direct reanastomosis or replacement with a graft.[28, 29] We consider 5 to 8 years of age the optimum age for surgery. Unremitting congestive failure during infancy would necessitate surgical repair, regardless of age.

INSUFFICIENT VALVES

Ebstein's Malformation

Ebstein's malformation of the tricuspid valve is an uncommon congenital defect in which portions of the tricuspid valve are displaced into the right ventricle. The valve leaflets, usually the septal and posterior leaflets, are attached to the right ventricular wall rather than to the fibrous annulus. The right ventricle thus is divided into a collecting chamber and a pumping chamber, causing tricuspid insufficiency and relative hypoplasia of the right ventricle. Occasionally, there may be some degree of tricuspid stenosis.

There may be a wide variety of symptoms, depending on the severity of the malformation. There may be evidence of right-sided failure and cyanosis. Paroxysmal tachycardias are seen in many patients. Physical findings are not striking. A soft systolic murmur may be heard low along the left sternal border. In addition, diastolic murmurs and triple or quadruple rhythms may be noted.

X-ray studies usually show evidence of cardiac enlargement. The pulmonary vascular markings are normal or decreased. Right atrial enlargement often is seen. Electrocardiogram reveals a Wolf-Parkinson-White syndrome, type B, in about 25 per cent of the patients. Most patients have tall, peaked P waves. Cardiac catheterization may reveal evidence of a right-to-left shunt at the atrial level and elevated right atrial pressure. There usually is evidence of tricuspid insufficiency. Angiocardiography usually reveals an enlarged right atrium and may demonstrate the abnormal attachments of the tricuspid valve leaflets.

Patients with mild forms have few or no problems, while patients with cardiac enlargement develop exertional dyspnea, fatigue, and episodes of paroxysmal tachycardia. Seventy per cent of these patients die before the age of 20 years.

Surgical repair of the tricuspid valve or replacement of the valve with a prosthesis has been reported to aid these patients.[30, 31, 32] Significant cardiac enlargement, cyanosis, or symptoms are the indications for surgery.

COMBINATION OF OBSTRUCTIONS TO FLOW AND INTRACARDIAC COMMUNICATIONS

Tricuspid Atresia

This is an unusual disorder that occurs in about 2 per cent of patients with congenital heart disease.[7] This abnormality prevents flow of blood

314

from the right atrium to the right ventricle. The right ventricle usually is hypoplastic, but access to the right ventricle may be possible through a ventricular septal defect. The systemic venous blood must flow through an atrial septal defect or patent foramen ovale; in addition, there must be access to the pulmonary circuit through a ventricular septal defect or patent ductus.

These patients usually have symptoms early in infancy. The mortality rate is high. Fifty per cent die within the first 6 months. The survivors are poorly developed and undernourished. They have cyanosis and clubbing, exertional dyspnea, and easy fatigability.

The second heart sound usually is single, and only the aortic component is audible. In the presence of a ventricular septal defect, a widely split second sound may be noted. The murmurs depend on the associated abnormalities.

The electrocardiogram usually reveals left axis deviation, left ventricular hypertrophy, and the peaked P waves of right atrial enlargement. X-ray features vary with the size of the atrial septal defect and the character of the pulmonary arterial supply. If the atrial communication is small, the right atrium is very prominent. The pulmonary conus segment is concave. Cardiac catheterization demonstrates a right-to-left shunt at the atrial level. Angiocardiography demonstrates an obstruction at the tricuspid valve.

Corrective procedures are not available. Surgery is aimed at providing adequate pulmonary blood flow and adequate emptying of the right atrium. A superior vena cava to right pulmonary artery anastomosis (Glenn procedure)[33] often provides satisfactory pulmonary blood flow and decompresses the right atrium; but during infancy, the results of this procedure are not satisfactory. The creation of an atrial septal defect by the Rashkind procedure and creation of an arterial systemic-pulmonary shunt appear to be the procedures of choice for the newborn.[34] Indications for the latter surgery are impaired emptying of the right atrium and diminished pulmonary blood flow. At present, it seems advisable to consider removal of the arterial shunt when the patient is large enough to tolerate a superior vena cava to pulmonary artery anastomosis.[35]

Tetralogy of Fallot

Tetralogy of Fallot is seen in about 10 per cent of patients with congenital heart disease.[7] It is the most common type of cyanotic heart disease seen after age 2. The condition consists of pulmonary stenosis, ventricular septal defect, dextro-position of the aorta, and hypertrophy of the right ventricle. The pulmonary stenosis usually is infundibular or combined infundibular and valvular. Twenty-five per cent of the patients have valvular pulmonary stenosis. A right aortic arch is present in 25 per cent of the patients.[36]

The clinical picture is dependent on the combination of pulmonic obstruction and ventricular septal defect, which produces a right-to-left shunt at the ventricular level but does not prevent complete emptying of the right ventricle. At times, the relative pulmonary-to-systemic resistance may change suddenly, causing hypoxic spells because of decreased pulmonary blood flow. The degree of cyanosis is dependent on the pulmonary blood flow. Patients commonly are noted to have exertional dyspnea, easy fatigability, cyanosis, and history of squatting. Examination reveals a long, harsh, systolic ejection murmur, loudest along the lower left sternal border. The second heart sound is single. The pulmonary valve component often is greatly diminished and sometimes is delayed. A thrill may be associated with the murmur. Patients usually are small and thin.

X-rays reveal the heart to be small or average in size; the right ventricle is prominent; occasionally, the right atrium is enlarged. The pulmonary conus segment usually is concave, and vascular markings may be diminished. The electrocardiogram reveals evidence of right ventricular hypertrophy. Cardiac catheterization reveals elevated pressures in the right ventricle, with a pressure gradient across the obstruction at the infundibular region. There is evidence of a right-to-left shunt through the ventricular septal defect. Angiocardiography demonstrates the ventricular septal defect and outlines the location, the severity, and the character of the outflow-tract stenosis. Angiographic demonstration of the left ventricle to rule out single ventricle and transposition are important in planning corrective surgery.

As they grow, patients with tetralogy of Fallot usually develop increasing pulmonary outflow obstruction and increasing right-to-left shunt. Increasing hypoxemia is reflected by increased symptoms and limitation of activity, increasing hematocrit, and hypoxic spells that may be life-threatening.

Surgical correction of tetralogy of Fallot involves repair of the ventricular septal defect and correction of the right ventricular outflow obstruction. This procedure requires the use of a pump oxygenator. At 5 to 8 years of age, the presence of a right-to-left shunt associated with this defect is an indication for corrective surgery. At an earlier age, evidence of severe hypoxia, marked cyanosis, or severe hypoxic spells are indications for a palliative operative procedure. A systemic-pulmonary shunt improves the condition by providing an adequate pulmonary blood supply. A Blalock-Taussig[37] anastomosis, which creates a subclavian to pulmonary artery shunt, appears to be the most useful. The Potts [38] anastomosis, which connects the descending aorta and the pulmonary artery, and an anastomosis between the ascending aorta and the right pulmonary artery have been valuable, especially for the small infant.[34, 39] The palliative procedures are associated with relatively low risks. The risk of corrective surgery is appreciable, but the results appear to be good. The optimum time for surgical correction of tetralogy of Fallot is 5 to 8 years of age.

COMPLEX ABNORMALITIES

Truncus Arteriosus

Truncus arteriosus is an unusual lesion (Fig. 4). It was present in 0.42 per cent of Keith's series.[7] The common arterial trunk results from the failure of the spiral truncoconal ridges to create an aorta and a pulmonary artery. A ventricular septal defect invariably is present. The number of semilunar valve leaflets varies from two to six. The entire circulation, including systemic arteries, pulmonary arteries, and coronary arteries, arises from the common trunk.[40]

The systemic venous blood enters the right ventricle and is pumped into the common trunk. The pulmonary venous blood returning from the left atrium and left ventricle also is pumped into the common trunk. Most patients with truncus arteriosus have large pulmonary blood flows, limited only by the pulmonary vascular resistance. In most patients with truncus arteriosus, the large pulmonary blood flow causes congestive failure and death early in infancy.

Dyspnea, fatigue and cyanosis, poor weight gain, and prominence of the left hemithorax are common findings. A continuous murmur and thrill may be detected high along the left sternal border. The degree of cyanosis varies, depending on the pulmonary blood flow and the general status. A wide pulse pressure may be present if the pulmonary blood flow is large. The first heart sound is normal. An aortic click is present in about half the patients. The second sound is accentuated. The expected single second sound is not invariably present.

The electrocardiogram often shows left ventricular hypertrophy or combined left and right ventricular hypertrophy. X rays may reveal absence of the main pulmonary artery from its usual location, increased pulmonary vascular markings, and enlargement of both ventricles. The "aorta" usually is large, and 25 per cent have a right aortic arch.

Cardiac catheterization demonstrates increased oxygen content in the right ventricular outflow tract. Arterial desaturation is always present. The right ventricular pressures are equal to systemic pressures. It often is difficult to distinguish a true truncus from a pulmonary window, and occasionally, a ventricular septal defect may offer a diagnostic problem. Angiocardiography proves the diagnosis and outlines the origin of the pulmonary arteries.

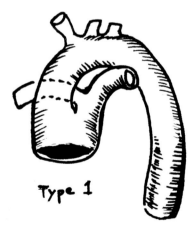

Figure 4. Truncus arteriosus, type I.

Type 1

Surgical banding of the pulmonary arteries has been reported to have moderate success.[16, 41] In addition, operative techniques have been reported that could correct these conditions.[42, 43] Since the mortality rate is high, most patients do not survive beyond 6 months; banding is indicated when there is evidence of congestive failure or deterioration of the clinical status. Surgical correction, which aims at closing the ventricular septal defect, creating a right ventricular outflow tract, and establishing a separate pulmonary blood flow with the use of homografts or prosthetic devices, should be considered in older children. These procedures offer hope, although they still are in the developmental stage.

Transposition of the Great Vessels

Complete transposition of the great vessels is an abnormality commonly seen during the newborn period. It has been reported in 18 per cent of the babies dying of congenital heart disease during the neonatal period,[7] although it is seen in only 5 per cent of children with congenital heart disease. Transposition is a malposition of the two great vessels relative to the ventricles or to each other at their origin (Fig. 5).[44] Many types have been described, with variations in the degree of malposition of the aorta and the pulmonary artery and variations of the anatomy of the ventricles. The presence of additional malformations also changes the clinical picture. Typically, two parallel circulations exist, in which the systemic venous blood returns to the right side and is pumped from the right ventricle to the aorta, while the pulmonary venous blood returns to the left atrium and is pumped from the left ventricle to the pulmonary artery and back to the lungs. Unless there are defects that allow mixing, the survival time is extremely limited. The foramen ovale and the ductus arteriosus permit survival for a short time. About 50 per cent of the cases have associated defects that permit longer survival. Transposition occurs in males more than twice as often as in females.

Cyanosis usually is noted shortly after birth but occasionally remains undetected for several months. Exertional dyspnea, feeding difficulties, poor weight gain, and slow motor development are common. Respiratory infections are frequent, and spells of hypoxia may occur. Murmurs are lacking in about 30 per cent of the patients. Hypoxia and congestive failure cause the deaths of most patients before 7 months of age.

The electrocardiogram usually reveals right axis deviation and right ventricular hypertrophy. Chest X rays in the immediate newborn period may appear relatively normal. In older children, the heart may have a narrow waist and resemble an egg on its side. The pulmonary vascular markings usually are increased.

Survival requires the delivery of oxygenated blood to the body and desaturated blood to the lung. Provision of an adequate bidirectional shunt is mandatory. This aim can be accomplished by the Rashkind procedure,[45, 46] creating an atrial septal defect by means of a balloon catheter.

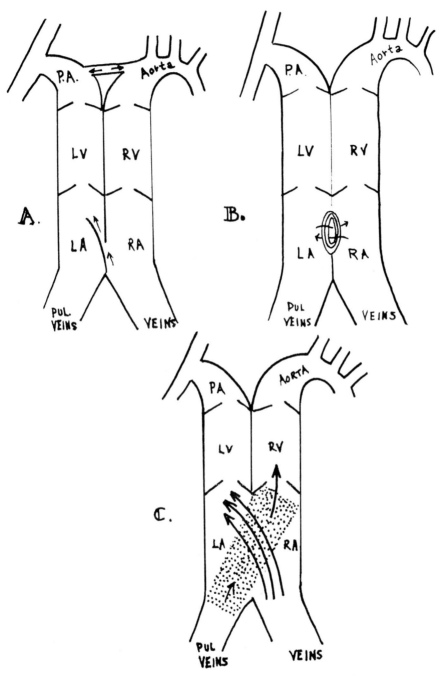

Figure 5. A, complete transposition with patent ductus arteriosus and patent foramen ovale. B, complete transposition following creation of an atrial septal defect. C, complete transposition following a Mustard procedure.

The results are immediate. When the patient has grown large enough to be considered for an elective open-heart procedure, one must consider the Mustard procedure,[47] which rechannels the venous return so that the pulmonary venous return is shunted into the right ventricle, while systemic venous blood passes across the mitral valve to the left ventricle and thereby into the pulmonary arteries. A pericardial graft is used to reroute the blood within the atrium. The Mustard procedure should be planned as early as possible, usually at 2 to 3 years of age, because cyanosis and increased pulmonary blood flow [48-50] cause the early development of permanent pulmonary vascular changes.

SUMMARY

The surgical correction of congenital malformations provides the solution to many abnormalities. The optimum time for surgical correction depends on the character and the severity of the malformation and the nature of the operative procedure. In addition, the size and clinical status of the patient must be considered. Indications for surgery must be weighed for each individual, carefully balancing the risk of his disease against the risk of surgery. For some conditions, surgery in childhood can be considered an elective procedure. For other conditions, surgery in the face of adverse conditions is the only hope for salvaging critically ill infants.

References

1. GROSS, R. E., AND HUBBARD, J. P.: *Surgical ligation of a patent ductus arteriosus: Report of first successful case.* J.A.M.A. 112:179, 1939.
2. SWAN, H.: *Hypothermia for general and cardiac surgery.* Surg. Clin. N. Amer. 36:1109, 1956.
3. GIBBON, J. H.: *Application of a mechanical heart and lung apparatus to cardiac surgery.* Minn. Med. 37:171, 1954.
4. KAHN, D. R., STRANG, R. H., AND WILSON, W. S.: *Clinical Aspects of Operable Heart Disease.* Appleton-Century-Crofts, New York, 1968.
5. VARGHESE, P. J., CELERMAJER, J., IZUKAWA, T., HALLER, J. A., JR., AND ROWE, R. D.: *Cardiac catheterization in the newborn: Experience with 100 cases.* Pediatrics 44:24, 1969.
6. KROVETZ, L. J., SHANKLIN, D. R., AND SCHIEBLER, G. L.: *Serious and fatal complications of catheterization and angiocardiography in infants and children.* Amer. Heart J. 76:39, 1968.
7. KEITH, J. D., ROWE, R. D., AND VLAD, P.: *Heart Disease in Infancy and Childhood.* The Macmillan Co., New York, 1966.
8. EDWARDS, J. E.: *Functional pathology of the pulmonary vascular tree in congenital cardiac disease.* Circulation 15:164, 1957.
9. EVANS, J. R., ROWE, R. D., AND KEITH, J. D.: *Spontaneous closure of a ventricular septal defect.* Circulation 22:1044, 1960.
10. BLOOMFIELD, D. K.: *Natural history of ventricular septal defects in patients surviving infancy.* Circulation 29:914, 1964.
11. SIMMONS, R. L., MOLLER, J. H., AND EDWARDS, J. E.: *Anatomic evidence for spontaneous closure of ventricular septal defect.* Circulation 34:38, 1966.

12. ASH, R.: *Natural history of ventricular septal defects in childhood lesions with predominant arteriovenous shunts.* J. Pediat. 64:45, 1964.

13. KIRKLIN, J. W., AND DuSHANE, J. W.: *Indications for repair of ventricular septal defect.* Amer. J. Cardiol. 12:75, 1963.

14. CARTMILL, T. B., DuSHANE, J. W., McGOON, D. C., AND KIRKLIN, J.: *Results of repair of ventricular septal defects.* J. Thorac. Cardiov. Surg. 52:486, 1966.

15. HOLLMAN, A.: *Ventricular septal defect.* Brit. Heart J. 28:813, 1967.

16. MULLER, W. H., AND DAMMANN, J. F.: *The treatment of certain congenital malformations of the heart by the creation of pulmonary stenosis to reduce pulmonary hypertension and excessive blood flow.* Surg. Gynec. Obstet. 95:213, 1952.

17. DAMMANN, J. F., McEACHEN, J. A., THOMPSON, W. M., SMITH, R., AND MULLER, W. H., JR.: *Regression of pulmonary vascular disease after creation of pulmonary stenosis.* J. Thorac. Surg. 42:722, 1961.

18. AINGER, L. E., AND PATE, J. W.: *Ostium secundum atrial septal defects and congestive heart failure in infancy.* Amer. J. Cardiol. 15:380, 1965.

19. HASTRITER, A. R., WENNEMARK, J. R., MILLER, R. A., AND PAUL, M. H.: *Secundum atrial septal defects with congestive heart failure during infancy and early childhood.* Amer. Heart J. 64:467, 1962.

20. CAYLER, G. C.: *Spontaneous closures of symptomatic atrial septal defects.* New Eng. J. Med. 276:65, 1967.

21. CRAIG, R. J., AND SELZER, A.: *Natural history and prognosis of atrial septal defects.* Circulation 27:805, 1968.

22. HOFFMAN, L. E., KROVETZ, L. J., VAN MIEROP, L. H. S., CRESSNER, J. H., WHEAT, M. W., BARTLEY, T. D., AND SCHIEBLER, G. L.: *Secundum atrial septal defects in children.* Ann. Thorac. Surg. 7:104, 1969.

23. GASUL, B. H., ARCILLA, R. A., AND LEV, M.: *Heart Disease in Children.* J. B. Lippincott Co., Philadelphia, 1966.

24. BROCK, R. E.: *Surgery of pulmonary stenosis.* Brit. Med. J. 2:399, 1949.

25. GERSONY, W. M., BERNHARD, W. F., NADAS, A. S., AND GROSS, R. E.: *Diagnosis and surgical treatment of infants with critical pulmonary outflow obstruction.* Circulation 32:172, 1965.

26. GERBODE, F., ROSS, J. K., HARKINS, G. A., AND OSBORN, J. J.: *Surgical treatment of pulmonary stenosis using extracorporal circulation.* Surgery 48:58, 1960.

27. MOSS, A. J., AND ADAMS, F. H.: *Heart Disease in Infants, Children, and Adolescents.* The Williams & Wilkins Co., Baltimore, 1968.

28. GROSS, R. E., AND HUFNAGEL, C. A.: *Coarctation of the aorta: Experimental studies regarding its surgical correction.* New Eng. J. Med. 233: 287, 1945.

29. CRAFOORD, C. AND NYLIN, G.: *Congenital coarctation of the aorta and its surgical treatment.* J. Thorac. Surg. 14:347, 1945.

30. BARNARD, C. W., AND SCHIRE, V.: *Surgical correction of Ebstein's malformation with a prosthetic tricuspid valve.* Surgery 54:302, 1963.

31. KAY, J. H., TSUJI, H. K., REDINGTON, J. H., YAMADA, T., AND KAGAWA, K.: *The surgical treatment of Ebstein's malformation with right ventricular aneurysmorrhapy and replacement of the tricuspid valve with a disk valve.* Dis. Chest 51:637, 1967.

321

32. PEREZ-ALVAREZ, J. J., PÉREZ-TREVINO, C., GAYIOLA, A., AND RETA-VILLALOBOS, A.: *Ebstein's anomaly with pulmonic stenosis. Implantation of a tricuspid valvular prosthesis.* Amer. J. Cardiol. 20:411, 1967.

33. GLENN, W. W. L., AND PATINE, J. F.: *Circulatory bypass of the right heart. Preliminary observations on the direct delivery of vena caval blood into the pulmonary circulation by azygos vein-pulmonary artery shunt.* Yale J. Biol. Med. 27:147, 1954.

34. WALDHAUSEN, J. H., FREIDMAN, S., TYERS, G. F. O., RASHKIND, W. J., PETRY, O., AND MILLER, W. W.: *Ascending aorta, right pulmonary artery anastomosis.* Circulation 38:463, 1968.

35. GLENN, W. W. L., GARDNER, T. H., TALNER, N. S., STANSEL, H. C., JR., AND MATANO, I.: *The approach to the surgical management of tricuspid atresia.* Circulation 37–38 (Suppl. II):62, 1968.

36. TAUSSIG, H. B.: *Congenital Malformations of the Heart.* New York, Commonwealth Fund, 1967.

37. BLALOCK, A., AND TAUSSIG, H. B.: *The surgical treatment of malformations of the heart in which there is pulmonary stenosis or pulmonary atresia.* J. A. M. A. 128:189, 1945.

38. POTTS, W. J., SMITH, S. AND GIBSON, S.: *Anastomosis of aorta to pulmonary artery.* J. A. M. A. 132:627, 1946.

39. HALLMAN, G. L., YASHER, J. J., BLOODWELL, R. P., AND COOLEY, D. A.: *Intrapericardial aortic-pulmonary anastomosis for tetralogy of Fallot.* Surgery 95:709, 1967.

40. COLLETT, R. W., AND EDWARDS, J. E.: *Persistent truncus arteriosus. A classification according to anatomic types.* Surg. Clin. N. Amer. 29:12, 1949.

41. GOLDBLATT, A., BERNHARD, W. F., NADAS, A. S., AND GROSS, R. E.: *Pulmonary artery banding: Indications and results in infants and children.* Circulation 32:172, 1965.

42. RASTELLI, G. C., TITUS, J. L., AND McGOON, D. C.: *Homograft of ascending aorta and aortic valve as a right ventricular outflow.* Arch. Surg. 95:69, 1969.

43. WALLACE, R. B., RASTELLI, G. C., ONGLEY, P. A., TITUS, J. L., AND McGOON, D. C.: *Complete repair of truncus arteriosus defects.* J. Thorac. Cardiov. Surg. 57:95, 1969.

44. ABBOTT, M. E.: *Atlas of Congenital Cardiac Disease.* New York, American Heart Association, 1936.

45. RASHKIND, W. J., AND MILLER, W. W.: *Creation of an atrial septal defect without thoracotomy.* J. A. M. A. 196:991, 1966.

46. RASHKIND, W. J., AND MILLER, W. W.: *Transposition of the great arteries: Results of palliation by balloon atrioseptostomy in 31 infants.* Circulation 38:453, 1961.

47. MUSTARD, W. T.: *Successful two-stage correction of transposition of the great vessels.* Surgery 55:469, 1964.

48. FERENCZ, C.: *Transposition of the great vessels. Pathophysiologic consideration based upon study of lungs.* Circulation 33:232, 1966.

49. WAGENVOORT, C. A., NAUTA, J., VANDER SCHOAR, P. J., WEEDA, H. W. H., AND WAGENVOORT, N.: *The pulmonary vascularity in complete transposition of the great vessels judged from lung biopsy.* Circulation 38: 746, 1968.

50. VILES, P. H., ONGLEY, P. A., AND TITUS, J. L.: *The spectrum of pulmonary vascular disease in transposition of the great arteries.* Circulation 40:31, 1969.

Index